AF552698

The American Dentist

A Pictorial History with a Presentation of Early Dental Photography in America

by Richard A. Glenner, D.D.S
Audrey B. Davis, Ph.D.
Stanley B. Burns, M.D.

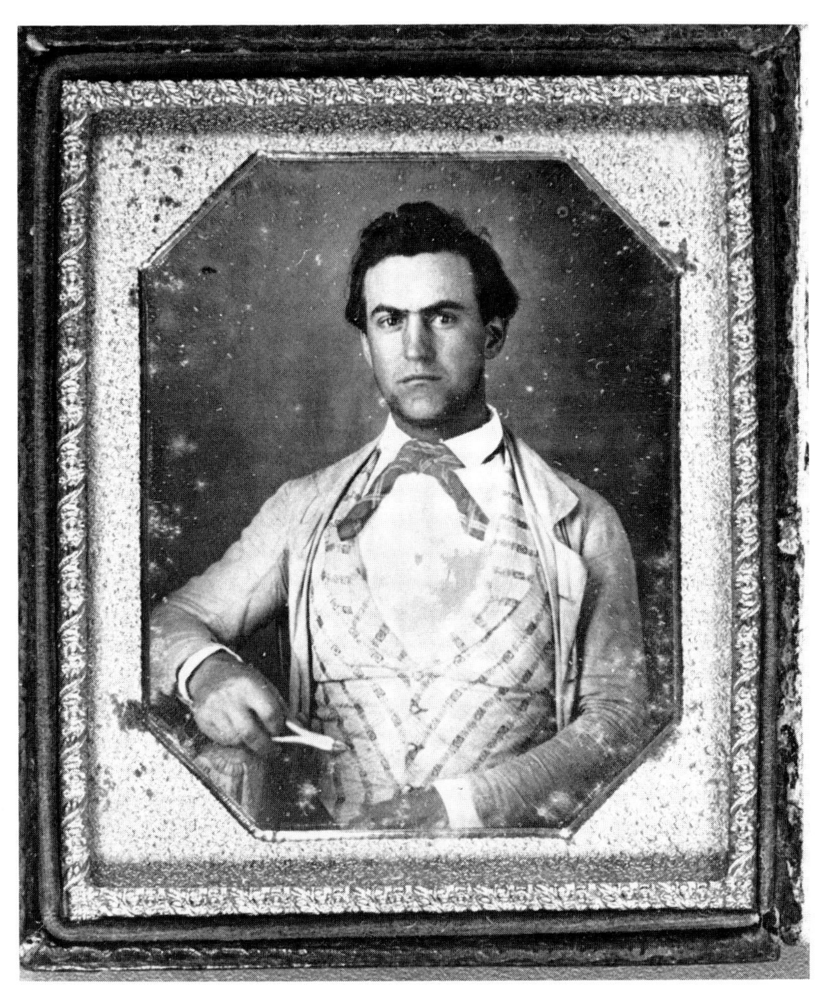

PICTORIAL HISTORIES PUBLISHING CO.
MISSOULA, MONTANA

LIBRARY OF CONGRESS
CATALOG CARD NO.
90-60363
90-60364

ISBN 0-929521-05-6

First Printing: January 1990
Second Printing: October 1994

Printed in U.S.A.

This image circa 1844, is perhaps the earliest photograph extent of a dentist. The head on confrontational pose is typical of early daguerreotypes, and there is a folk art aura about the picture. The demeanor of the subject presents a powerful image of strength of character in America's era of territorial expansion. He looks squarely at us, grasping his dental forceps as a symbol of his occupation. (Burns Archive)

PICTORIAL HISTORIES PUBLISHING COMPANY
713 South Third Street West, Missoula, Montana 59801

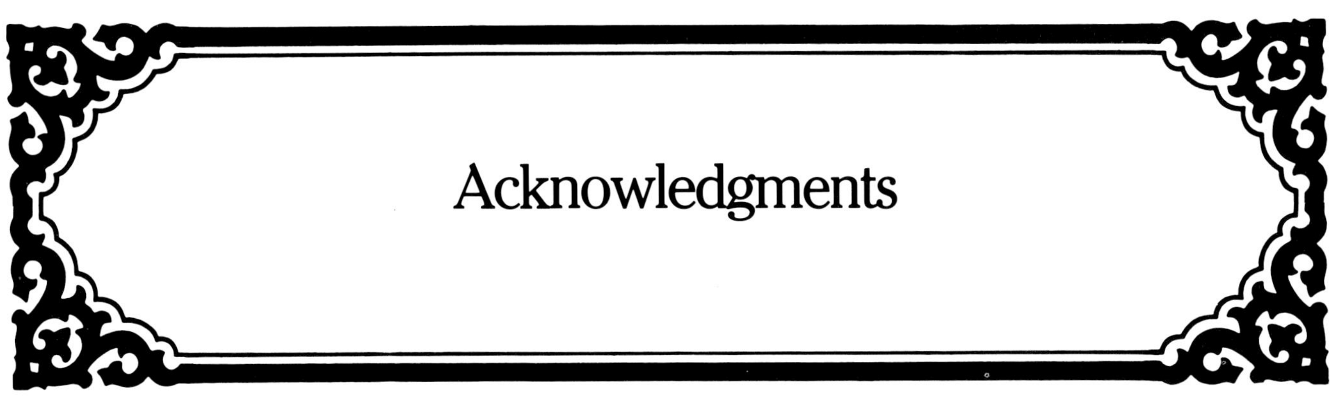

Acknowledgments

This book is an equal collaboration between Richard Glenner and Audrey Davis with the exception of the Introduction which was written by Stanley B. Burns.

We thank all our friends who have taken an interest in our study. Our special gratitude is offered to those who responded to our requests for books, articles, photographs, etc., especially Aletha Kowitz, director, Bureau of Library Services, American Dental Association Library, who provided the index; John Whittock Jr., librarian emeritus, School of Dental Medicine, University of Pennsylvania; Bud Friedman; J.P. Roan, librarian, National Museum of American History; the staff of the Smithsonian Institution Photographic Division including Mary Ellen McCaffrey, Richard Hofmeister, Eric Long, John Steiner and Louie Thomas; the curators and librarians of historical societies, university libraries and archives, who are many and who were most helpful in identifying, selecting and sending photographs; Dr. Milton B. Asbell; Dr. J. Henry Clarke; Dr. Gordon Dammann; Dr. Jack Gottschalk, curator of Bainbridge Museum of Dentistry; Dr. Maynard K. Hine, chancellor emeritus, University of Indiana; Dr. Frank J. Orland; Dr. Malvin E. Ring; Matthew Isenberg and Linda Amster, news research manager, *The New York Times*.

Also our sincere thanks to Stan Cohen, publisher, and Leslie Over, editorial assistant, for all their help and support.

The Authors

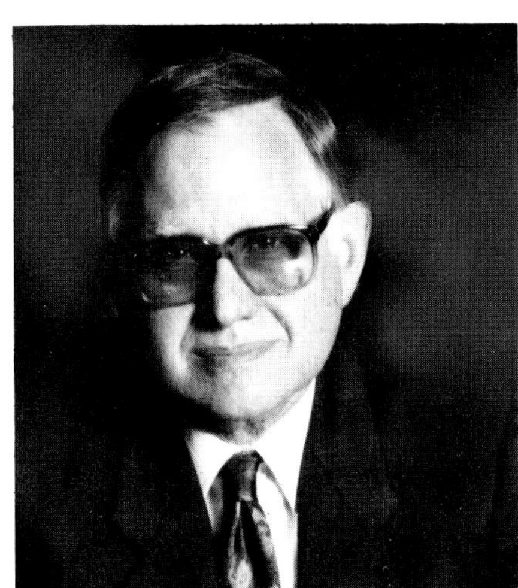

RICHARD GLENNER, D.D.S.

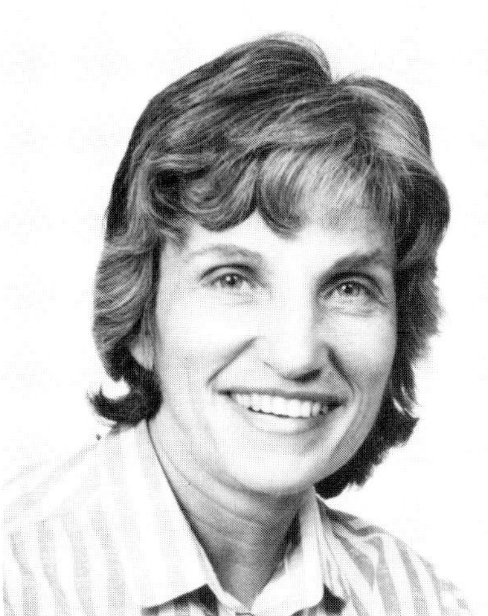

AUDREY DAVIS, PH.D.

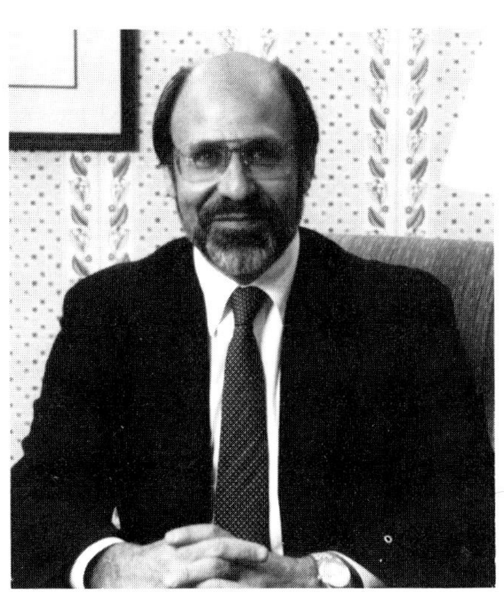

STANLEY B. BURNS, M.D.

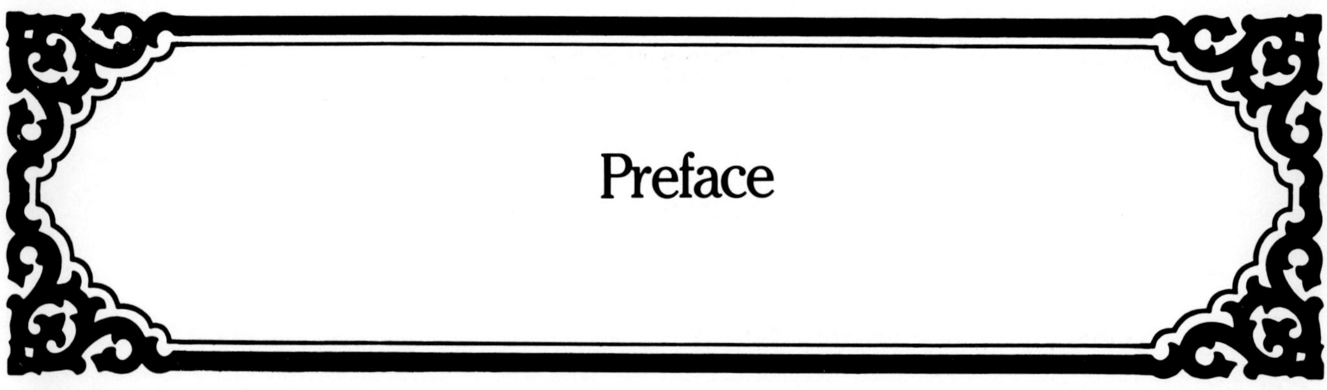

Preface

American photography and dentistry celebrated 150th anniversaries in 1989. The birth and growth of these two professions reveals interesting parallels and interactions. Dentistry started on a new path to become a scientifically based practice with specific educational standards. Photography was brought to the U.S. and quickly developed into an art and a science of value to many people, industries and professions. Photography played an important part in establishing and maintaining the image of dentistry over the past century and a half.

Photography and dentistry developed other links through outstanding individuals who worked as both photographers and dentists, in the use of photography by American dentists to advertise their skills, and later, to perfect dental diagnosis through X-ray photography. Advancements in both fields growing out of America's "mechanical ingenuity" were labeled "American" and considered the best available in their respective fields. "American dentistry" and the "American process" of daguerreotypy (earliest form of photography) grew in the 19th century to become the most desired in the world.

Photographs of dentists with patients provide the earliest pictorial evidence of a medical professional treating a patient. Studying photographs and understanding the people, fashions and processes associated with photography provides another major source of data to enlarge the scope of the history of American dentistry.

From photographs we see similarities in the ambiance of both the dentist's and photographer's work places. Natural light required in both professions led to the placement of the dental office and the photographic studio on the top floor beneath a skylight. Both the dentist and photographer decorated their entry rooms to attract the public and keep them pleasantly occupied while waiting for service. The dentist's and photographer's waiting rooms in the 19th century were designed to resemble a well-furnished home to make their middle and upper class clients feel comfortable in surroundings with which they were familiar. Later, as the equipment of both professions became elaborate and artificial light was employed, attention to professional duties divided the professional's interest in the details of climate, atmosphere and environment in which the service was delivered.

Both professions serve people with the result that often enhances the appearance, which could be immediately perceived and acknowledged by the client-patient. This one-on-one relationship created a bond between the professional and the public which stimulated reactions that were advertised for perspective purchasers of their services.

One could emphasize the history of American dentistry and photography without including other important factors in the development of dentistry, however, a book limited to these subjects would not satisfy the general reader who wishes to learn more about the heritage of a medical-dental system which he/she relies on today. Understanding the important discoveries, trends, techniques, people, institutions, etc., which shaped a health profession lays the ground work for a more enlightened evaluation and response to its current practices. American dentistry evolved as a profession by taking into consideration those who required, insisted upon and paid for its services. Social changes impinged on the practice of dentistry, revealing its strengths and weaknesses. These turning points are significant because they show us that all health related practices are primarily social endeavors that depend on the interaction of provider and patient-recipient. Photographs and the history of photography add a special dimension to the sociological perspective of the American dentist.

This historical-sociological account is intended to introduce the reader to major components of a dentist's career and how it grew out of American society, as well as contributing to this society over the past century and a half.

Contents

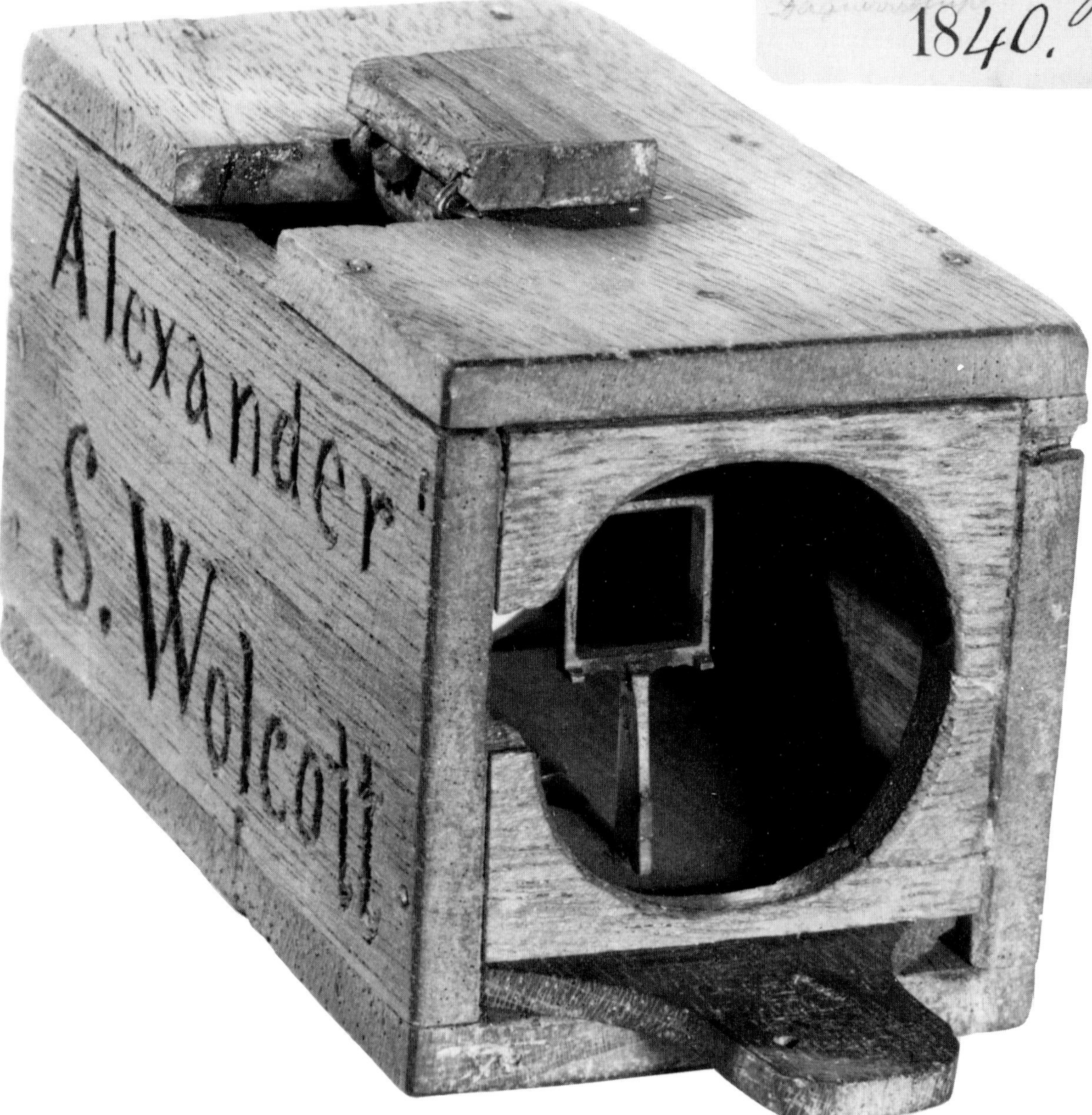

First U.S. Patent for camera by Alexander S. Wolcott, 1840. Wolcott, a dentist, designed a mirror camera which used a concave mirror instead of a lens to form an image on the photographic plate. This was popular with early daguerrotype portrait photographers for several years, but his patent model, one fifth the size of the working camera, is the only example known to have survived intact. From the Smithsonian Institution, Neg. Nos. 76-4208, 31432.

INTRODUCTION

Pictorial History of Dentistry with a Presentation of Early Dental Photography in America*

*Photographs except as noted courtesy of Stanley B. Burns, M.D. and the Burns Archive. Written by Stanley B. Burns, M.D.

This chapter on the earliest era in American dental photographic history grows out of 12 years of study and search for the photographs both of dentists as subjects and of dentists who were pioneer photographers. The major thrust has been to fill a void in dental photographic history. 1989 is the 150th year of photography's beginning; therefore, it is appropriate to review and examine how various professions were affected by, and how they affected, early photography. American dentists were among the first medical practitioners to use photography in the 1840s to document surgical results. The important role of dentists in the early years of photography has not previously been addressed.

Early photographs (the earliest photographs were called daguerreotypes) give us an opportunity for better understanding and new insight into 19th century dentists, their patients, their practices, and their role in the development of American photography. Abundant photographic illustrations reveal for the first time, the nature and extent of early dental portraiture in America. These portraits in combination with a variety of photographs taken by dentists and of dentists in the office provide the widest range of dental photography ever published.

The daguerreotypes and other early photographs in this monograph open a window into dentistry's past that has been closed for almost a century and a half. These images were taken at a time when the profession was struggling for an understanding of itself and seeking a place in the scientific and public eye. Many of the photographs which document early dentistry now are considered works of art and thus offer the dental community a proud place in the history of art, as well as in the history of medicine and science.

It is hoped that this chapter will enhance appreciation of early dental photography, not only as unique historical pictures, but also for preserving our dental and visual heritage. Other individuals and institutions are encouraged to preserve, collect, and further study dental photography. This study only exposes the tip of the iceberg of this promising and significant subject. Most of the early photographs are from the Burns Archive, which contains the largest collection of the earliest dental photographic images in the U.S.

Crucial years 1839-40

1839 was a birth year, both in photographic history and in dental history. In that year, the first practical process of photography was presented to the world, and the world's first dental journal was inaugurated. Each episode started a chain of events that would affect us all. Within a few short years these fledgling professions would change the nature of American life; photography became an American obsession that influenced our perception of the world. In dentistry the pioneer anesthetists and dentists Wells and Morton, introduced in 1846 a method to make surgery and dentistry painless with their discovery and promotion of the general anesthetics, nitrous oxide and ether.

The following year, 1840, was a turning point in American photography and in American dentistry. In this year, stimulated by a professional journal, the world's first dental school and the world's first national dental society were organized. In New York City the world's first photographic gallery was opened and operated by a dentist turned photographer.

American dentists in the mid-19th century were divided into two general groups. There were "mechanical dentists," who made the tools of dentistry, such as instruments, artificial teeth, etc. and there were "operative dentists," or those who treated patients. Some practiced both mechanical and operative dentistry. Operative dentists fell into three categories based on their training: those who were medically trained but preferred to practice dentistry, those who learned their craft by studying with established dentists (preceptorship), and those who were self-taught. Among the self-taught were those who attempted to practice professional dentistry and those who were quacks.

"Itinerant" practitioners included dentists of all qualifications, but many were quack tooth-pullers and tooth-carvers who duped an unsuspecting public. The quack, anxious to disguise his lack of skill, was drawn to the career of itinerant dentist, since he need never confront the patients he mistreated after leaving town. The image the public had of dentists, and the image they had of themselves is an interesting study in the iconography of a profession, an endeavor that was not attempted before because sufficient early photographic images were not assembled.

The roots of dentistry began in medicine. The first dental educators were physicians who specialized in the practice of dentistry. Prior to the early 19th century the public looked upon dentistry disparagingly, considering it a craft and not a health service. During the 19th century the question of whether dentistry was an autonomous profession or was a branch of medicine and surgery was often debated. The position taken had a direct effect on the training of dentists. At the time it was established in 1859, the American Dental Association's greatest concern was how dentists were to be educated—in preceptor programs, by studying with established dentists, or in special dental colleges linked to medical schools.[1] Photographs of dentists often reveal their method of training and degree of education.

Early Photography and Dental Portraiture

The discovery of photography in 1839 offered a chance to record the world more faithfully. Until the invention of photography all visual representations including prints, paintings, drawings, sculpture, etc. were subjective interpretations. To the pre-photographic mind the idea of permanently recording what could be seen was a fantastic notion. Photography allowed for exactly reproducible visual images and a new sense of credibility. One early observer described the photographic phenomena as if one held up a mirror to the world and whatever is imaged in that mirror will be preserved forever![2] The daguerreotype, the first practical photograph, a one-of-a-kind image on a silver-coated copper plate, seemed like that mirror. Dentists soon were spotlighted in that magic mirror.

Early photographic portraits employed conventions that had been used by painters for centuries. In paintings, physicians were depicted as scholarly men of science and were posed with books, skulls and bones, or with the tools of their trade.[3] American dentists, who were physicians, adopted these conventions. Dentists, who were not physicians, but were trained by preceptorship, also used photography to project the occupational image of "educated scholarly dentists." In contrast, itinerant tooth-pullers, were portrayed as workmen pulling teeth. Both physician and preceptor trained dentists occasionally also posed extracting teeth. This may have been done to make a statement about their preference for the practice of dentistry over that of medicine. These dental extraction photographs depict the first scenes of active intervention on the part of any medical professionals. American dentists in the act of treating patients were unique in having their photographs taken. No photographs are known of European dentists in occupational poses from photography's earliest era.[4]

The images included here represent the spectrum of all dental images that have survived. There are three types of poses: 1. dentists beside props such as books, dental tools and teeth, 2. dentists at work on patients—most of these demonstrate extractions in various stages, 3. normal portraits without props which are of interest when the subject is identified as a dentist. Dental occupational portraiture can be viewed as an ongoing visual language in which the dentist projected himself, his patient, and the science of dentistry.

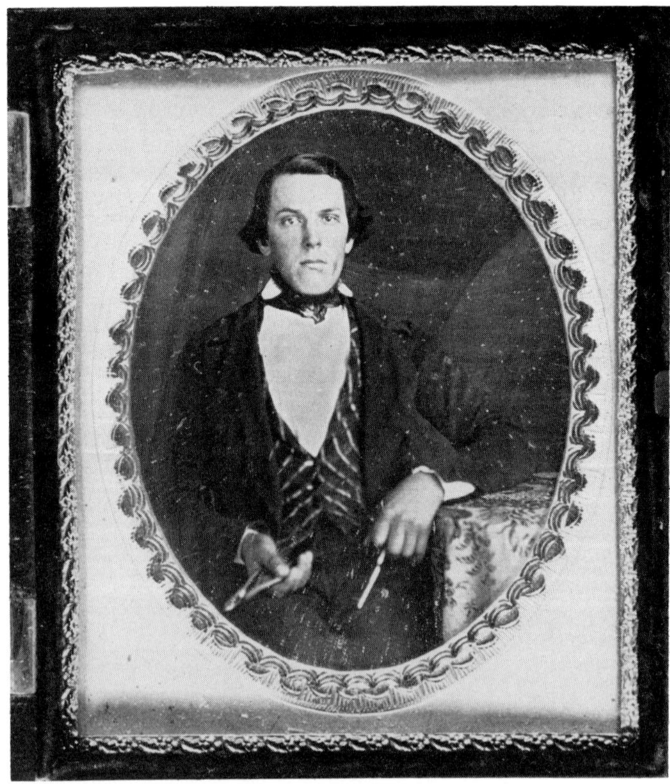

Dentist with Key and Forceps Daguerreotype 1848
This daguerreotype illustrates a similar pose as the cover photo. The dentist holds two of the tools of his trade, a key and a forceps.

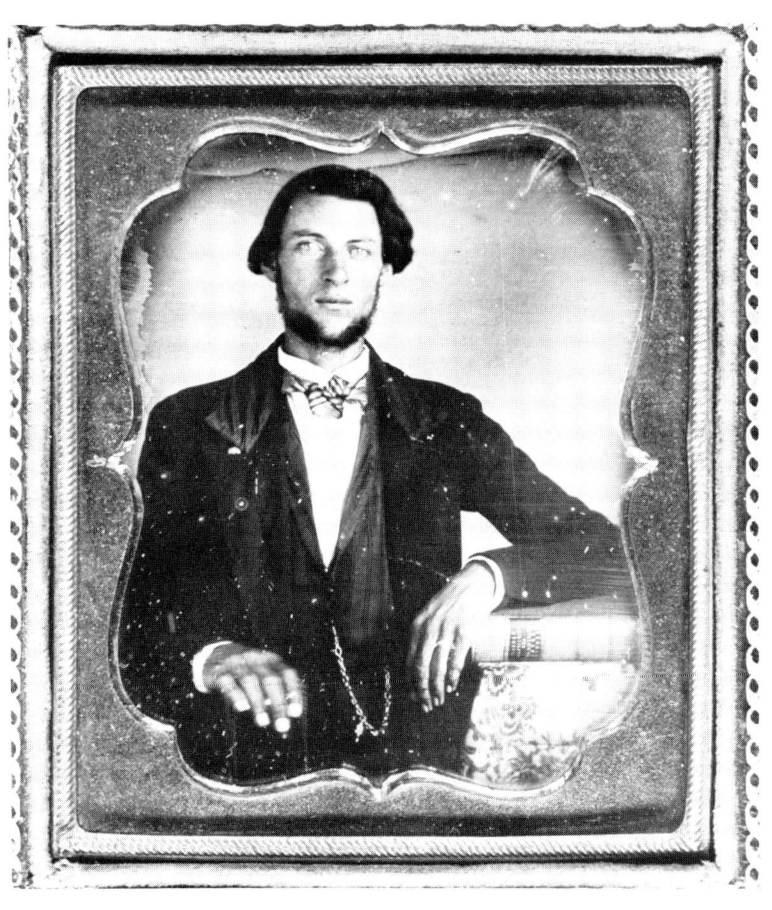

Dentist and Dental Surgery Book Daguerreotype 1847
This daguerreotype illustrates the classic convention of the educated scholar. Rather than pose with dental tools, which any one might pick up and practice with, this dentist wants to let us know that he is trained. Perhaps one of the graduates of an early dental school or even the first, Baltimore College of Dental Surgery, he poses with Chapin Harris' *Principles and Practice of Dental Surgery*. The print is always reversed in daguerreotypes, unless a special prism was used to take the picture.

Dentist and Woman Patient Daguerreotype 1847
This daguerreotype is highly unusual for its era, in that the patient is female. Most likely she is the dentist's or photographer's wife. By including a woman, calmly sitting in the dental chair, the dentist telegraphs a mannered, non-frightening image of "painless dentistry." The image also contains a prop, a complete dental operating kit of considerable quality. This is the only photograph of such a set from photography's earliest era. Because of the props and poses there can be no doubt this dentist was a serious professional. Note the toothbrushes displayed in the case which do not appear in other photographs. Courtesy Matthew Isenberg.

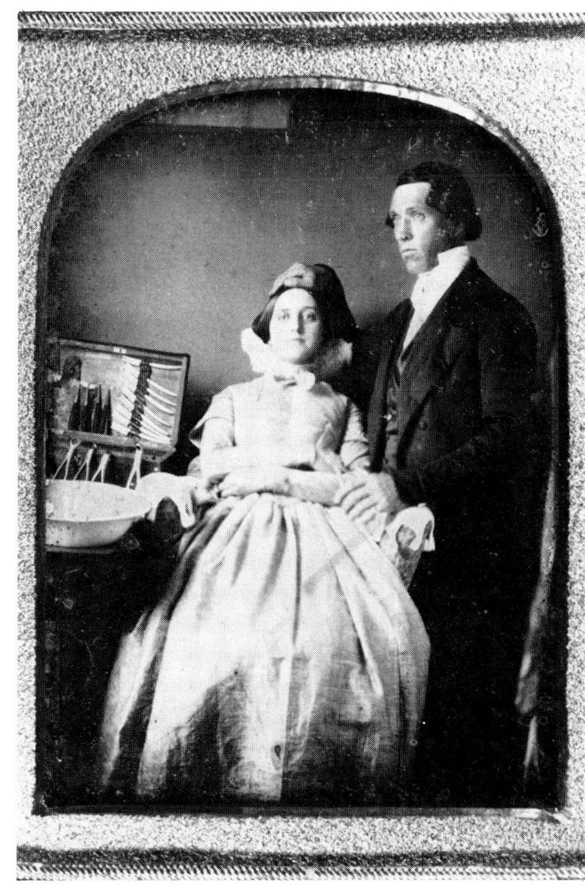

Plyers of their Trade

One category of images that has not received historical study and preservation is early photographs (1840-1870) of dentists pulling teeth. No one has assigned them a place in dental and photographic history. This has happened as a result of the rules of artifact survival. One of them is that we tend to forget and/or destroy that which seems erroneous or embarrassing. A new interest in the social and historical importance of vintage photographs has led to the preservation of all images, including those of dentists, which make new interpretations possible. Certainly photographs may be re-interpreted by future generations. C.W. Ceram observed in 1965 that early photographers tended to discover "reality" in the lower strata of society. Horrifying scenes also held a fascination for photographers, especially those who produced the first documentary images. They photographed corpses lying on the Civil War battlefields.[5] Later, historians studying these photographs found new social interpretations.

Photographs of dentists pulling teeth revealed an image which dentists in later periods were anxious to forget. The photographs are primitive and the subject often unprofessional. These dentists pose in the style of the craftsman, an image dentistry was fighting to change. Hence these advertising photographs of tooth-pullers have been largely ignored by dental historians, dental schools and museums. Photographic dealers have a relatively plentiful supply of these occupational portraits of tooth-pullers and itinerant dentists.

Identification of these images as photographs of itinerant and small town dentists rests on the evidence that these images are mainly produced as tintypes. The tintype was a less expensive form of photograph that was popular in small town galleries and was made by itinerant photographers. A tintype, because of its cheapness and availability in small towns and developing areas, was the type of photograph chosen by the average rural American. The primitive nature and pose of tintype images give them a folk art quality, rather than, a professional artistic character. Recently it has been discovered that many folk artists became photographers, and as a corollary, small town photographers emulated folk paintings in arranging the subjects of their photographs. In cities photographic galleries preferred the paper albumen print and almost all portraits of city dwellers were made in this format. Images of dentists displayed in city galleries do not portray them extracting teeth, but instead, in the stately and conventional manner of the physician. It is thus my conclusion that the tintypes of dental extractions are for the most part the images of grass roots dentistry in America, the itinerant tooth-pullers, as well as, the small town practitioners. Further research and study may unequivocally show that these images are indeed tooth-pullers plying their trade.

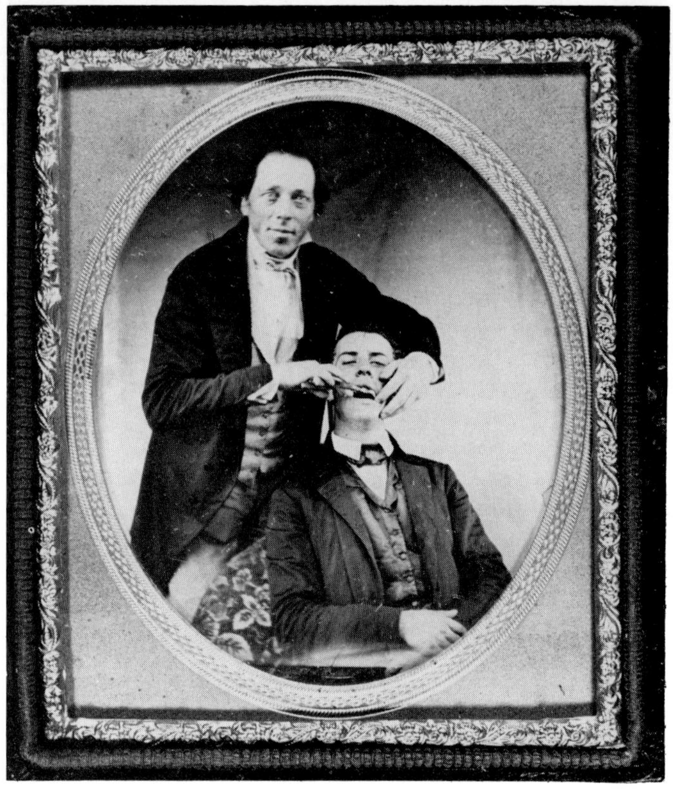

Extracting Tooth Daguerreotype 1847
This photograph came from the collection of Leo Steffens, Chicago's revival daguerreotypist of the 1890s. Steffens tried to bring back the art of daguerreotype portraiture, and used this image as part of a widely exhibited collection of "Great Images of Daguerrean Art of the 1840s and 1850s."

Although the position of the dentist and his patient are typical, only a handful of daguerreotypes feature dentists posed this way. Most photographs depict them in the classical physician-style imagery holding a tool of their trade, usually a key tooth-extractor or a pair of pliers. There are no known daguerreotypes showing a physician examining or posing with a patient. The dental extraction image was a specialized genre, and most often in photography's earliest years, the convention of the itinerant and quack tooth-puller.

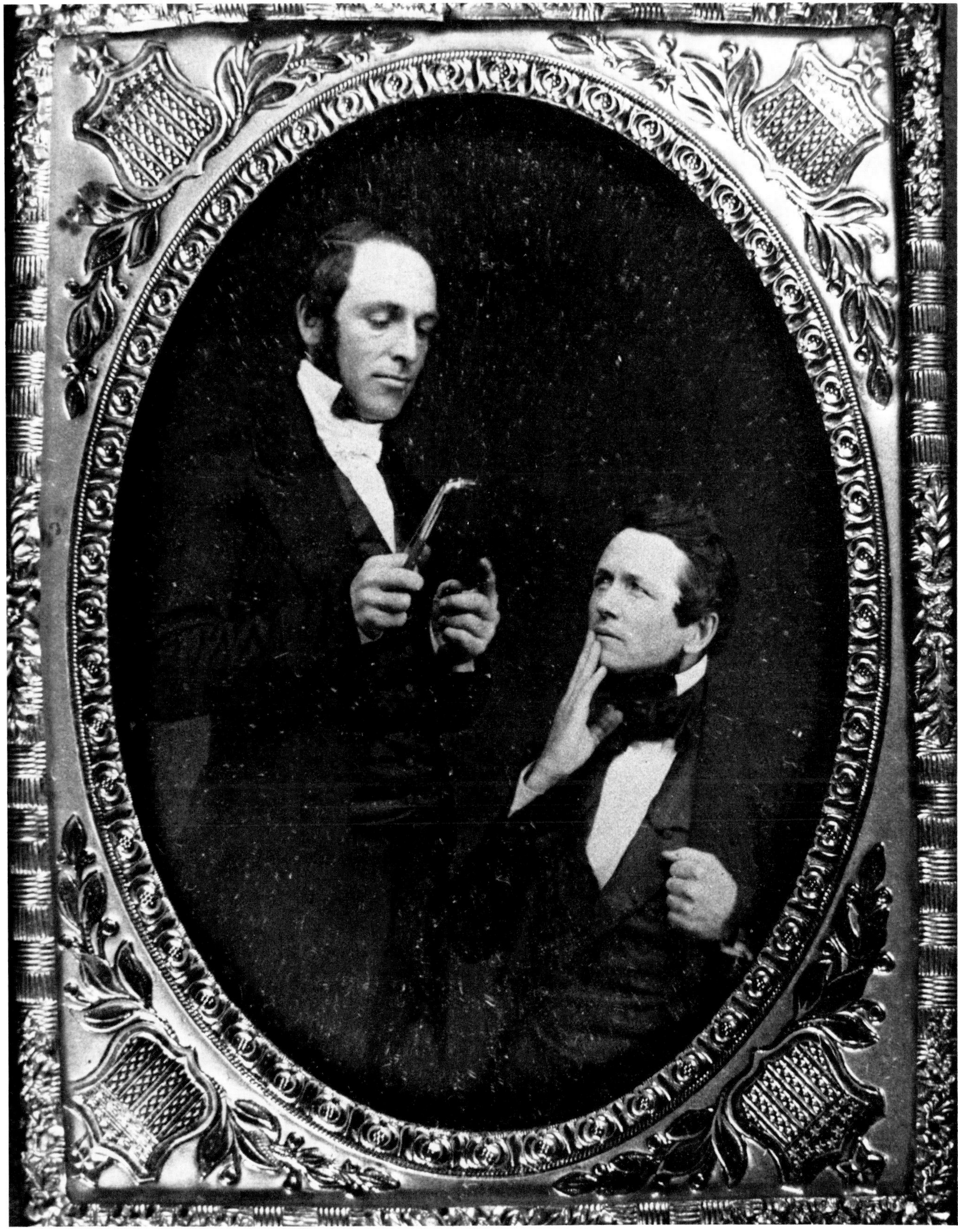

Amazed Patient Dental Extraction Daguerreotype 1850
In this 1850s photograph the dentist subtly demonstrates the image of painless dentistry. The dentist holds up his forceps and examines the tooth he has just removed. The patient appears not only calm but amazed. He holds his jaw in disbelief that his tooth is gone. The dress and demeanor of these subjects suggests that a professional dentist is at work.

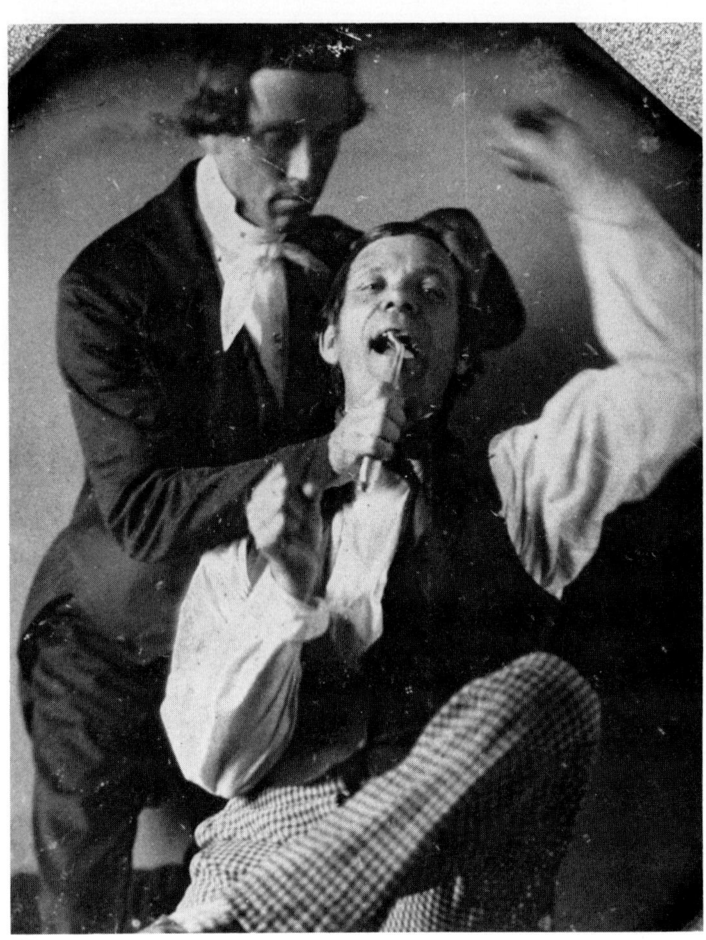

Dentist Extracting Tooth
Daguerreotype 1852
This dramatic picture shows a patient waving his arms about to protest the dentist's invading forceps. A classic photograph of the itinerant quack dentist who was more interested in showing off his prowess with the pliers than the professionalism of the educated practitioner.
Courtesy Matthew Isenberg.

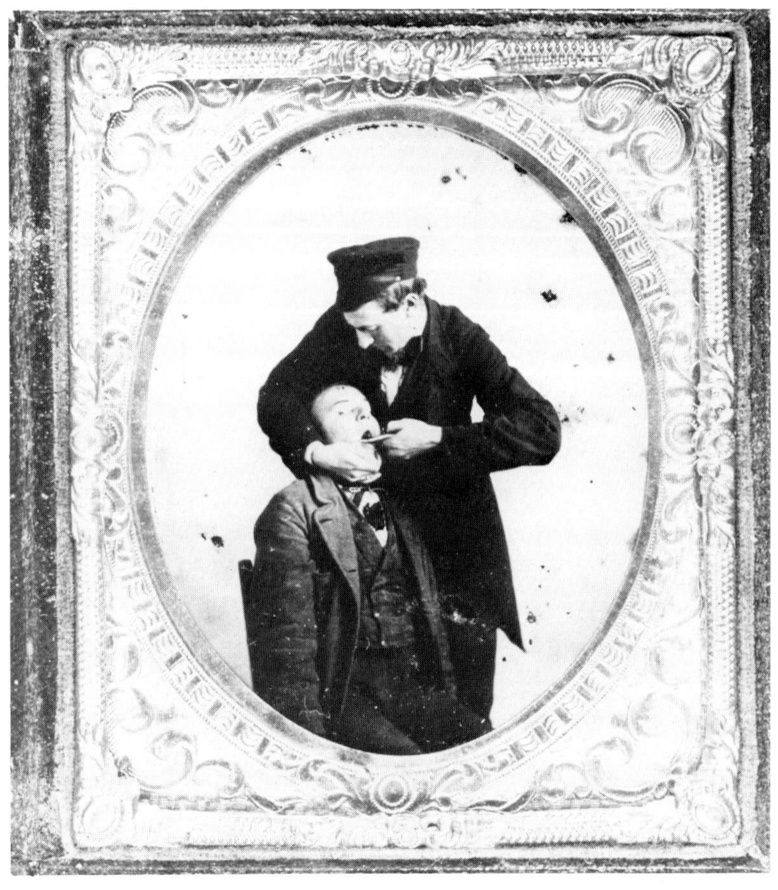

Dental Extraction
Ambrotype 1857
This ambrotype is typical of the extraction images of the time. The hat the dentist wears makes him seem like more of a workman than a professional dentist and he may, in fact, be a quack dentist.

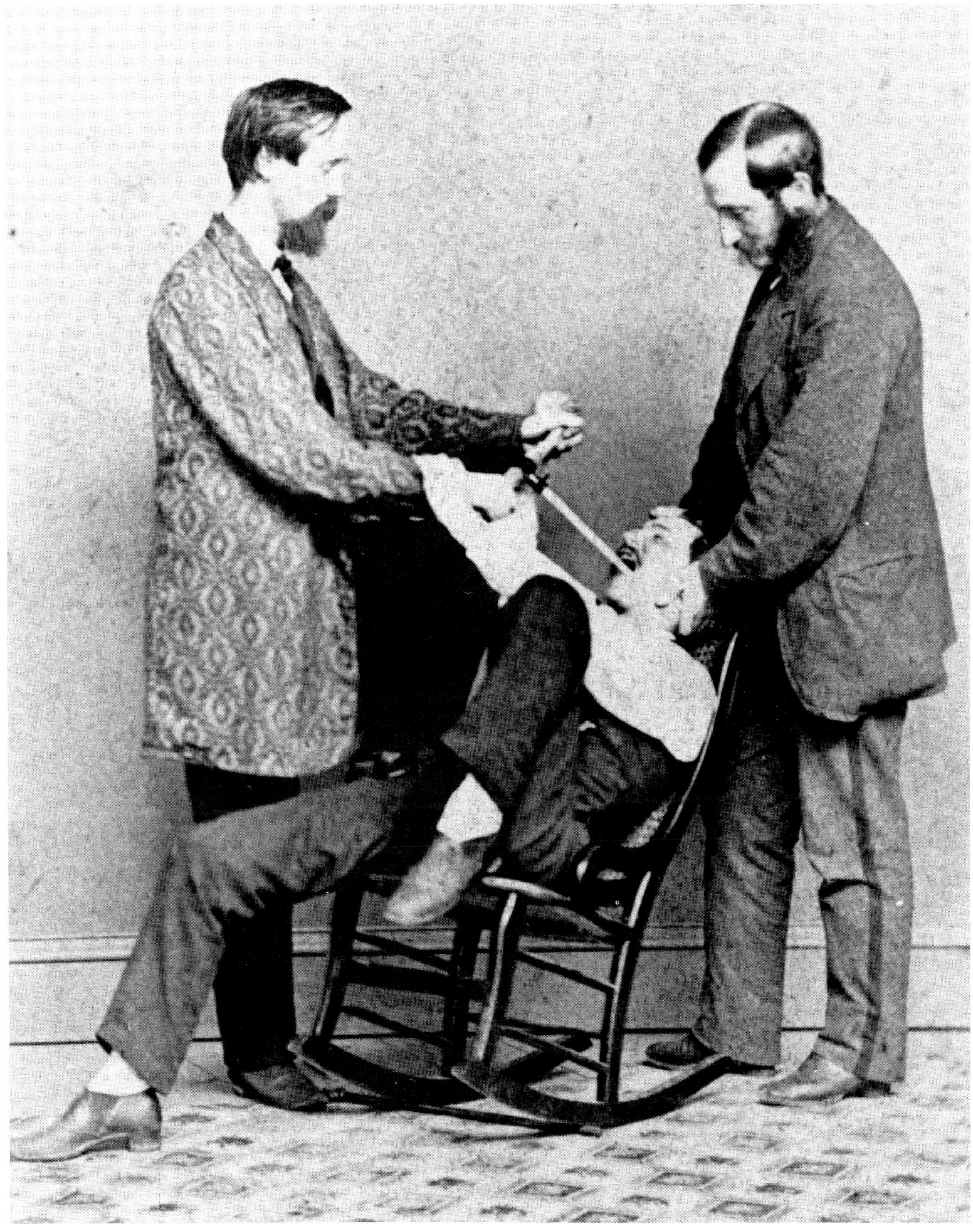

Extraction with Huge Key Carte de visite 1860
This 1860 *carte de visite* is quite unusual, because of the large key that is depicted extracting the tooth. A frequent first response to the image is that it is a comic scene. However the serious expression of everyone argues against this interpretation. In comic scenes someone is always laughing. This may be the announcement of a new dental device. The multicolored coat the dentist wears, although seen in comic images, was very popular in anatomy and dissecting laboratories of the period.

The Dental Image 1870-1900

The American dentist made his statement to the world with his "occupational portrait." These images changed in arrangement and style not only as the profession progressed but as the photographic process developed. Posing as physicians decreased after the dental profession separated from the medical profession. With the establishment of dental colleges and professional organizations dentistry became a separate profession.

By the 1870s, more dentists, proud of their profession and independence, had their photographs taken during the practice of extracting teeth. In the 1880s when the dry plate photographic process came into general use, allowing pictures to be taken "instantly" (exposure times were now 1/25 of a second), photographs in offices became practical, and thus, ensued the common dental image of the era. Dentists were now shown in their offices working with the latest equipment. The images made a good advertisement and a statement of their own high professional standards.

The surgical photographs of the first decade of the 20th century are quite different. These images portray the surgeon as the focus of attention, in the center of his operating amphitheater, dressed in sterile white, separated from his audience; a multitude of eager students watching a delicate procedure, or new miracle device being employed.[6] The master surgeon and his audience had its counterpart image in dentistry. Dental surgeons followed their medical colleagues' examples and took similar styled photographs to herald the new modern dentistry and its mechanical and surgical marvels. By mimicking surgery dentists sought to gain some of the prestige that this profession acquired. A good example of such a photograph is the 1902 image of Matthew H. Cryer, D.D.S., M.D. (1840-1921), professor of Oral Surgery at the University of Pennsylvania Dental College. (See photo page 18.) Cryer demonstrates a new electric drill capable of 5,000 rpm to a packed amphitheater at Philadelphia's Medico-Chirurgical Hospital.[7] Photographs such as these were framed and hung on hospital and clinic walls to show the public the emergence of dentistry as an important part of health care.

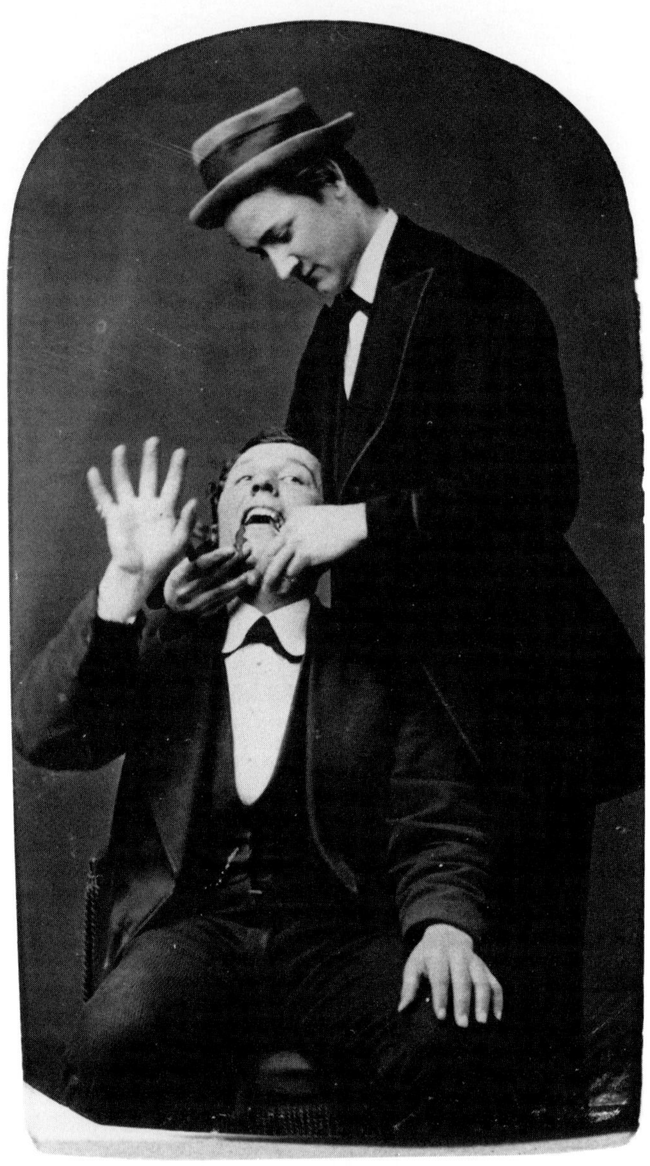

Dental Extraction 1864 and 1870s
These tintypes illustrate the itinerant dentist/quack dentist type of photograph. The patient in most of these images gestures with his hands up, to stop the extraction. It often looks like the patient is praying. Photographs such as these were not the type of public image the professional dentist was anxious to present. The photographs are representative of the craftsman roots of dentistry. They have not been significantly studied or appreciated.

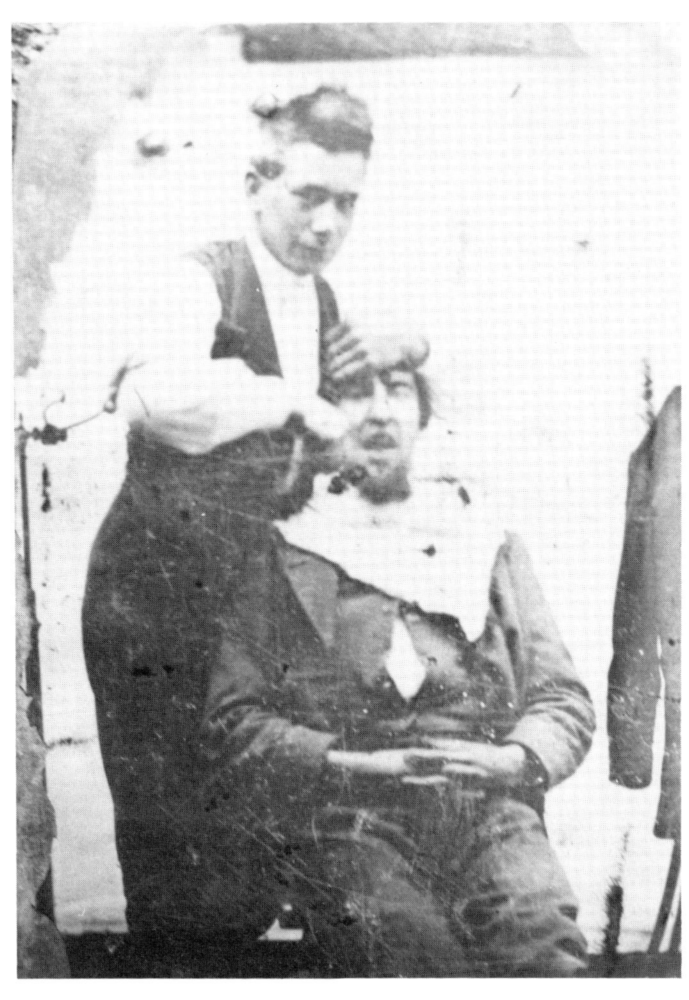

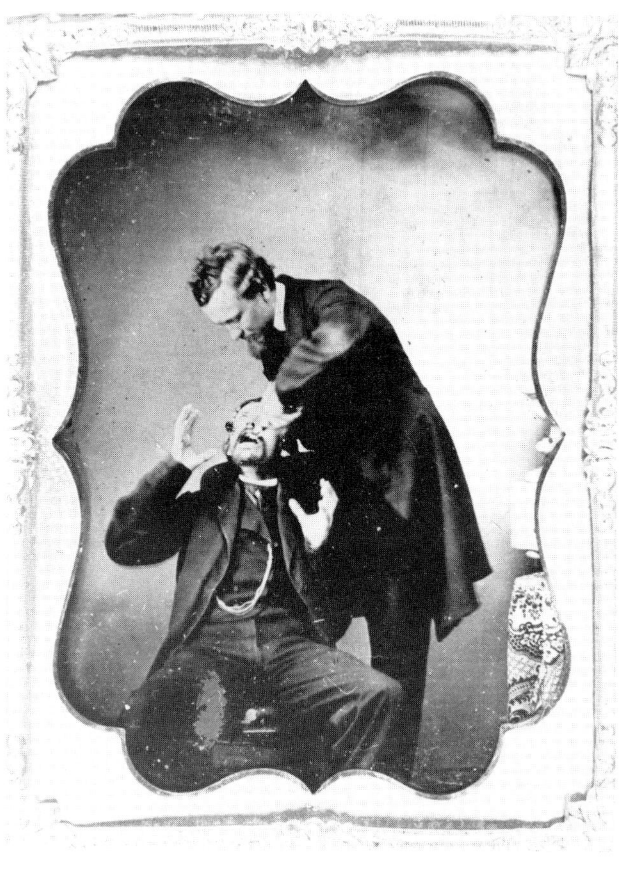

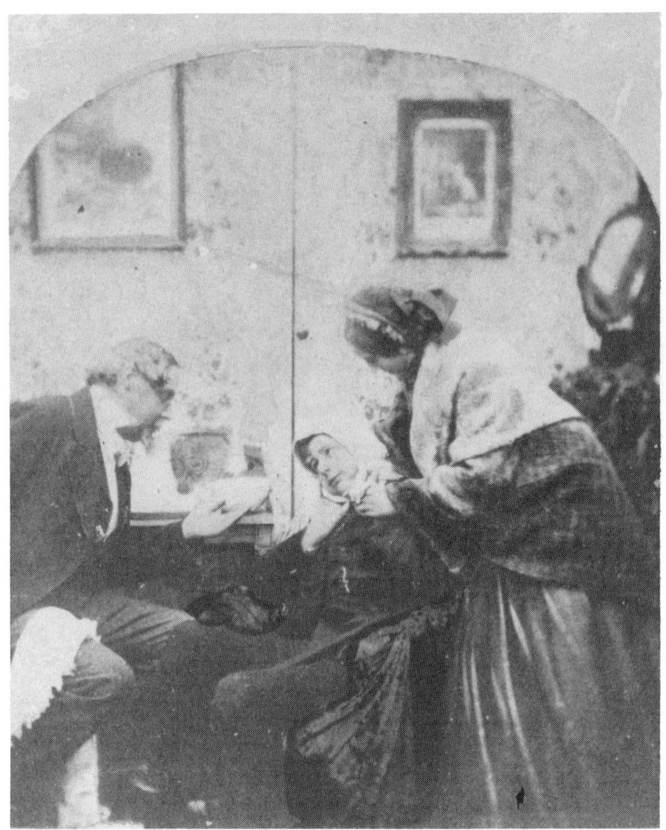

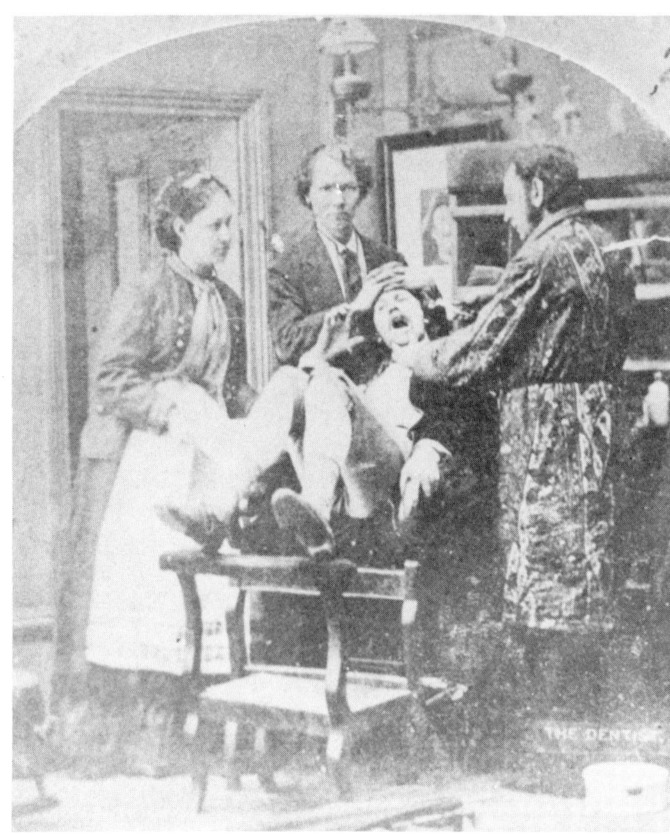

Top Right: Dentist and Preceptee Extracting Tooth Stereoview 1860s
Despite the magnitude of anesthetic and surgical discoveries, old concepts died hard. The pain of tooth extraction remained a frequent subject in 19th century photography. Perhaps the popularity of such images, almost sadistic in their portrayal of suffering, reflected a need for the public to confront their fear of the inevitable trip to the dentist. This stereoview shows an unusual dental operating chair and two assistants holding the patient's head who might have been a preceptor dentist in training.

Top Left: The Toothache Stereoview late 1850s
This stereoview is particularly interesting since it portrays a poignant scene of a patient presenting herself to a physician-dentist to remedy her condition. The professional demeanor of all participants is in striking contrast to comic views and could only elevate the professional image of the dentist. The patient's mother weeps as if her daughter were dying from some fatal disease, giving the impression that dental disease and pain is perhaps as important as other "serious" diseases. None of the dental engravings of the time portray such a realistic, believable, empathetic picture of everyday dental disease.

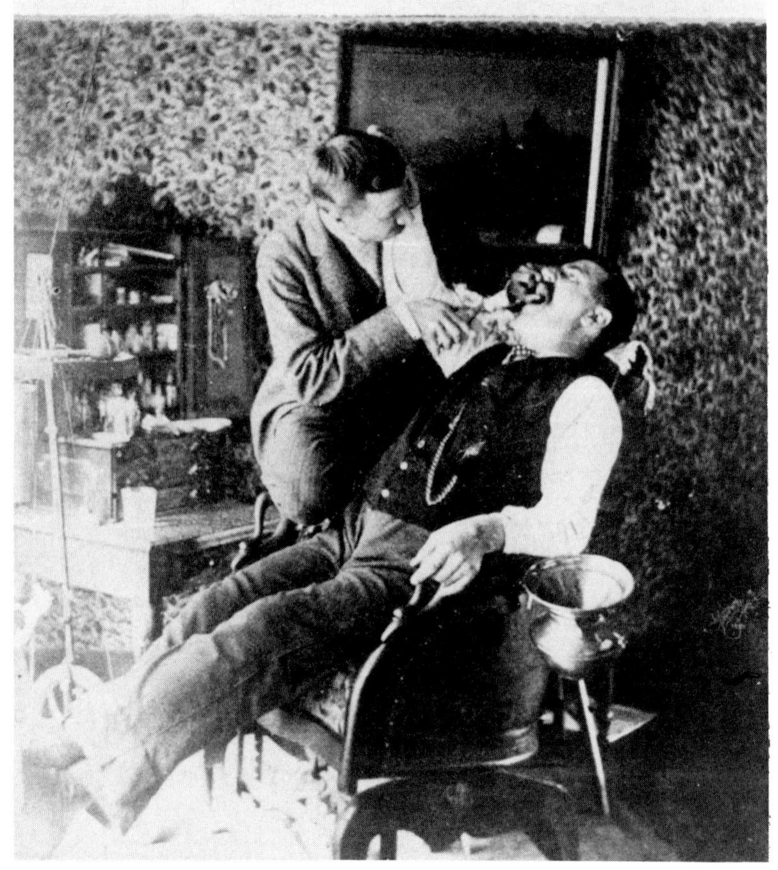

Bottom: Dental Extraction circa 1880
By the 1880s, dental extraction photographs depicted a professional scene. The dentist is shown in his office, which is filled with the latest equipment standing in the background. The patient sits in a commercial dental chair.

Dentists as Photographers

Dentists, as well as physicians, not only faced the camera, but became pioneer photographers. Dentists had the chemical and mechanical knowledge as well as scientific interest to pursue photography. An unrecognized and unheralded part of dental history is the role dentists played in early photography.

Alexander S. Wolcott (1804-1844), America's trail blazing photographer was a mechanical dentist who practiced in New York City. Wolcott's place in photographic history is monumental. He took the first successful photographic portrait in the U.S. on October 7, 1839 and obtained the first photographic patent for his invention of a camera on May 8, 1840. He also developed a system of photographic studio lighting in February 1840 and on March 13, 1840 opened the world's first commercial photographic studio. Wolcott made dental instruments and equipment with his partner, John Johnson, at 52 First Street in New York City.[8]

To understand Wolcott's place in photographic history a recapitulation of early daguerreotypy is necessary. On January 7, 1839, Louis J.M. Daguerre announced his discovery and showed his photographs to the French Academy of Arts and Sciences. On August 19, 1839 the process of taking a daguerreotype was presented. D.W. Seager, who had carried the first photographic manuals with him from Europe when he arrived on September 20, 1839, worked with Samuel F.B. Morse, the inventor and president of the National Academy of Art and Design, who had seen daguerreotypes while on a trip to Europe. Seager produced the first daguerreotype in 1839 and exhibited it on September 30. On Saturday, October 5, Seager gave a lecture on the process, attended by John Johnson, Wolcott's business partner. On Monday October 7, Johnson told Wolcott about the process.[9] They immedi-

Kings Chapel Burying Ground, Boston by Dr. Bemis
This image, dated April 19, 1840, is the first image taken by Dr. Samuel Bemis, America's first amateur photographer. Over the next few years, using his whole plate (6½- by 8½-inch photo size) daguerrean camera, Dr. Bemis continued to photograph Boston scenes. From the International Museum of Photography, George Eastman House.

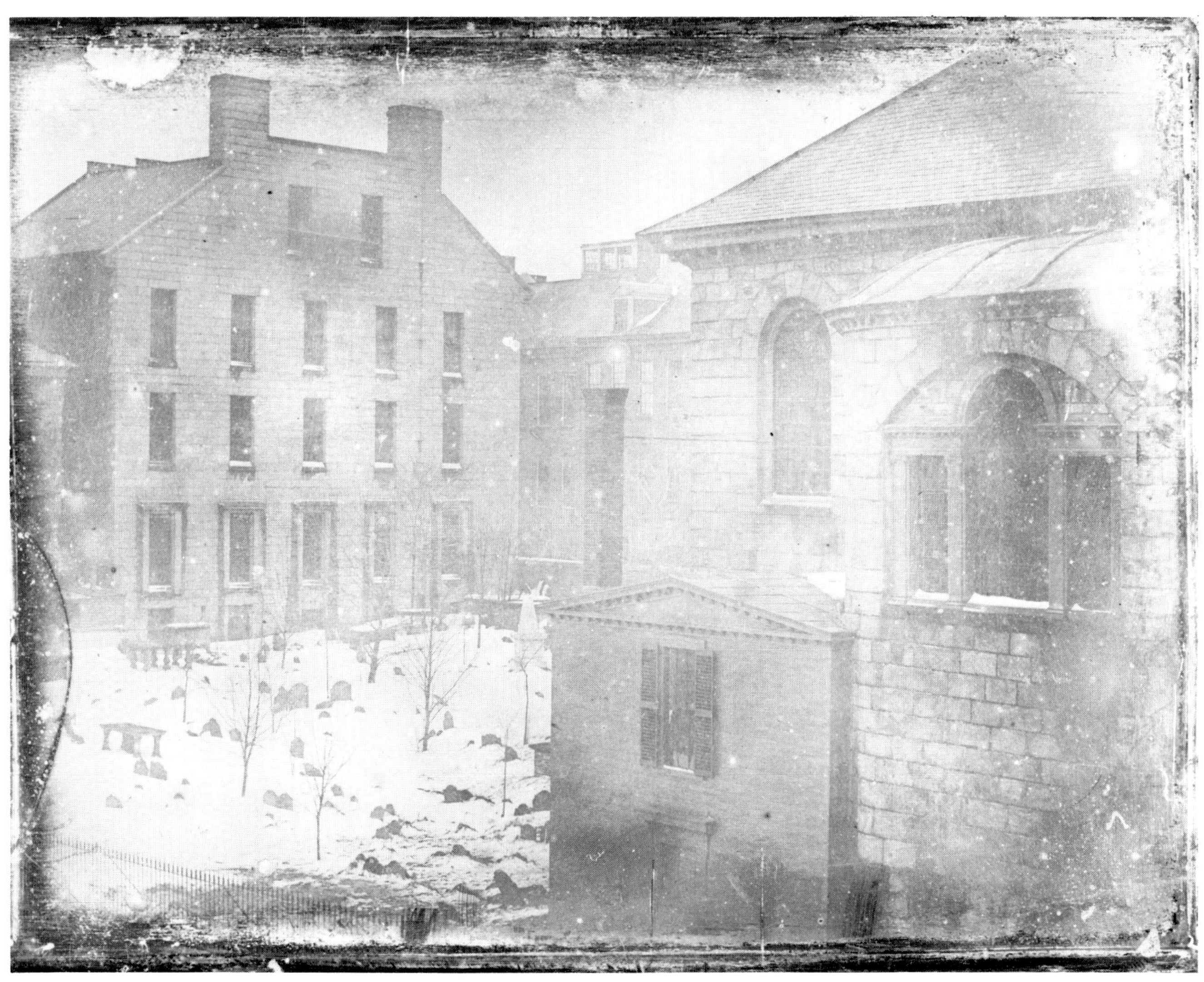

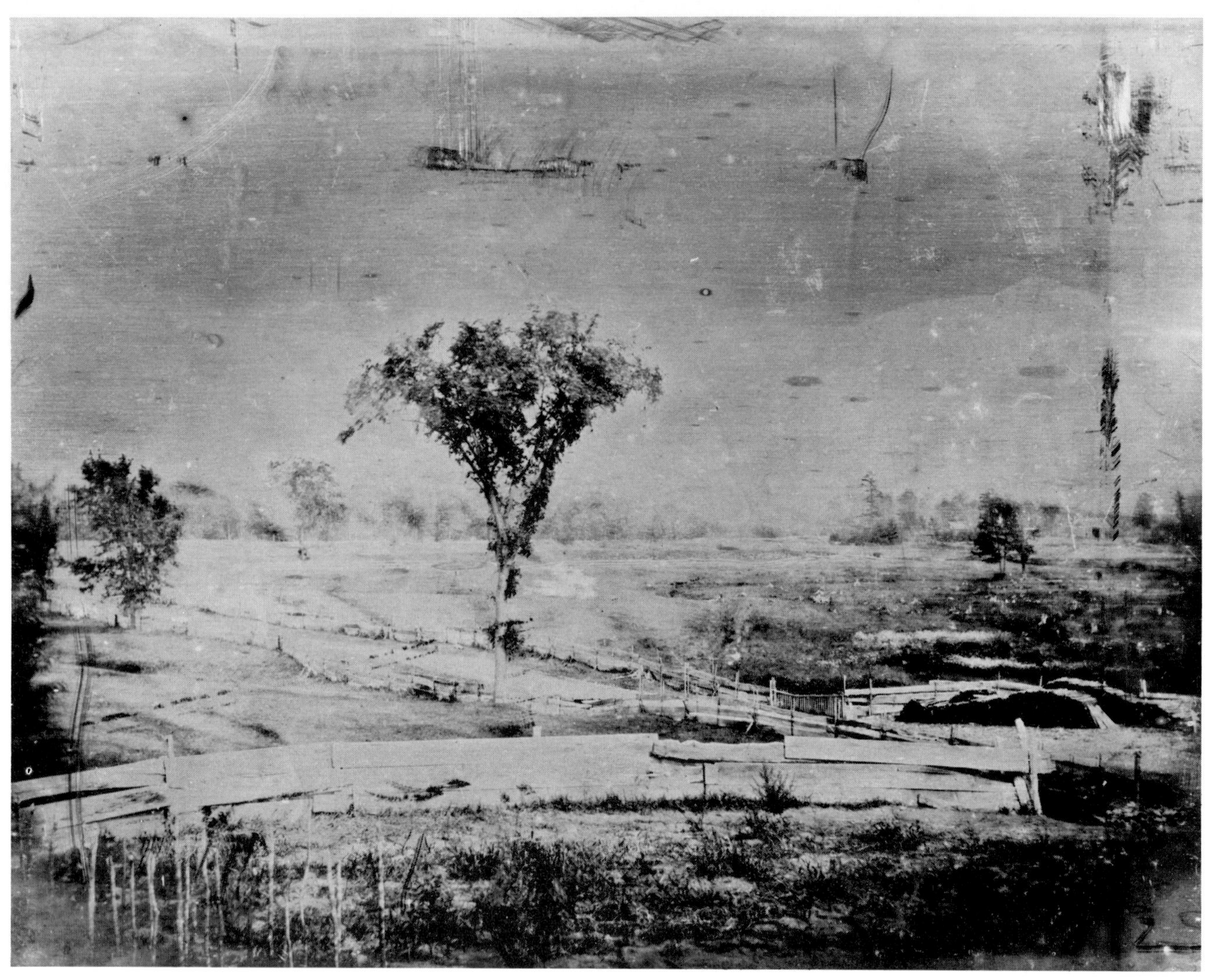

Crawford Notch, New Hampshire by Dr. Bemis
Dr. Bemis' artistic views of the New Hampshire countryside are considered the pioneer effort in American pictorial photography. This particular image is often compared to artist Thomas Cole's painting of the same area. From the International Museum of Photography, George Eastman House.

ately began to make a camera, which was the prototype of the patented camera. The patent model resides in the National Museum of American History. A second example was donated by Johnson in 1866 to the York Institute of Saco, Maine, which he established.[10]

Wolcott took photographs of Johnson. Although now lost, they were the first successful pictures taken of anyone in the United States.[11] The successes of Johnson and Wolcott in America led them to operate with English pioneer, Richard Beard, one of the first photographic studios in England in November 1841. Samuel Morse attempted unsuccessfully to get Wolcott to join him in the further development of the daguerrean art.[12] Wolcott's death, at age 40, in 1844, put an end to a career that contributed much to the development of photography. His association with the practice of dentistry has not been generally appreciated.

Dentists intrigued by photography bought cameras to record their world. Some practitioners gave up the practice of dentistry to become full time photographers and others did photography as a sideline to supplement their income. One of the most noted early American photographers was a practicing dentist—Dr. Samuel Bemis (1789-1881). Bemis is known as America's first landscape and pictorialist photographer.[13] His 1840 daguerreotypes of the New England landscape are now considered works of art and are frequently compared to esteemed paintings of the same scenes. Many of Bemis' images have survived and they represent the world's largest collection of early photographic outdoor scenes.

Bemis bought his camera on April 15, 1840 and started taking views of Boston four days later. It took him 40 minutes to expose his plate of Kings Chapel Burying Ground. Soon afterward he traveled to New Hampshire, pointing his camera at the landscape around Crawford Notch.[14] Dozens of his views of the countryside survive. Only a handful of American scenic images remain that are earlier than Bemis'. Another dentist who began to use a camera in 1840 was a Philadelphian, Dr. J.E. Parker, who turned his lens on the city. Unfortunately, none of his original daguerreotypes survive, but copy prints of them are intact.[15] Another New Yorker, a physician-dentist, M. Villers, opened a photographic studio at 233 Broadway in November of 1841.[16]

Southern practitioners also followed the heliographic art. In Tallahassee, Florida, Sterling McIntyre advertised in January 1845 that he is "taking colored Daguerreotype Likenesses in the latest style and will continue, as heretofore, the practice of Dentistry in all its branches." McIntyre was an itinerant photographer traveling around Florida and adjacent states. Although little is known of his dental practice, McIntyre practiced photography in Charleston, South Carolina (1847-48), New York City (1850-51), and even, traveled to California during the gold rush, where he took panoramic daguerreotypes of San Francisco in 1851.[17]

Isiah W. Taber (1830-1912) was another photographer who also practiced dentistry. He traveled to California during the gold rush. In 1849 he became an associate of Robert Vance, the famed daguerreotypist of gold mining camps. Taber returned to the East in 1854 to practice dentistry in his native town, New Bedford, Massachusetts. Photography was his calling, however. He moved to Syracuse, New York and opened one of the first galleries there, but returned to California in 1864, when he was invited to join the prestigious San Francisco gallery of Bradley and Rulofson. He opened his studio in 1871 and, four years later, introduced the "promenade" sized photograph, a 4-by 7-inch print that became quite popular as its greater length permitted a more congenial portrait. Taber went on to become one of California's noted photographers. He photographed Queen Victoria's Jubilee in 1887 and was named a commissioner of Yosemite Park in 1888.

By 1906, after 57 years of photography, Taber had accumulated an extensive collection of images of California estimated at 80 tons of portrait negatives and 20 tons of scenic view negatives. The earthquake and fire of 1906 destroyed all of these items, an irreplaceable loss of the visual record of early California.[18]

European dentists also became photographers. Among the most noted was James Robinson, D.D.S. of Dublin, Ireland, a distinguished dentist and the namesake of one of England's leading practitioners. Robinson took up photography in the late 1840s and became one of the most important European medical photographers of the 1870s. In 1853 Robinson became official photographer to the British Army. At the end of the Crimean War, he opened a photographic studio in his shop at 65 Grafton Street, Dublin. During the next 20 years Robinson was called upon by his medical colleagues to record their surgical cases, pre- and post-operatively.[19] A pioneer in scientific photography, in 1849 Robinson attempted unsuccessfully to daguerreotype the moon. He concluded that since the moon could not be photographed the moon must not radiate actinic rays which were believed necessary for photography.[20] Several of the photographs he took were published as engravings in the *Dublin Journal of the Medical Sciences*. Much of Robinson's collection of medical photographs, now in the Burns Archive, has been recognized by art and photographic historians as masterpieces of medical photography.[21] Robinson was active in photographic circles and was a founding member of the Dublin Photographic Society. His sons continued his photographic business until the end of the century.

Photography in America

Photography became an American pastime that helped to solidify the country as a nation, by promoting a national spirit. It allowed Easterners to see the magnificence of the American west, and everyone to see how the country was developing and expanding. Photography permeated American life. Everything was expected to be photographed and it was. Dental offices appear in streets photographed all over the U.S.

Photography, unlike painting, was available to the poor, as well as the affluent. Because photography was moderately priced and daguerreotypists traveled the countryside plying their craft between 1840-60, almost every town and village had an opportunity to have its inhabitants photographed. Itinerant photographers brought their cameras to every corner of America on horseback, in covered wagons, down rivers in flatboats and on mules through the mountains.

Americans have been enthusiastic about photography since its inception. It is estimated that between 30 and 40 million daguerreotypes were taken in the two decades after 1840. Many of these images survive. Importance alone has not guaranteed that an image would be preserved. Entire subjects may be lost. For example, in the 1850s, there were over 100 daguerreotypists in Manhattan. Indeed New York City was the center of daguerreotypic photography in America. Thousands of views of the city were taken, which is proved by the engravings made from the daguerreotypes, yet not one original daguerreotype of Manhattan survives from this period.[22]

Early Photographic Processes

Images of dentists survive in all of the early photographic processes used in America. For a better understanding of the images and the eras in which they were taken, a brief outline of these photographic processes is in order. The daguerreotype, popular from 1840-1860, is a one-of-a-kind

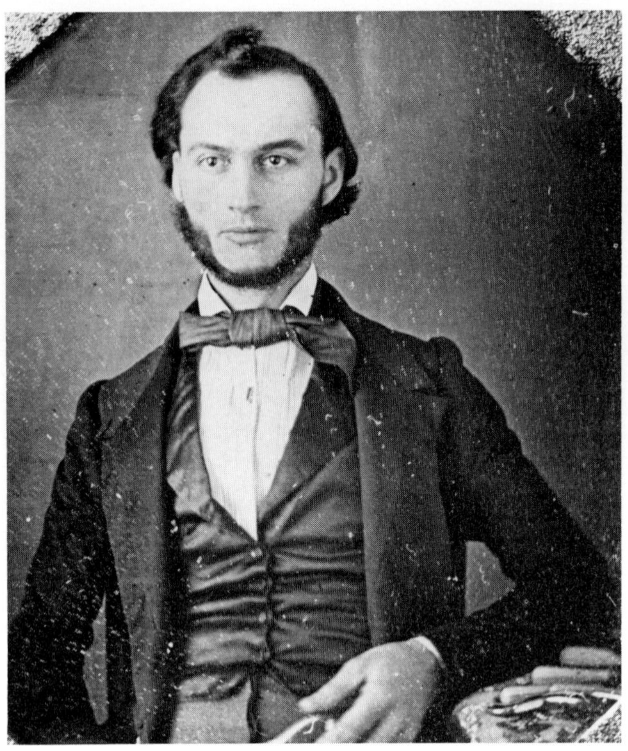

Henry Daniel Cogswell D.D.S. Daguerreotype—1850s
This is the only identified daguerreotype of a dentist, Dr. Henry D. Cogswell (1818-1900), who was reported to be the first dentist in California to use chloroform in oral surgery.

Cogswell practiced in a tent on lower Washington Street in San Francisco and later moved into an office at 219 Washington Street, where he displayed a golden tooth sign. In the 1860s James L. Cogswell joined him in practice at the Cogswell Building located at 610 Front Street.

Dr. and Mrs. Cogswell founded the Cogswell Polytechnic College in 1887. In 1975 it was renamed the Cogswell College.

This daguerreotype shows the pioneer dentist beside a set of extraction tools. In his hands he holds a forceps with an extracted tooth. The original daguerreotype is now lost. Copy print courtesy Richard Rudisill.

image on a silver-coated copper plate. Because of their fragility they were housed under glass and placed in cases. The daguerreotype possesses a clarity of detail, brilliance, three-dimensionality and flesh-like color that is unmatched by any other type of photograph. Millions of daguerreotypes were destroyed over the years. Some owners attempted to clean the picture that had tarnished and ended up wiping it away. Other images were thrown out by people who wanted the cases for other pictures.

The wet plate process was discovered in 1851 by the Englishman Scott Archer, and ultimately, replaced the daguerreotype. It involved coating glass or almost any other substance with an emulsion containing collodion as the vehicle to hold the photosensitive chemicals. If glass was used, it became a negative from which to print photographs. Many different kinds of images were possible. Ultimately, the discovery of an albumen based paper allowed for development of the reproducible paper photograph. The wet plate process received its name from the fact that the photographer had to prepare his plate, expose it in the camera, and develop it, all while the plate was still wet. This meant trotting around with cumbersome equipment and made it an unattractive hobby for an amateur.

The ambrotype, popular from 1854-1865, is a one-of-a-kind wet plate photograph on a glass plate. Instead of using the glass as a negative to make paper prints, in this form of the wet plate, the glass negative itself was used as a positive picture by placing it on a black background and then, mounting it in a case, as had been done with daguerreotypes. Most ambrotypes are dark and display poor contrast.

The tintype, popular from 1856-1910 (they were taken until the 1940s) is a one-of-a-kind positive photograph on a thin sheet of iron. The name came from the fact that they were cut from the sheet of iron with tin snips. Tintypes were cheap, and they were not fragile. The surface could not be rubbed off, as could a daguerreotype or ambrotype.

The calotype, perfected in England by William Fox Talbot in 1841, was a paper print from a paper negative. The photograph required a long exposure time and had a lack of clarity and a mistiness. Calotypes were rarely taken in America, as taking them required a license from the inventor and Americans preferred the detail and clarity of the daguerreotype. There are no known photographs of dentists in the calotype format.

The carte de visite, popular from 1850-1870s is a small paper print 2½- by 3½-inches, pasted on a mounting card 2¾- by 4-inches. Due to its reproducibility and low cost the carte de visite brought about the demise of the daguerreotype. Printing houses were soon making and selling thousands of photographs of notable people and events. Collectors were able to familiarize themselves with the world in a way that had been heretofore impossible. Collecting these photo cards necessitated the placement of them in a photographic album.

The Cabinet card, popular from 1870-1900 is 4- by 5½-inches mounted on cardboard 4¼- by 6½-inches. The larger size allowed photographers greater leeway in posing, lighting and background. The negatives were easily retouched.

The Dry Plate, developed in the 1870s, became the American standard in 1881. It permitted instantaneous photographs, but most importantly, it freed the photographer from being the platemaker. All the other photographic processes demanded that the photographer prepare his own plates and develop them himself. With the dry plate one purchased prepared plates, took the pictures, and then, was able to send them off to a company to develop the images. The dry plate allowed for the expansion of photography to anyone. Amateur photography began to proliferate. The modern age arrived in 1889, when George Eastman introduced his Kodak camera to be used with flexible film in a roll holder. All the owner had to do was point the camera and shoot.

The Stereograph, was a popular form of photography in the 19th century and a form that included all the different processes of photography. The stereograph consists of two pictures shot at a slightly different angle: when placed in a special device called a stereoscope the viewer sees a three-dimensional illusion that makes it appear as if he is actually in or witnessing the photographed scene. Viewing stereographs in the parlor was a popular entertainment of the 19th century comparable to television. Stereographs were sold in America until the 1930s. Dental scenes abound in this format.

Mechanical photographs, the making of a permanent photograph by a printing press was developed in response to the demand to illustrate publications. Paper prints could be used in publications but they had to be hand pasted or tipped-in. It was expensive, time consuming, and the prints faded. Prior to development of the modern halftone in the 1880s, two types of permanent mechanical prints were perfected that were used for illustrations in America: the woodburytype and collotype.

The woodburytype, patented in 1866, was one of the most pleasing photographs ever created. Its tonal quality is wide and its clarity is excellent. It has fine definition and an absence of grain or halftone effects, and most importantly, does not fade. Its one disadvantage was that the picture had to be printed on a different press than the publication, and then, trimmed and mounted on the page.

The collotype, brought to America in 1869, had numerous variations and names (artotype), albertype, heliotype). The tones of a collotype are less bright and have poorer definition than woodburytypes. The great advantage of the collotype is that it can be printed directly on the page with easily pre-set margins, thus eliminating the problems of margination and the labor involved in pasting the print on the page. Woodburytypes were popular in the 1870s and collotypes in the 1880s. Halftones replaced them in the 1890s.[23]

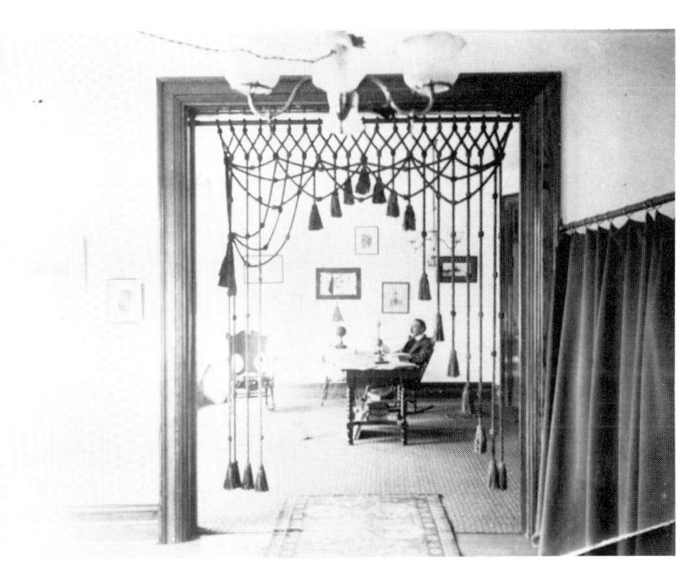

During the late 1880s it was one of the fashions of the times to take photographs in the home framing the subject in the type of cord drapes you see here. Dentists were popular subjects in these views. In one image we see the dentist in the background with his patient, in the other he sits at his desk in a contemplative mood. In both photographs the predominant object is the drapes. Artistic considerations in this era now seem more important than the documentary.

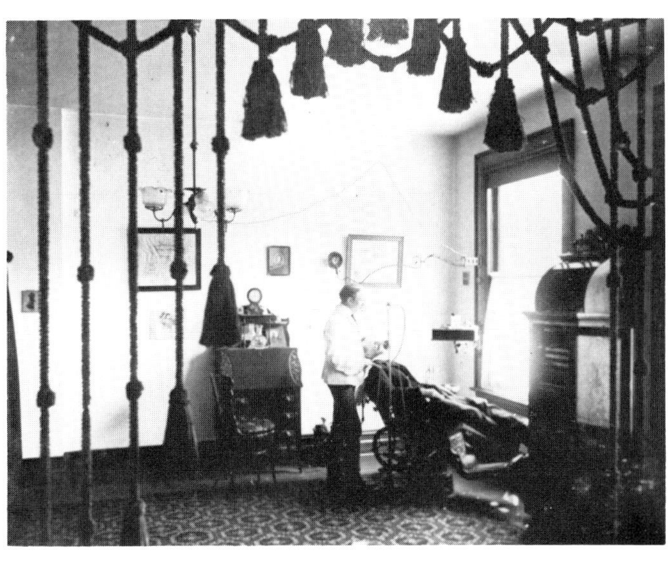

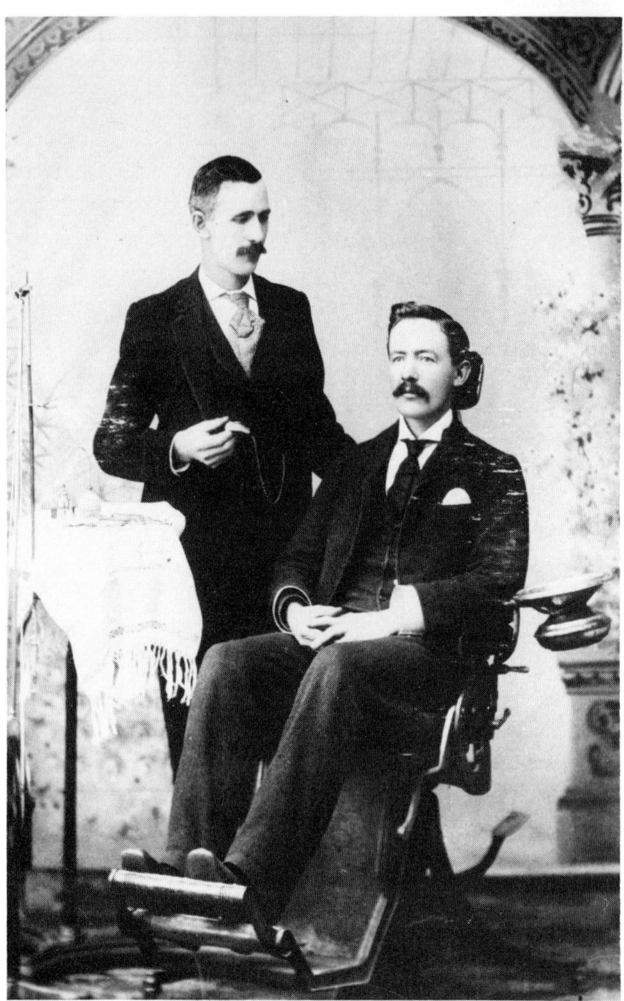

Dr. Ambrose.
Cabinet card, circa 1880, is unusual in that the dentist is identified by his name printed on the towel that covers his instrument stand. It is also unusual in that the main focus of the picture is the artificial teeth which the dentist holds in his hand. This picture most likely was taken for advertising purposes as it was taken in a photographic studio, rather than, his office. The lighting and composition is perfect for the era. The dentist would have had to bring his equipment to the studio which may have been near his office, since both offices usually were found on the second or upper floors to take advantage of sunlight.

Photographic Record of Dentistry's Most Important Discovery

The pain and discomfort of dental work and extractions is legendary. The suffering which accompanies so common a procedure prompted the search for an effective desensitizing agent. The desire for "painless dentistry" led American dentists to discover and promote the use of general anesthesia, in the opinion of many, America's greatest gift to medicine.

New England dentist, Horace Wells and the physician-dentist, William Morton, discovered and promoted the earliest effective anesthetics. John M. Riggs extracted the tooth of his partner, Wells, a Hartford, Connecticut dentist on December 11, 1844. Sedated with nitrous oxide, as instructed by Wells, the operation was a painless success. Later, Riggs, Charles Jackson and the Boston physician-dentist, William Morton, who was most interested in lessening the pain of preparing teeth to be filled, replaced the anesthetic, nitrous oxide with sulphuric ether. Then, on September 30, 1846, in the Massachusetts General Hospital's amphitheater, Dr. Morton performed a completely painless tooth extraction.[24]

On October 16, 1846, Morton administered anesthesia for the first public demonstration of the effects of sulfuric ether.[25] Dr. John Collins Warren removed a tumor from the neck of the unconscious patient, Gilbert Abbott. This event occurred only six years after the founding of America's first Dental College in Baltimore. Surgery and dentistry would never again be the same and without the pain associated with an operation. Surgeons and dentists could now undertake longer and more specialized operations which the unconscious patient could endure. As a result, by the early 20th century, surgery would become a most respected medical specialty.

Photographer Josiah Hawes was present and was prepared to take a photograph of the first operation under anesthesia on October 16, 1846, but the sight of the blood unnerved him and the plate was never made. He returned, however, to photograph subsequent ether operations. The images remain a legacy of a major achievement—the conquest of pain. Morton is not in this picture and the anesthetist is unidentified. These two views of the same early ether operation are presented side-by-side for the first time. Most photographic historians are not even aware of the existence of two photographs that were taken of the same ether operation.

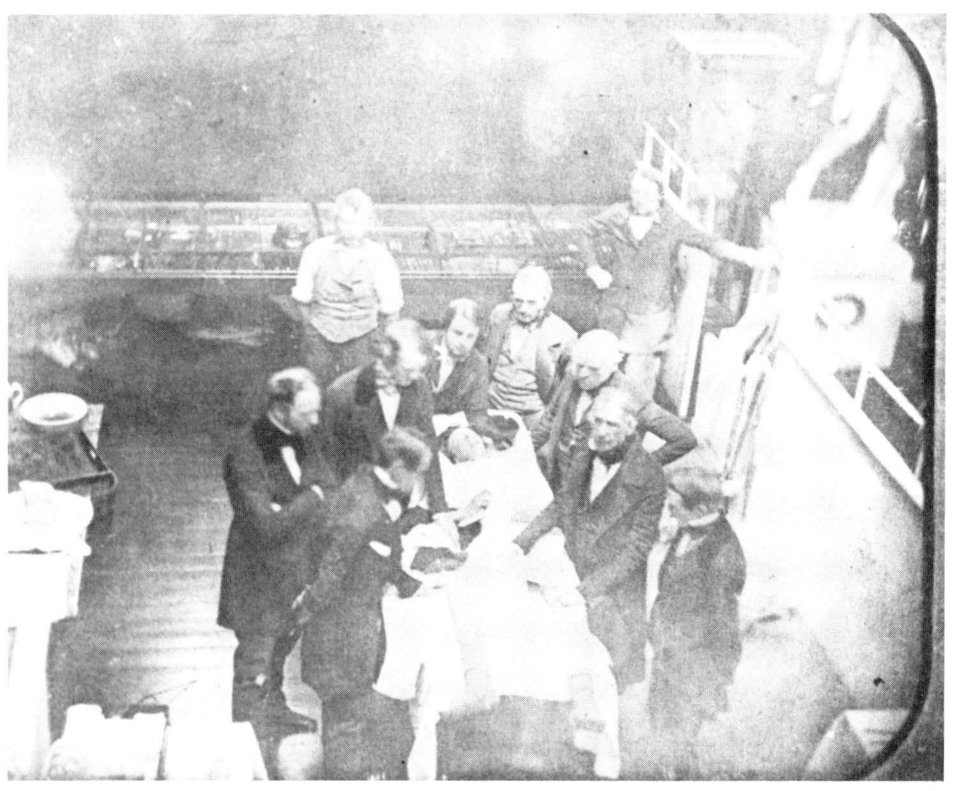

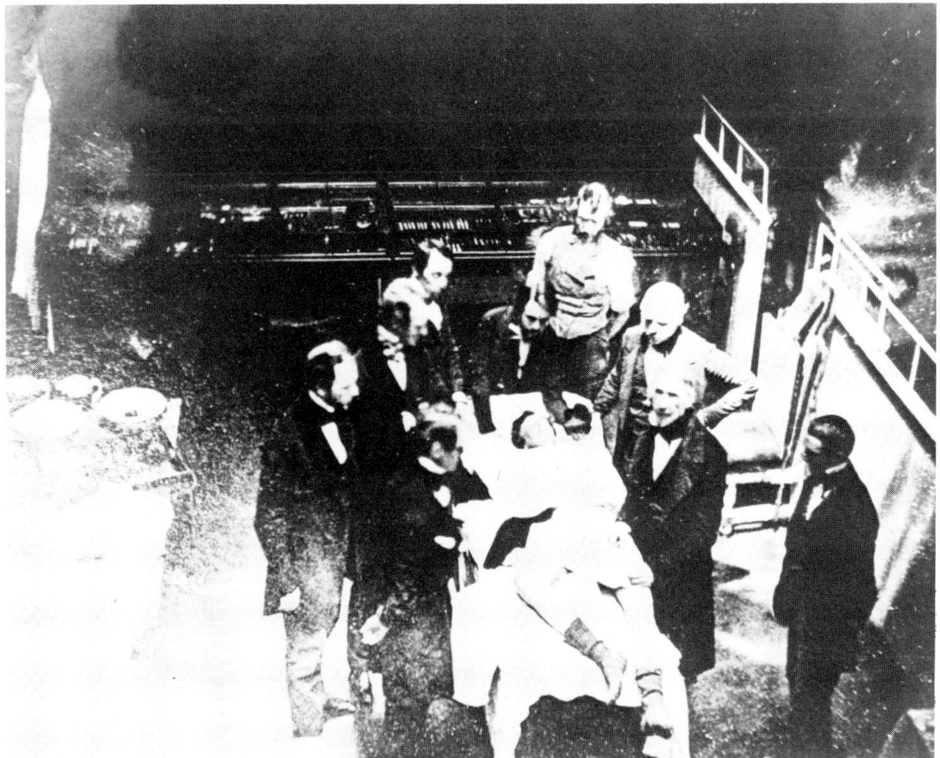

First Photographed Ether Operation
These daguerreotypes of an ether operation in the Massachusetts General Hospital amphitheater in 1846 document the discovery of general anesthesia and are the first American documentary photographs. Several daguerreotypes of early ether operations were taken in the winter of 1846-47 but these may be the first. This is the first time images taken at the same ether operation are published side-by-side. Most photohistorians do not know of the existence of two daguerreotypes recording the same operation. John Collins Warren who performed the first ether operation stares up at us. Henry Bigelow is opposite, only the two men at the top of the picture changed positions for the second image. The anesthesiologist is unidentified.

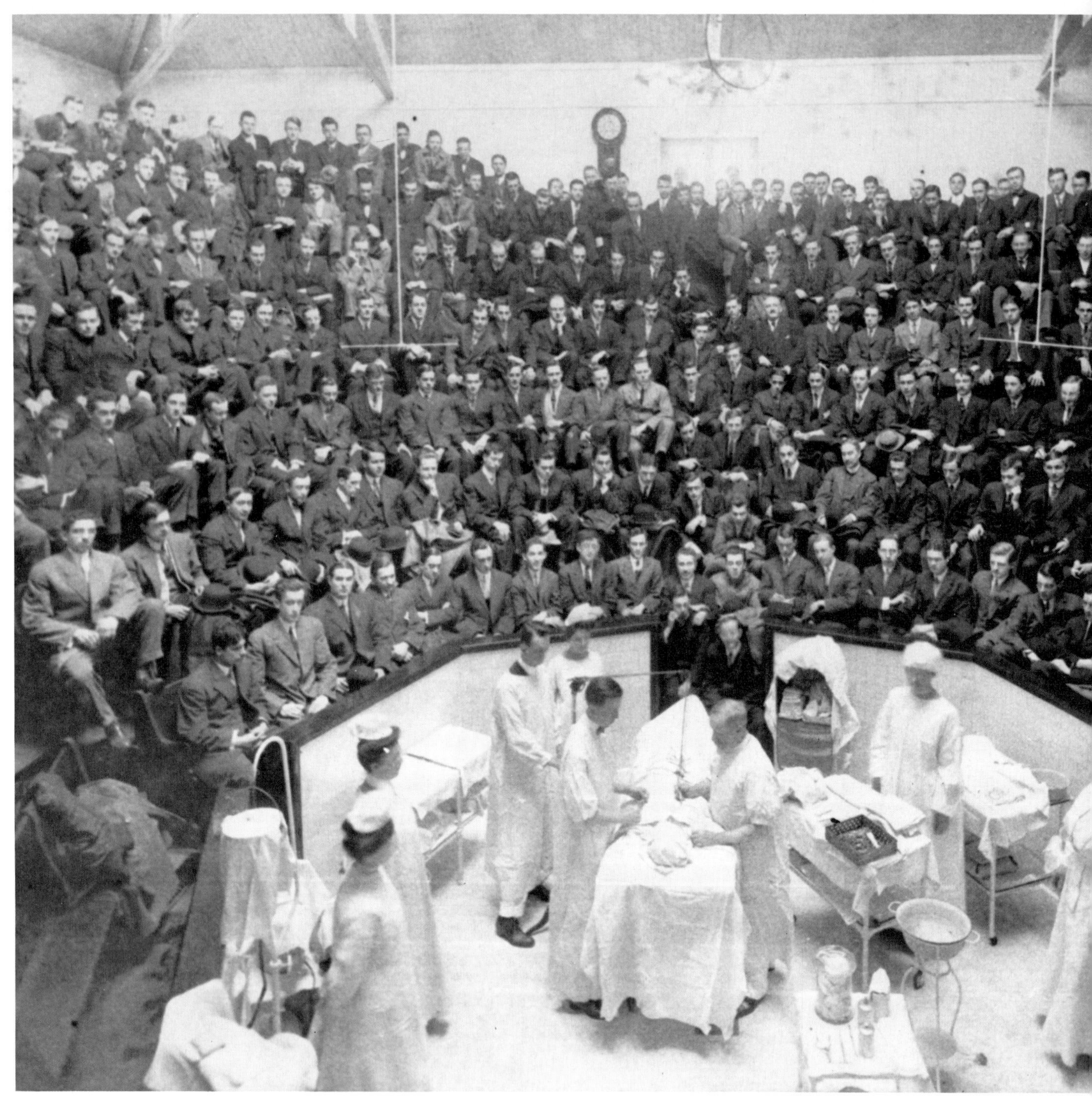

Changing Dental Image—The 20th Century

The image the physician chose to project changed dramatically in the 20th century. Included in this change were dental practitioners. Far from their image as barbaric tooth-pullers, dentists are pictured much closer in imagery to skilled dental and oral surgeons.

This photograph might well be called "The Master Dentist and His Student Hierarchy." This distinction between a trained professional and those still learning had become an important one in professional hierarchy. Gone were the days of the Jacksonian era and philosophy when anyone could enter any career. The photographs underscored the years of training and the many levels of achievement required before the ultimate goal of professional competence and recognition would be reached.

Symbolizing the dentist's recently acquired aura of expertise was this new model electric drill, developed just the year before this photograph was taken. Foot-powered drills had been around since the 18th century for laboratory use, as had crude electric drills, however this "modern-day" unit was capable of operating at 5,000 rpm.

This image was recorded at Dr. M.H. Cryer's clinic at the University of Pennsylvania's Hospital. It was taken April 5, 1902 by C.E. Waterman, a specialist in medical photography. The original is a 9- by 13-inch silver print.

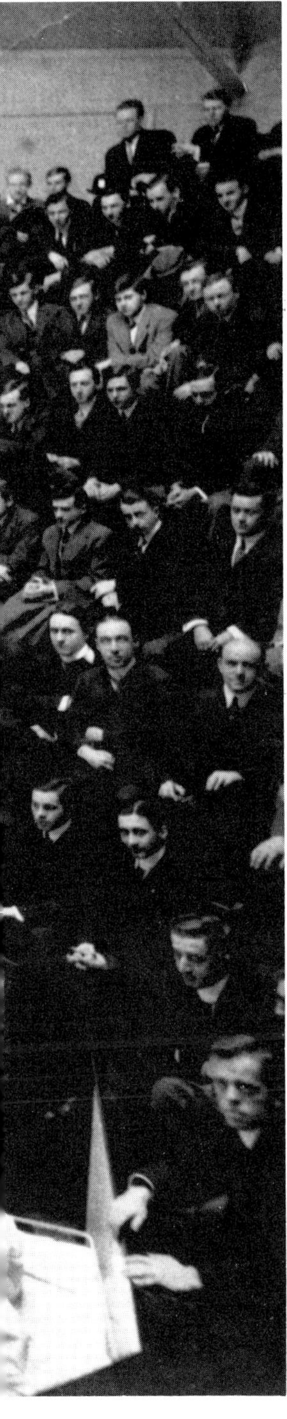

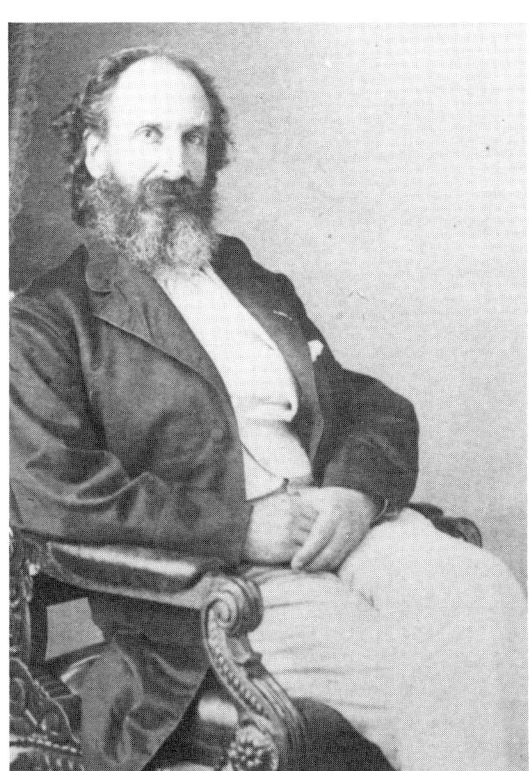

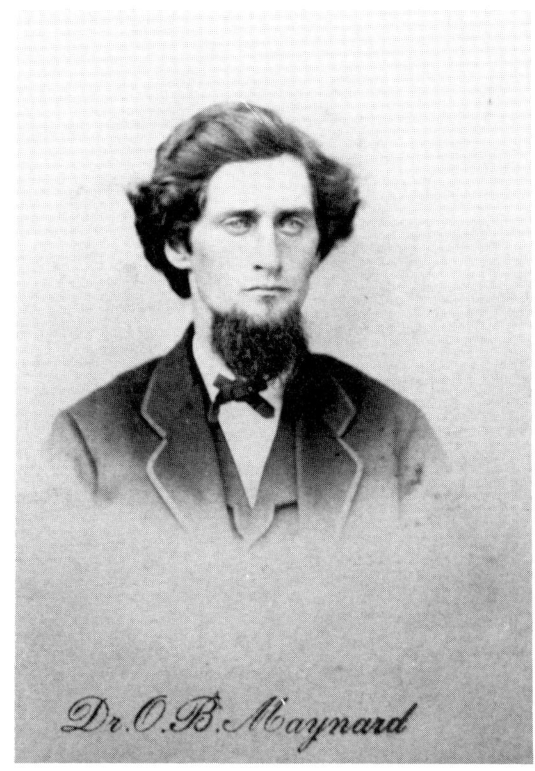

Dr. Edward Maynard (1813-1891) and Son

One of the 19th century's well-known dentists was Edward Maynard. Yet today he is almost forgotten by his dental colleagues. He is one of the few 19th century dentists whose picture is preserved at the National Portrait Gallery and much of his memorabilia is preserved at the Smithsonian Institution and Library of Congress. Maynard is remembered for his revolutionary firearm inventions, the importance of which overshadowed his dental work and discoveries. This is unfortunate because Maynard was a master dentist.

Maynard invented a system of firearm ignition in 1845, a roll of caps in a special holder, that replaced the percussion cap. The patent model for this invention is shown in photograph, Neg. No. 88-12793, taken by Richard Strauss, Smithsonian Institution. The system of caps employed in this gun, while too complex to use for military purposes, was modified and is used today in toy guns.

In 1851, Maynard patented a breech loading rifle, which when adapted, in 1859, to his 1856 invention of metallic cartridges, was the most advanced firearm of the time. Other firearm innovations followed. Some of his inventions were ultimately taken up by every major nation for their military forces. Maynard was honored by foreign nations.

In dentistry Maynard made significant contributions, among them was his announcement of the existence of dental fibrils, an improved drill to prepare cavities, and a system of non-cohesive gold filling. In 1838 he advocated removing the tooth-pulp and filling the pulp-canals with gold foil. He invented barbed broaches for pulp removal and enlarging the pulp canal. His exquisite operative dexterity earned him an invitation as Imperial Court Dentist to Nicholas of Russia. Maynard refused the offer and returned to Washington, D.C. in 1845 to resume his dental practice, which eventually included several presidents, senators and other government officials.

Maynard taught dentistry and became an associate editor of the *American Journal of Dental Science*. Maynard advocated the formation of an official dental corps, which was not established until 1901.

The *carte de visite* photographs pictured here were taken by Alexander Gardner in Washington, D.C. and are part of an album acquired by the Burns Archive from Maynard's descendants. Edward's son, John, carried on his dental heritage, practicing in New York City. Alexander Gardner is now recognized by many as the most important photographer of the time, surpassing Matthew Brady whose pictures were taken by hired personnel because of Brady's own poor vision.

Patients

Because the head and face are the most public and prominent parts of the body, disease of the area is usually brought to the attention of the physician and dentist early in its course. In the fearful pre-Listerian era, when surgery generally was avoided, the most frequent elective surgical procedures performed involved surgery of the face. Many facial disorders, which required an unusually skillful surgeon to repair, were allowed to deteriorate to a degree which seem unendurable today. Dentists played a prominent role in this surgery because many tumors involved the jaws and necessitated replacement of the teeth. Reports of removal of the jaw and tumors filled the medical and dental literature of the period. Many note the work of the dental surgeon in performing a stage of the operation or in restorative work, such as tooth reconstruction. Dentists also manufactured artificial parts for the face—even full masks—to hide the defects of the surgery. The illustrations here display some of the types of facial tumors patients exhibited.

Facial Prosthesis
During the 19th century disfigurements of the face due to diseases, war wounds, or surgical procedures were often managed by dentists. These practitioners artfully made parts of the jaw, teeth and any other type of prosthesis to make life more tolerable for these unfortunate patients. Talking and eating solid food was made possible by these pioneer prosthetic artists. Vulcanized rubber was the miracle product often used to mold facial arts.

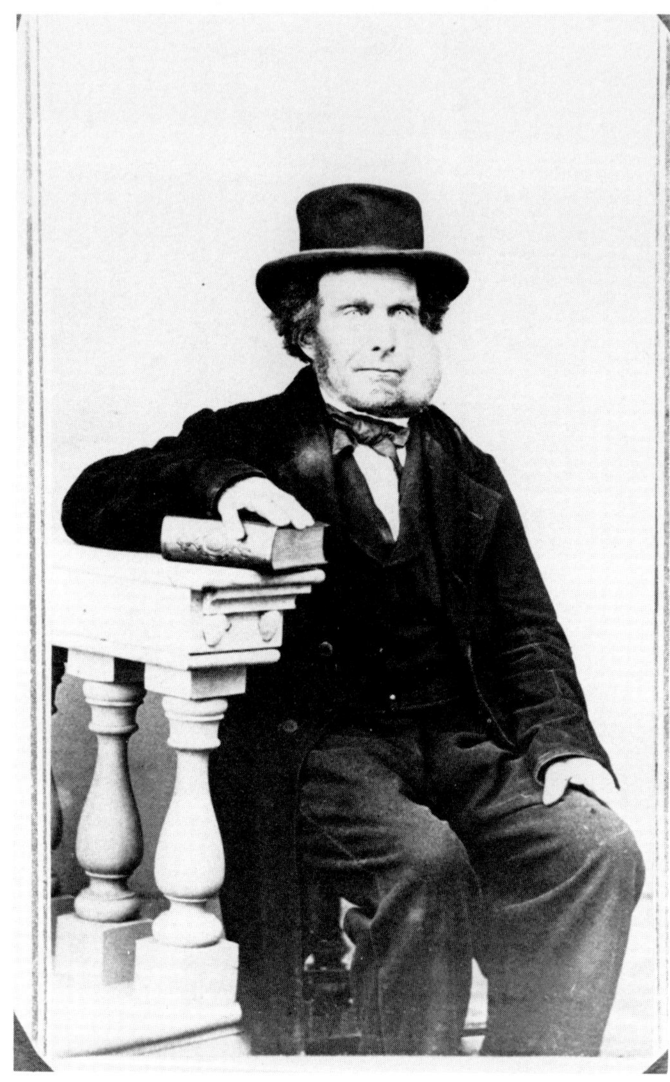

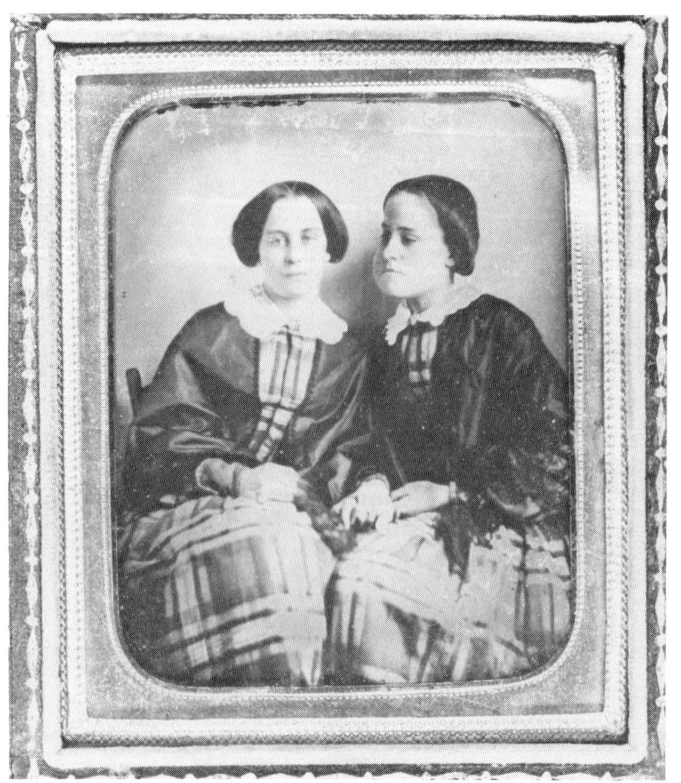

Patients with Jaw Tumors
These patients are typical of the many with tumors of the parotid, mandible or mouth that ultimately sought medical/dental attention. These photographs show the extent of tumor growth that some people lived with. Fear of surgery in the pre-antiseptic era was justified because even the most minor procedure could lead to death by infection. When eating became a problem however, surgery was resorted to, but by then, the tumor would have grown to huge proportions. In this 1858 ambrotype the young girl turns the afflicted side of her face away from the camera in an effort to hide her deformity. The elderly man similarly turns his lesion from the camera's prying eye.

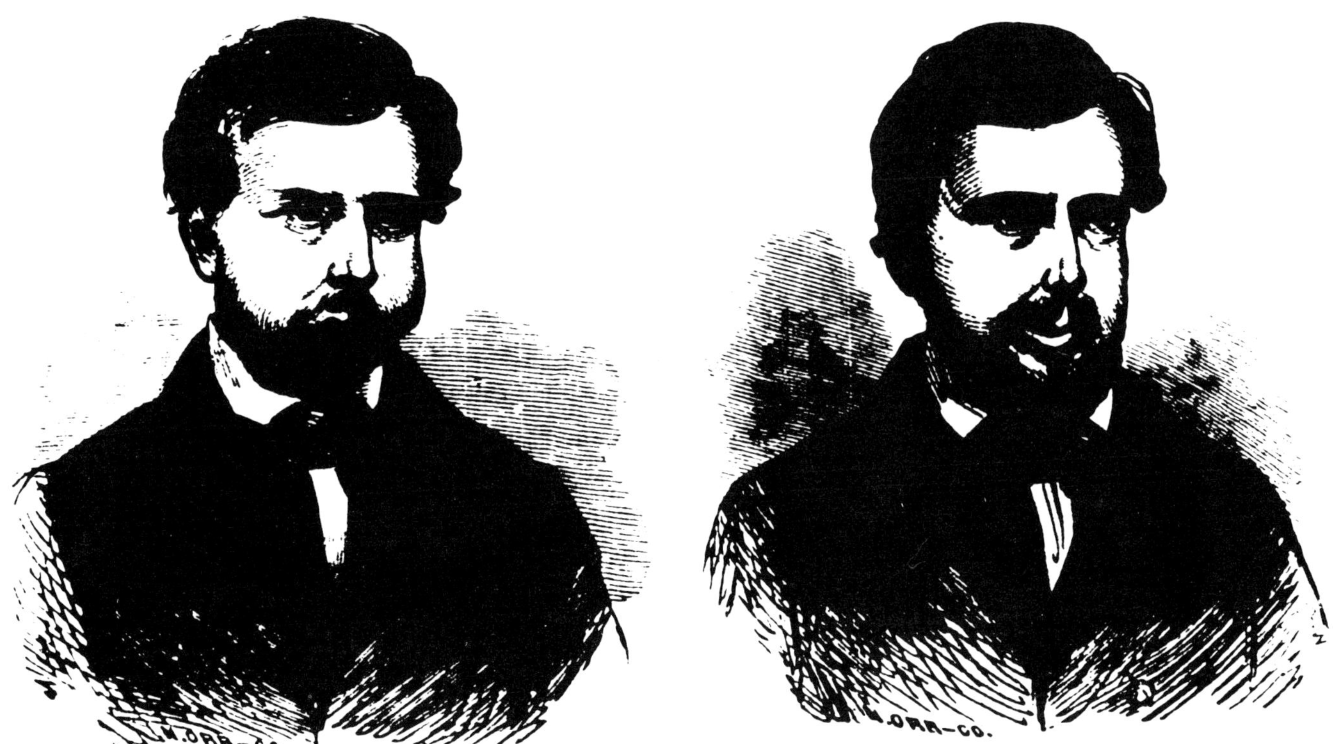

These engravings, published in the *American Journal of Dental Science*, April 1857, were sent by English colleagues. Edwin Sercombe presented in a photograph, his patient, with destruction of the entire palate, which he corrected with a prosthesis that allowed the patient to talk and appear in public.

Diseases such as syphilis and tuberculosis often caused massive destruction of the nose and associated facial anatomy. "These deformities of the face are particularly disgusting to the patient and the beholder," wrote H. Hoopes, D.D.S. in the July 1860, *American Journal of Dental Surgery*, Vol. 10. Dr. Hoopes presented this patient with syphilis, who had terrible destruction of bones and soft parts. The prosthesis he made consisted of a roof of the mouth made of gold, with teeth fitted in, then an artificial nose and lip made of vulcanized rubber which was inserted by bars into the palatine bone, an artificial mustache was added, and the prosthesis painted to match the skin. Glasses were placed at the upper nasal juncture to conceal the nose line.

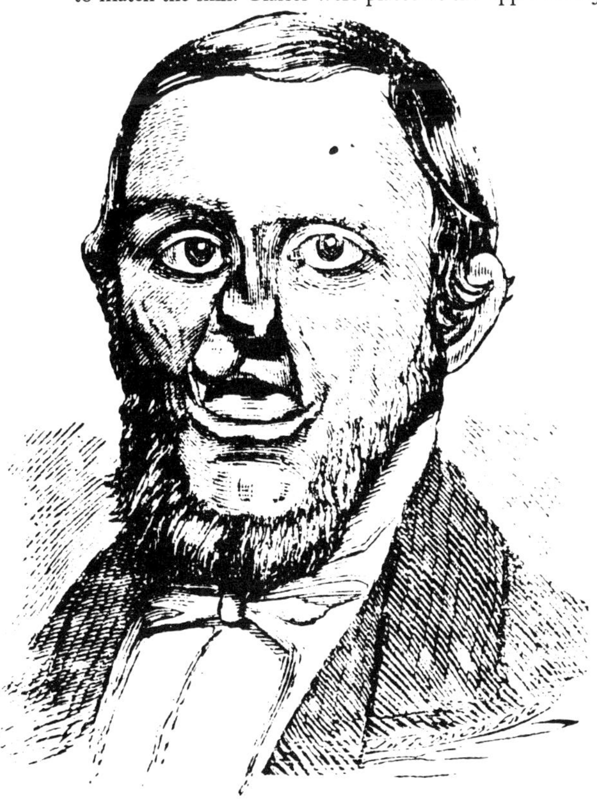

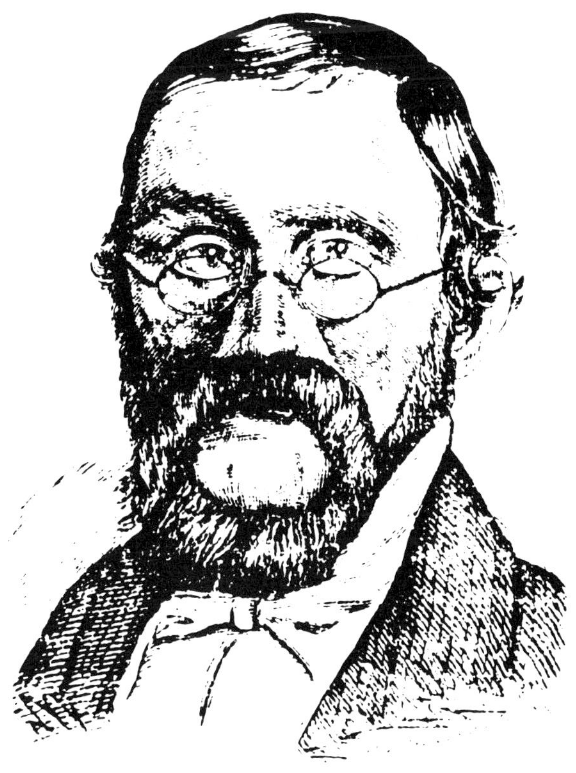

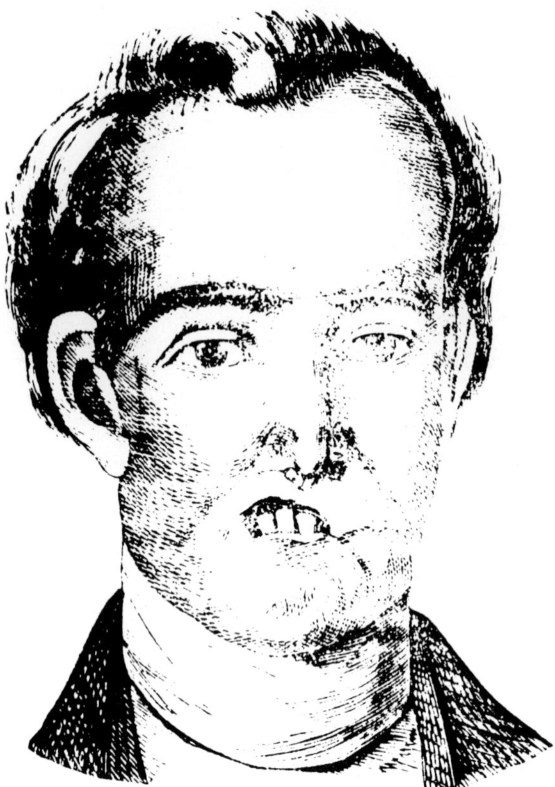

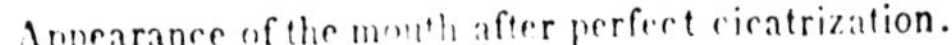

Appearance of the mouth after perfect cicatrization.

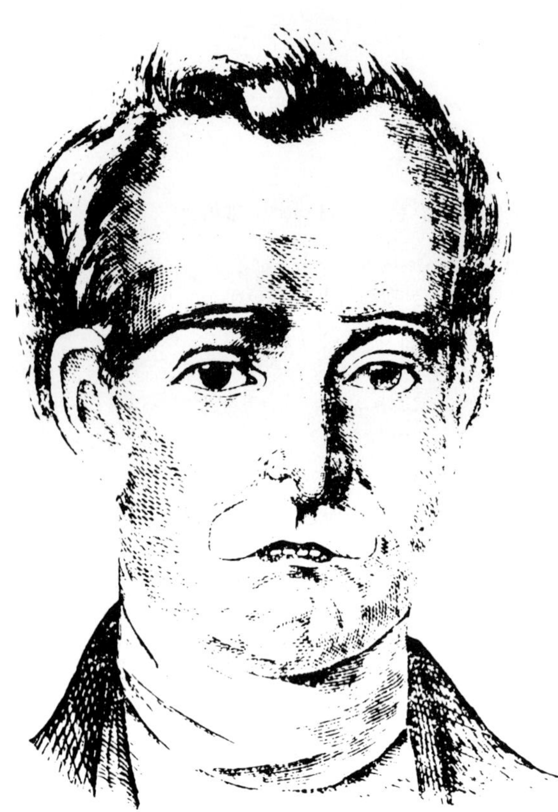

Appearance of the mouth with false lip adjusted.

Dr. L.D. Radzinsky reported in the *New York Dental Journal*, January 1860, on his interesting patient, who made fuses for matches and suffered from an industrially induced disease. The patient suffered necrosis and loss of the inferior maxillary bone by being exposed to phosphoric acid fumes. In November 1858, the entire lower jaw was removed. Necrosis continued and in October 1859 most of the upper jaw was removed. Dentist G. Dieffenbach made the artificial jaw including inset teeth. He devised a special "eccentric spring" that operated the jaw for chewing and made the "bones" out of a specially tinted amber resin that was lighter than other materials traditionally used.

Tooth In—Tooth Out 1880s

This photograph of the 1880s clearly demonstrates the result of dental treatment. The subject, a child, is quite happy with the results of her extraction and seems none the worse for it, as a matter of fact, she is much better. This type of photograph clearly presented to the public a positive image of dentistry.

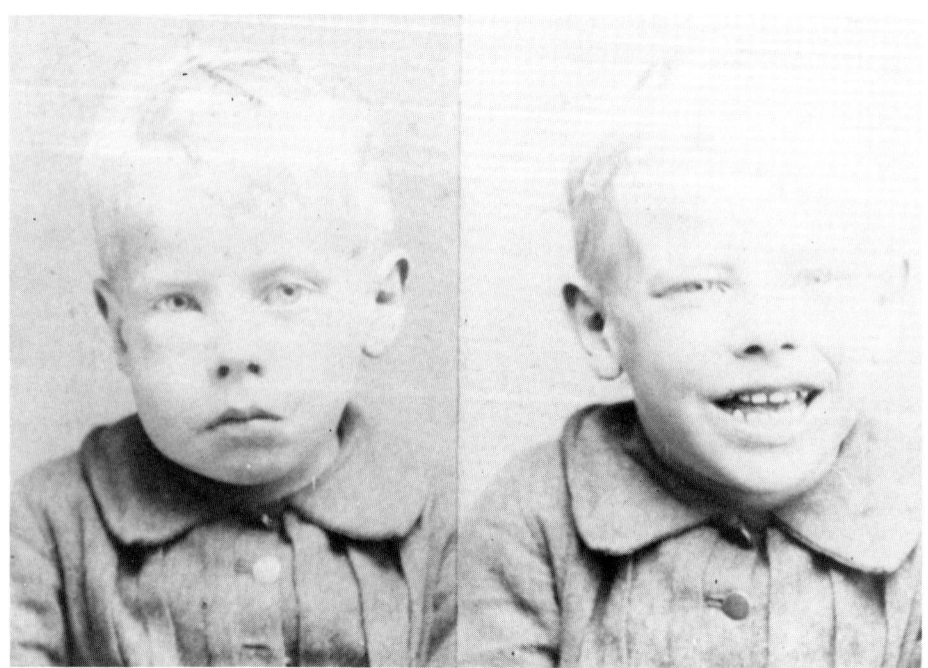

Clinical Photography

American dentists were among the first practitioners in the world to use clinical photographs of patients as a means of recording the results of surgical treatment. They used photography for such documentation before European physicians or dentists. In 1848, Dr. R. Thompson and Dr. W.E. Ide, of Columbus, Ohio removed the left superior maxillary bone along with a large tumor of the jaw, and repaired the defect with an oral prosthesis of gutta-percha. They photographed their patient pre- and post-operatively and used the pictures as engravings in an article in the *American Journal of Dental Science* of 1850 to document their treatment.[26] This was the first time in the world's literature that pre- and post-operative photographs were published. Only one prior publication of a clinical photograph is known, that of Gurdon Buck's operation in 1845 to straighten a leg.[27]

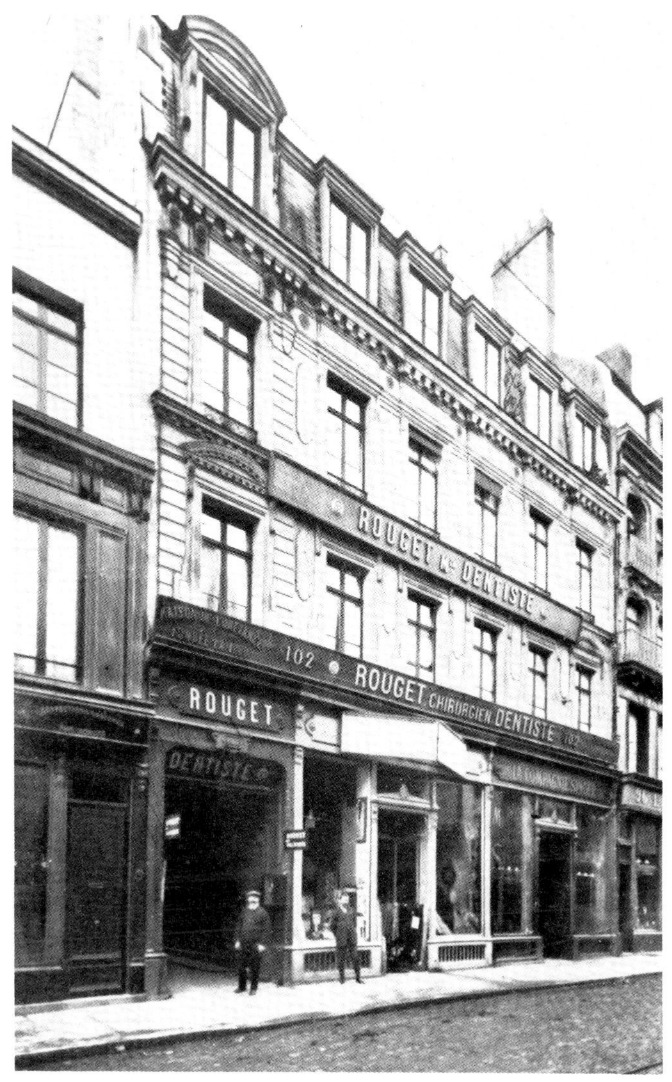

Special post card made as an advertisement for the dental offices of Dr. Rouget. "Founded in 1880." Dr. Rouget, a graduate of the Paris Dental School, mentions several locations of his dental clinics. This one being his main office.

European and American Dentistry

In the 19th century American dentists received worldwide acclaim for their innovative ideas and operative techniques. In medicine, Europe was the center of training and innovation, in dentistry the U.S. took the spotlight. As a result of America's leadership, European aristocrats and government leaders often consulted and engaged American dentists. One of the most famous dentists of the time was Edward Maynard, who was invited to become the "Actual Dentist to His Imperial Majesty" Czar Nicholas of Russia, if he would remain for a decade and teach his methods. Maynard chose to return to the U.S. to practice. Another dentist of world reknown was Thomas W. Evans, D.D.S. (1823-1897). Evans arrived in Paris in 1847, and by 1850, he was the personal dentist to Napoleon III. In 1856 he was appointed court surgeon-dentist by Czar Alexander II of Russia and also served Victor Emmanuel of Italy and Sultan Abdul Medjid of Turkey. During an emergency he was called upon to try to save the life of Crown Prince Frederick, heir to the throne of Germany when his physicians were unable to help him.[28] European physicians traveled to America to show their expertise, in dentistry the voyage was reversed.

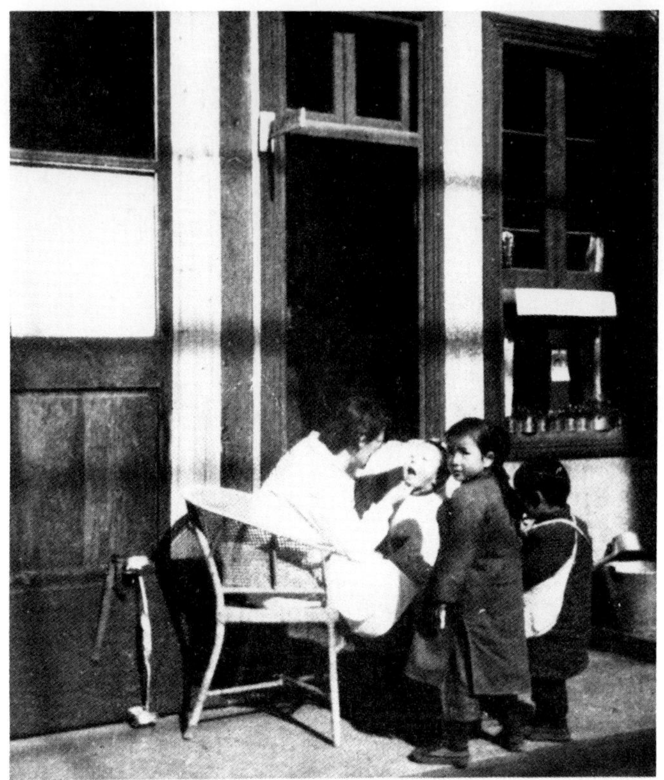

"Open your mouth wide"

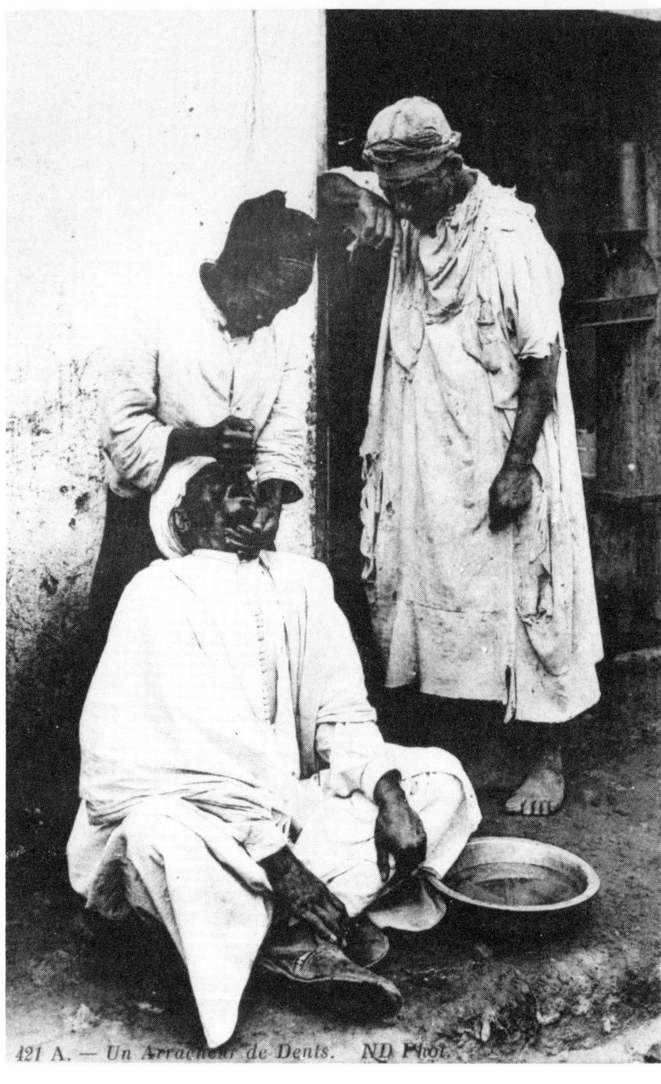

Prior to the mid-19th century, dentists often operated in the streets. Public surgery not only attracted attention to dentists abilities, but offered procrastinators immediate treatment. Although in the Western Nations street dentistry was a thing of the past by the end of the century in third world countries, the age-old tradition persisted. In one photo we see an Algerian street dentist extracting a tooth, in the other, an American missionary dentist examines children outside his storefront office in Hangchow, China.

Use of Photography in Dental Journals

American dentists started to use photography in their periodicals about the same time as their medical colleagues. In order to document and evaluate the use of photography by dentists, a study of dental journals of the era was undertaken. The following 13 journals were surveyed from their inception to 1883 or their last publication, if before this year.

Journal	**Year Began to Publish**
American Journal of Dental Science	1839
Der Zahnarzt uber Zahnheilkunde	1846
New York Dental Recorder	1848
Dental Newsletter	1847
Dental Register of the West	1847
Dental Obturator	1855
New York Dental Journal	1858
Dental Cosmos	1859
Transactions of the American Dental Association	1859
Pennsylvania Journal of Dental Science	1874
Transactions of the Penn. State Dental Society	1875
New York Odontological Society	1873
Independent Practitioner	1880

From 1850 to 1880, dental journals at one time or another, used engravings from photographs for illustrating operative results. Most of the patients illustrated suffered from tumors or wounds that required cosmetic surgery and involved reconstruction or replacement of facial or mouth parts. Dental periodicals carried numerous articles on repair of hare-lip and other aspects of facial surgery that now fall under the care of general, plastic, neurologic and otolaryngologic surgeons. Interesting illustrations also were republished from European journals.

Photographs were initially published as tipped-in paper prints: the calotype and albumin print. In Paris where the daguerreotype was invented, Alfred Donné was the first physician to photograph a microscopical section. In 1840 he made a photomicrograph of a bone section with his microscope-daguerreotype apparatus. The photographs were copied by an engraver and used to illustrate Donné's *Cours de Microscopie* which was published in 1845. After 1850 photomicroscopy was common.[29]

The first American medical texts to use albumin prints appeared in the 1860s. A European dental journal published a tipped-in carte de visite photograph in 1864. Volume 19 of *Der Zahnarzt uber Zahnheilkunde* contained a portrait of Dr. G. Blume as a frontispiece. In 1870 the first American medical journal to use tipped-in prints was published. None of the American dental journals surveyed published albumin prints. The first journal to use a tipped-in photograph was the *Transactions of the American Dental Association*. In 1875 in an article "Report on Histology and Microscopy," H.S. Chase of St. Louis illustrated his new ideas on the histology of dental tissues by including nine microphotographs. The photographs were prepared by Dr. O.C. Oliver of Chicago and reproduced as woodburytypes by the American Photo Relief Company. Woodburytypes were the first successful mechanical photographs with the distinct advantage that they would not fade as did albumin and calotype prints.

The first article to appear in a dental journal on the topic of photography was published in *The Dental Cosmos* of December 1866. Entitled "Microscopical Photography," it presented a method of taking microphotographs by Albert Leeds of the Philadelphia Dental College. The paper had originally been given, along with a demonstration of photography, at the Odontological Society of Pennsylvania on November 5, 1866.

The Dental Cosmos in its review of the literature regularly reported on photographic advances. In the July 1863 issue, it reported and reprinted parts of Dr. Oliver Wendell Holmes' article on photography that the editor thought contained "several valuable suggestions in a direction eminently interesting and practical in their character to the dentist." In the September 1870 issue it reported on the use of *Photography in Medical Instruction*, noting that

> leading medical hospitals and colleges in this country and Europe now regularly employ skilled photographers . . . to take . . . faithful representations of the general appearance of a patient . . . These may be . . . reproduced on glass . . . then . . . By means of the magic lantern, the pictures are thrown on a screen and magnified so that the most minute parts are rendered clearly visible to large audiences. For medical instruction, this method is of great value, by reason of its extraordinary accuracy and distinctness.

In the November 1871 issue the journal reported a "New Light for the Use of Photographers and Others," a combination of zinc in iodide of ethyl and hydrogen gas. This light was brilliant, but inferior to magnesium light. By the mid-1870s, dentists, like their medical colleagues, were using photography to record dental and oral disease.

A brief review of dental texts was undertaken. It was not until 1883 that a text was found with a photograph. In Marshall H. Webb, D.D.S.: *Notes on Operative Dentistry*, Philadelphia, S.S. White Dental Manufacturing Company, a frontispiece photograph of Dr. Webb was published. It is a collotype mechanical print and phototype. Philadelphia photographer Frederic Gutekunst took the image. Additional research is necessary to completely evaluate the role photography played in dental texts.

Bloodletting

Bloodletting, the backbone of medical therapeutics for thousands of years has not been generally recognized as part of the practice of American dentistry. Yet local and general bloodletting was the first thing many practitioners did before filling a decayed tooth. In Volume 1 of the *American Journal of Dental Science*, B.A. Rodrigues of Charleston, South Carolina explained the philosophy of bloodletting in his article "Of treating Caries of the Teeth . . ."

> The first step to be taken in the treatment of decayed teeth, should be to relieve the surrounding structures, and the teeth themselves, from all inflammation, whether idiopathic or symptomatic. To accomplish this, due attention should be paid to the state of the system. Local and general bloodletting, etc. . . .[30]

The photograph shown is of an itinerant physician, perhaps a dentist. The image documents the classic position of the patient for general bloodletting or venesection. The bowl is held between the legs and a wooden staff used to help the patient propel blood and steady the arm. These props had been used for centuries. There are no photographs of bloodletting in the dental literature.

Along with the use of the lancet and cupping, application of leeches was a standard dental treatment. The 1835 edition of Samuel Fitch's *Systems of Dental Surgery*, Philadelphia, Corey, Lea & Blanchard, describes such use in detail. In his important section on "Of the order in which Dental Operations should be Performed," Fitch notes "Leeches on the gums over inflamed teeth often have a happy effect. If the incisors or canine teeth are inflamed and tender, a few leeches will alleviate all pain and tenderness in a very short time. With proper prudence on the part of the patient, and a faithful performance of the foregoing directions, inflammation of any of the teeth, or their membranes and nerves, or of the lining membranes of these sockets will very rarely take place. If a disordered state of the general system is present whilst these operations are going on, it should be remedied as far as possible." By this Fitch meant the use of the then popular "Herioc Therapy." Bleeding, purging, vomiting and blistering a patient until the constitution was improved!

Bleeding was often used to the detriment of the patient. Fitch reports a case of H.G. Courtous, from *The Dental Observation*, Paris, 1775. The patient suffering from scurvy had a canine tooth extracted. Afterward bleeding from the socket could not be controlled by tampons, etc. A few days later on re-examination the patient was found to have a general ooze of blood from his scurved gums. After consultation with physicians it was decided to increase the "consistency of the patient's blood, that is thicken it, so it would clot: the treatment to thicken the blood—repeated bloodletting! The outcome, the patient died 10 days after the tooth extraction.

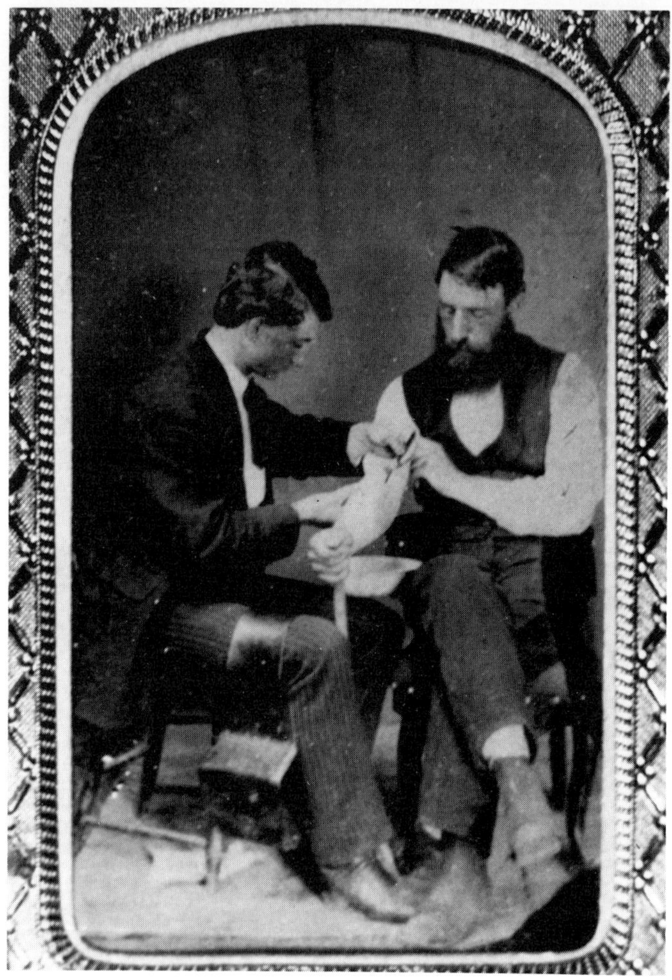

Bloodletting Tintype 1860
Bloodletting was the backbone of medical therapeutics for over 3,000 years and was a part of the dental art. It reached its zenith in America in the first half of the 19th century. Dentists routinely bled a patient as part of the therapeutic regimen for filling a tooth. Bloodletting preceded cleaning the tooth or gums. This tintype, circa 1860, is part of a set of three pictures taken by a country practitioner in the act of bleeding a patient. Despite the fact bleeding was so popular and ingrained in medical/dental practice, this series of pictures are the only ones that remain showing bloodletting in the 19th century.

Comic Dental Scenes

Fear of dentistry, and the claims of quacks to the nature and practice of the dental process, led satirists to parody dentistry. Photography aided the process. Dentists were frequently portrayed in a comic light, or shown extracting teeth by absurd methods. Although it is well established that one often jokes to reduce anxiety, some comic pictures seem to go beyond comedy and make a social statement about how deeply the public feared and recoiled from dentistry.

The images seen here demonstrate the range and style of "comic" dental views. Many of the photographs were made as stereoviews and were sold to the public to be enjoyed at home with the family. Some of the comic images were taken by dentists as testimonials to the art and folly of dentistry. Others were made by students as mementos of their initiation into the dental fraternity.

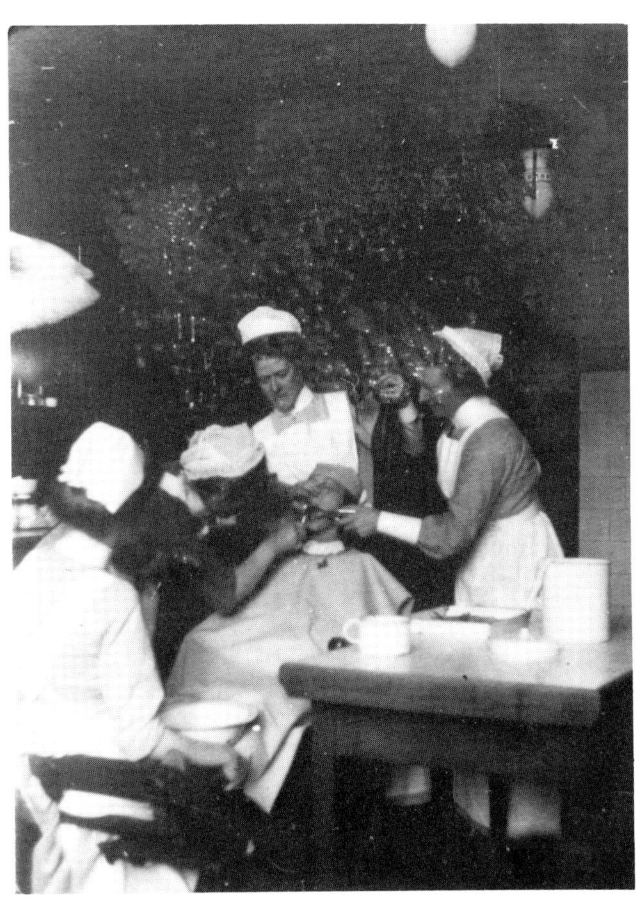

Nurses Extract Tooth
This series of photographs taken during WWI depict what may be a tooth extraction among a group of nurses. There are comic overtures to one of the images that may reveal relief that the procedure is over.

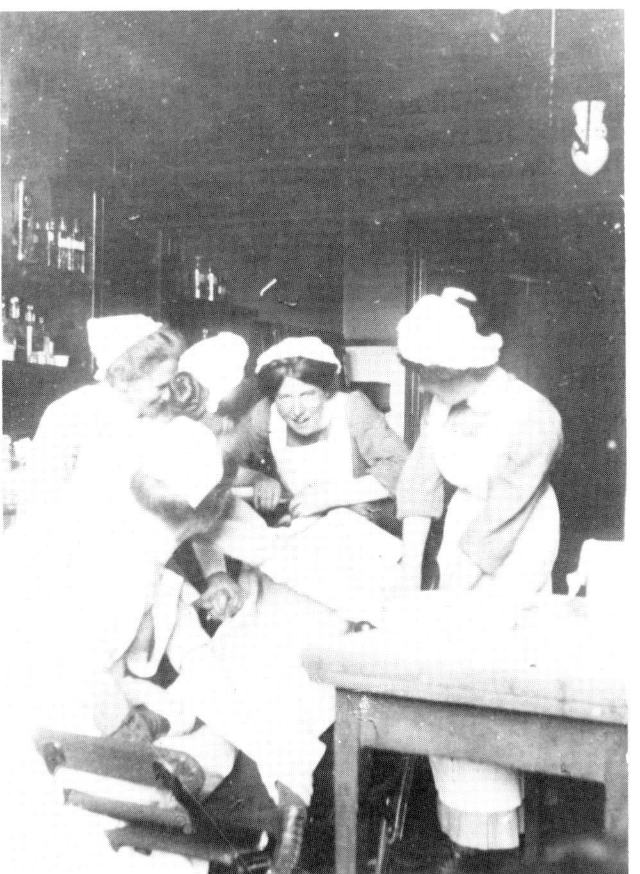

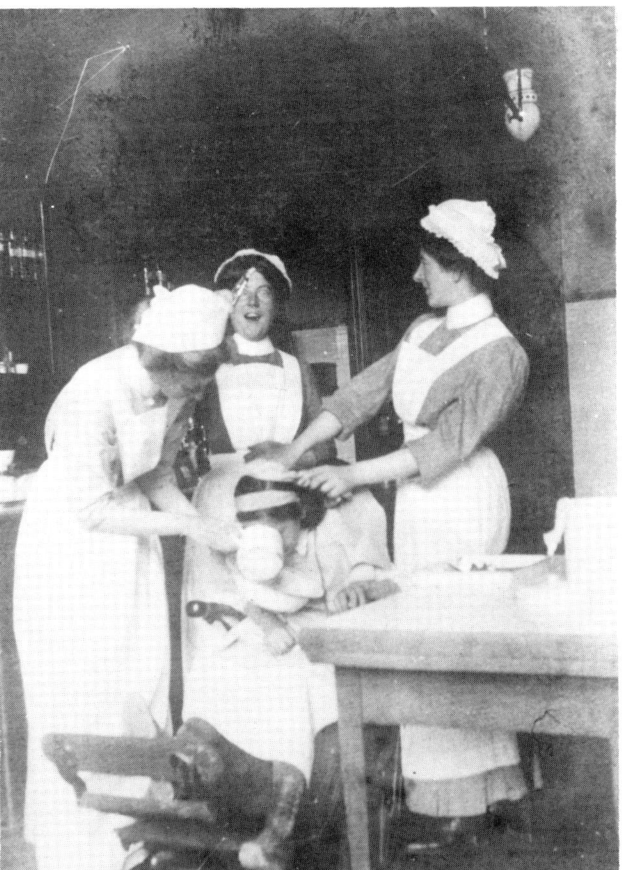

This comic pose is set in an English photographer's studio in Leeds, circa 1880s. What appear to be dental students, restrain the patient as in the style of comic views of the 1860s and '70s. A headrest interestingly is visible behind the patient. English photographs taken or set up by practitioners, depicting various aspects of medical or dental practice in a comic light are exceedingly rare.

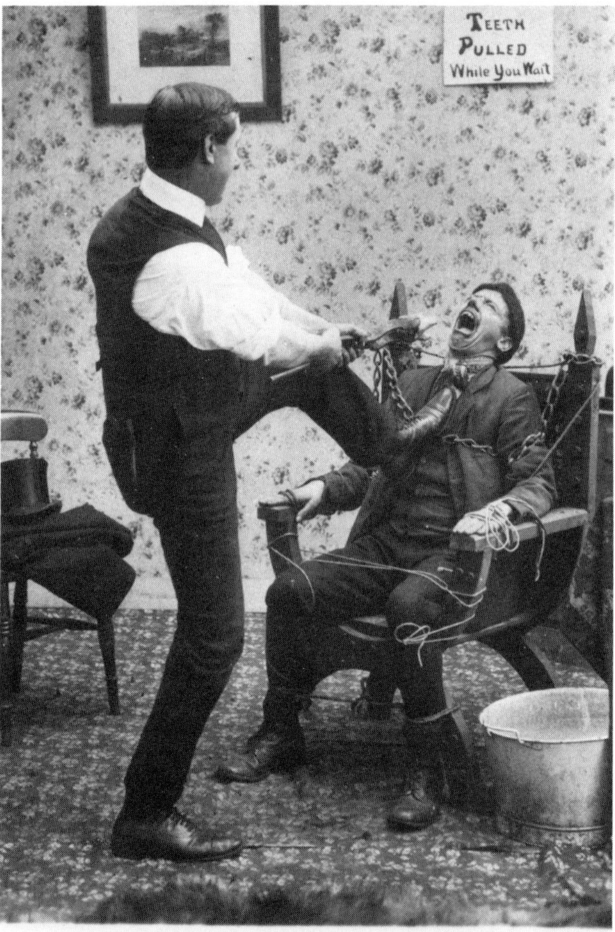

" PAINLESS EXTRACTION."

How nice

This card from a turn-of-the-comic-century series on tooth extraction continues the nineteenth century exaggeration and bufoonery of the hapless patient and "painless" dentist. Taken by New York City photographer Bamforth.

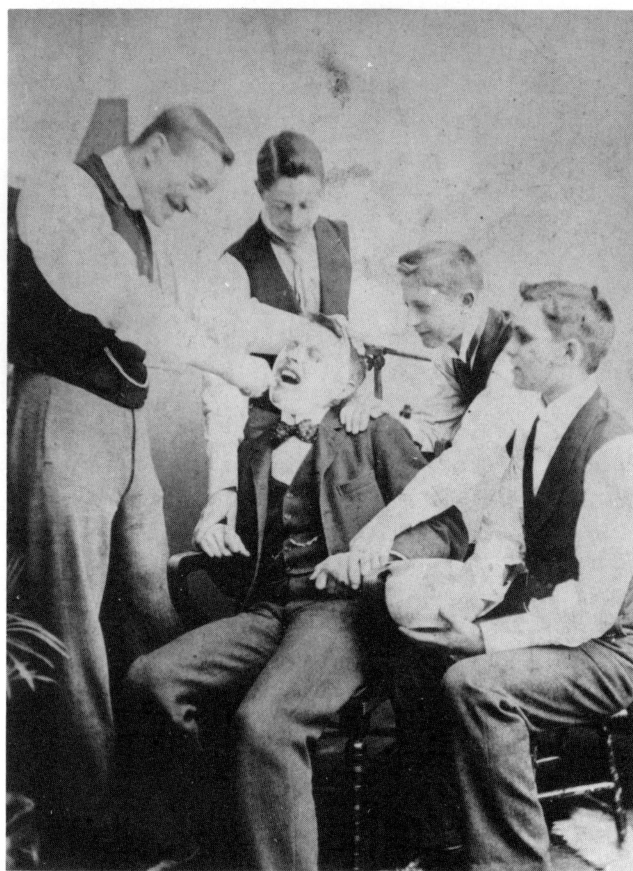

Comic Dental Extraction Series

These three "comic views" of a tooth extraction, circa 1872, were sold as a series to show an encounter with the dentist. The photographs were not taken during one session; the dress, props and background change in every image.

"Giving Gas" is particularly extraordinary since it is the only American photograph depicting the gas reservoir anesthesia delivery system popular with some anesthetists. In England there is a series of pictures taken of Dr. Clover, reknowned British anesthetist, using a gas reservoir system. This image shows dental tools spread out on a table, the dentist's sign hanging prominently on the wall above a medicine case and the patient wearing an apron. The dental assistant, often a young apprentice, holds up a bottle labeled ether, while unbelievably the dentist smokes a pipe, showing his unconcern for the highly flammable chemical.

In the second image "Extracting Teeth," the dentist's roots in blacksmithing are evident. The dentist extracts the hapless patient's tooth with a huge pair of forceps. Another large forceps lies on the table, which in the previous image, held proper dental tools. The anesthesia is also gone, and the patient is restrained by a scarf tied precariously across his neck. A spittoon is placed conveniently on a small stool. The dental sign is prominent.

In the last image "Oh What a Tooth," the patient examines the results of his operation. Curiously the extracting forceps are gone from the table and replaced by medicinal and anesthetic bottles.

These images were part of a large series of over 300 photographs lampooning various occupations and aspects of 19th century life. Although Weller, of New Hampshire, was the photographer of the series, the images can be found under several names. The practice of the time was for other photographers to buy the rights to the images, copy them, and sell them under their names.

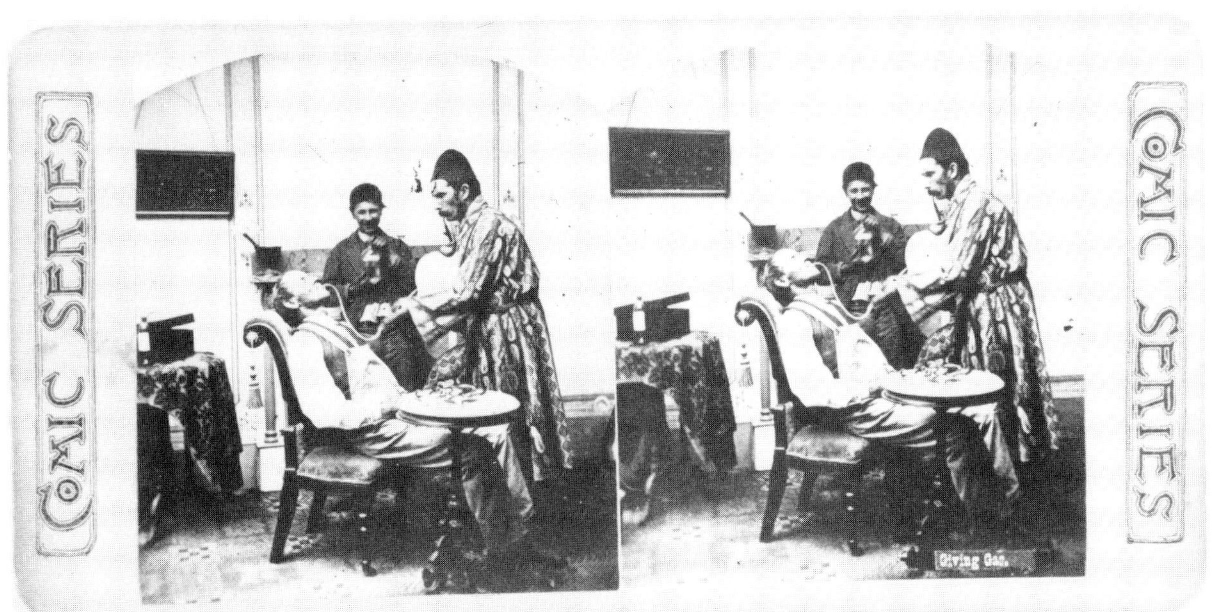
COMIC SERIES
Giving Gas.
COMIC SERIES

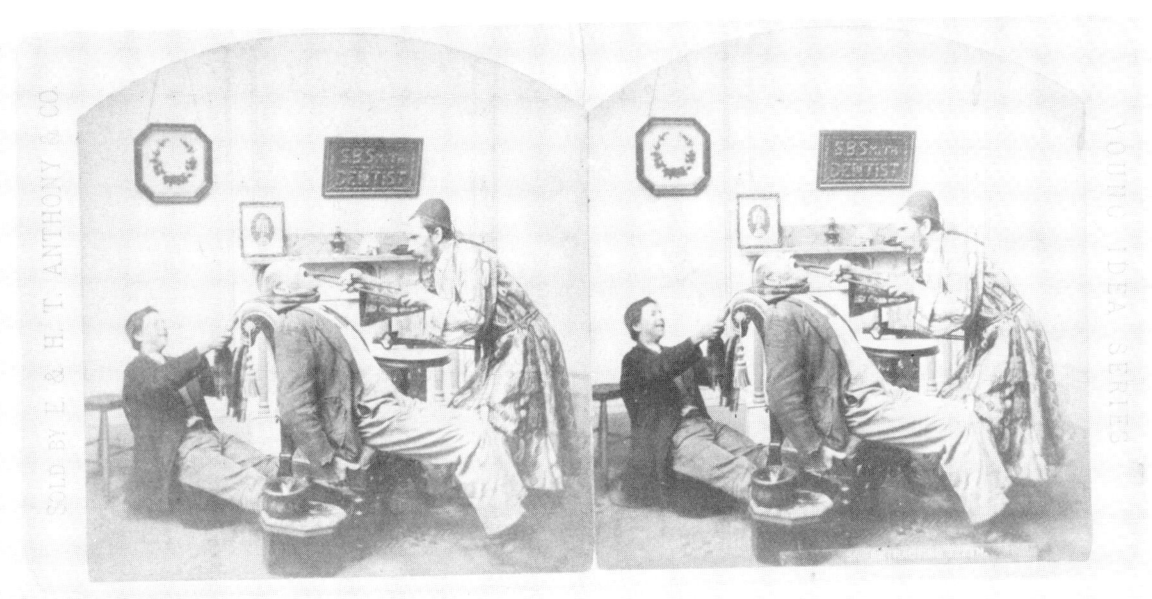
SOLD BY E. & H. T. ANTHONY & CO.
S.B. SMITH DENTIST
YOUNG IDEA SERIES

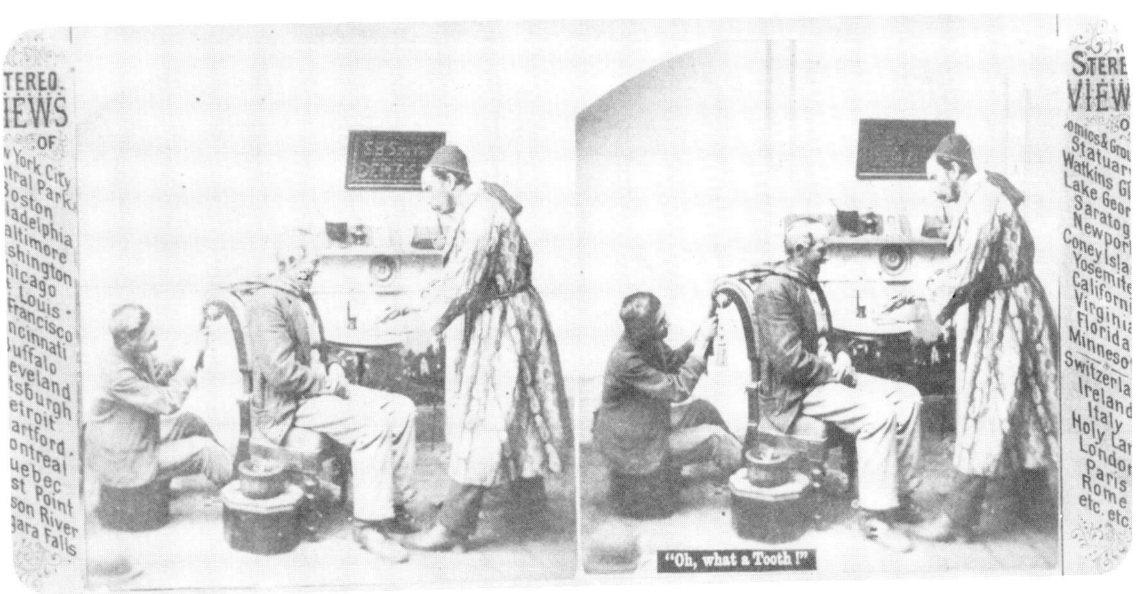
S.B. SMITH DENTIST
"Oh, what a Tooth!"

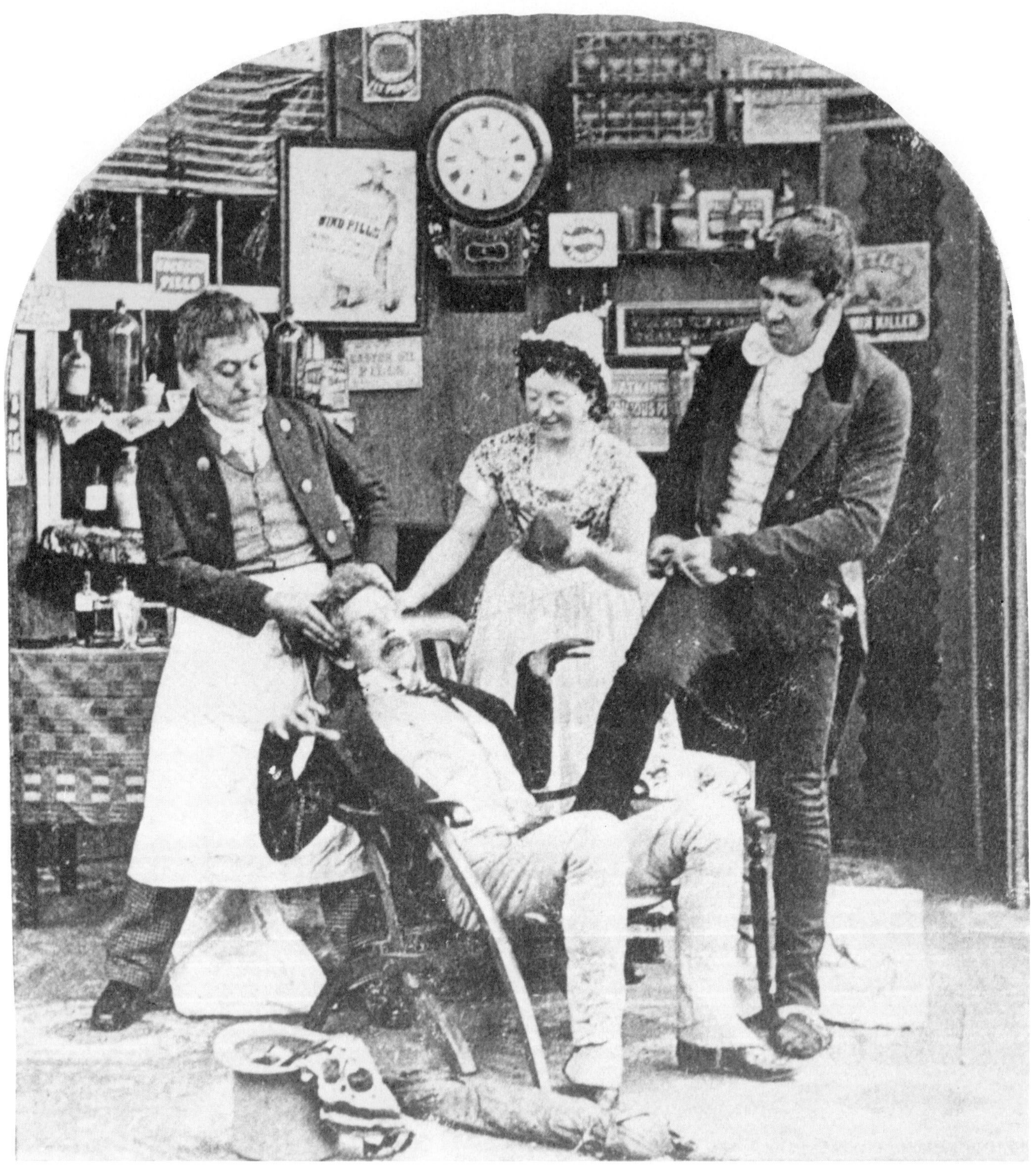

English Comic Dental Extraction
This view is part of an English series, circa 1858, lampooning various aspects of medical practice. Here there is no pretense of professionalism. The dental assistant steadies the patient, a string has been tied around the patient's tooth and the dentist is pulling on it.

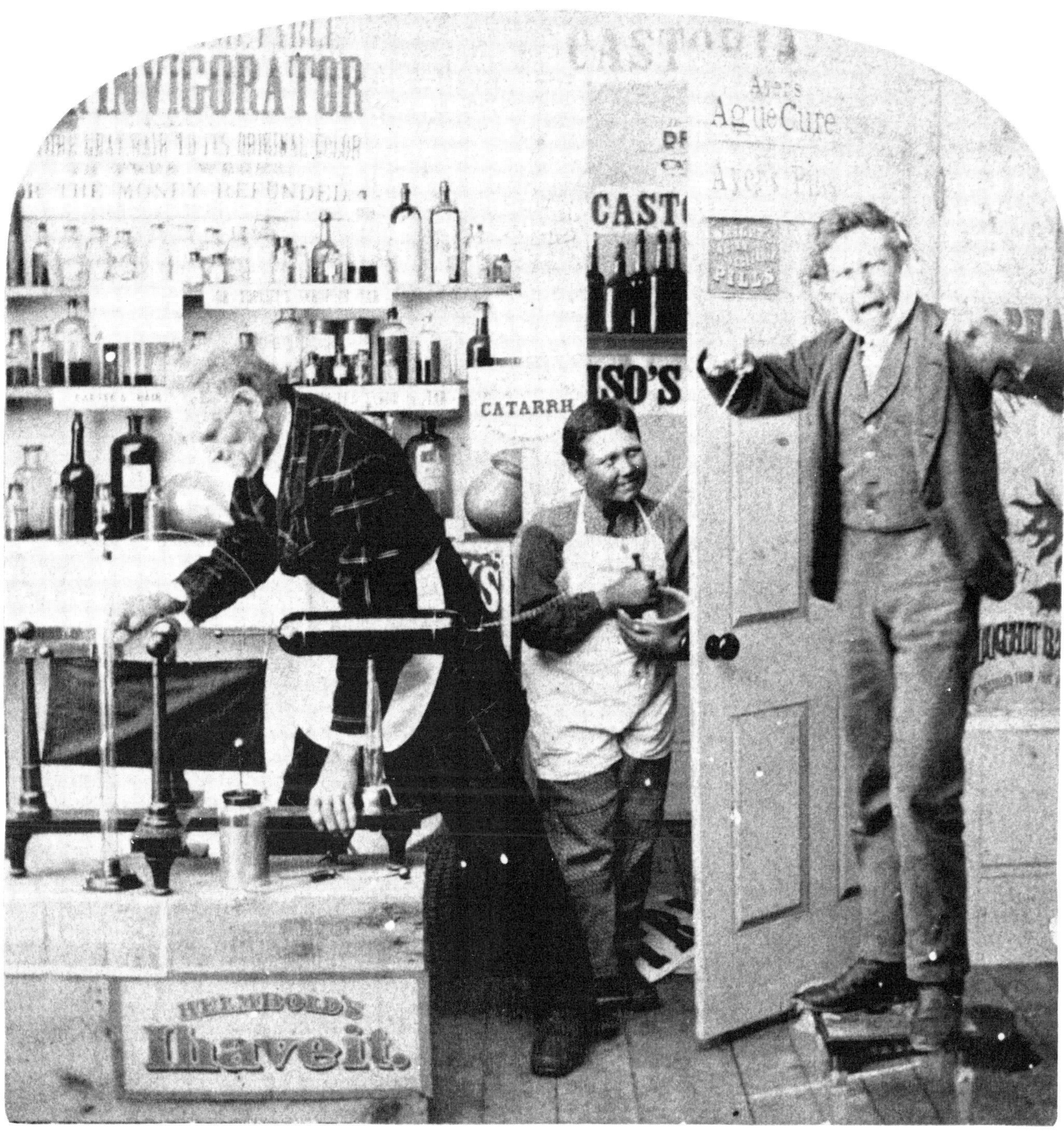

Electrical Therapy used to Alleviate a Tooth Ache comic stereoview 1872
This stereoview pokes fun at the electrical therapy practices of the time. Here in this image the hapless patient suffers from a toothache. The "good" doctor/dentist is rapidly turning the crank on his generator to supply voltage to the patient. The image is a testimonial to the efficacy of dentistry and electrotherapy.

The Impact of Social Structure on American and European Dentistry

In the 19th century dentistry was the only health care field in which Americans were world leaders. Although American ingenuity is generally credited with inspiring the advance of dentistry, another reason was a higher standard of living. Dentistry usually enhanced personal comfort and appearance, rather than saving lives. Consequently, dentistry held a low priority in poorer nations. Furthermore, the collegial support needed to exchange ideas and techniques was lacking in Europe. In Europe the separateness and jealousies of various nations did not allow for the ease of dissemination of ideas. The guild system and strict class hierarchy prevalent throughout Europe often restricted dentists and others from advancing or innovating. Inflexible social structures and cultural barriers were additional hindrances to professional change.

Dentistry's growth in the U.S. was nourished by egalitarian concepts, especially by placing dentists in the same class as physicians and surgeons.

In contrast, Europeans reserved the highest social status for physicians with university degrees and medical training. European surgeons were hampered by their less sophisticated image as "barber-surgeons." They ranked lower socially since they were considered educated tradesmen. European dentists were ranked the lowest of all medical groups.

In America, physician and surgeon were one and the same, usually the product of a non-university "medical school." Since these schools did not require prior university training, a medical degree was easily obtained. Many dentists attended medical schools, and by the 1840s, the better dentists had received degrees. American physicians and dentists benefited from a close cross-professional association. For example, at the Baltimore College of Dental Surgery, in 1847, a committee of five physicians and three dentists examined the school's candidates for the D.D.S.[31]

American dentists strengthened by American inventions, and unhampered by a closed society, offered the world important dental firsts noted above. Beginning with the first school established in 1840, American dental schools increased to 13 by 1880. These dental colleges set standards of education and expertise that erased the image of the dentist as a tooth-pulling quack. The "Doctor of Dental Surgery" replaced the "physician-dentist." These practitioners focused on saving, rather than extracting teeth.

Chapin Harris noted in his 1845 text *Principles and Practice of Dental Surgery* that American dentists were more skillfull than their European colleagues. In 1850, James Robinson, D.D.S., a noted London dentist addressed the Society of the Alumni of the Baltimore College of Dental Surgery, lecturing on "Dental Education in England." Robinson summarized his long lecture:

> The conclusions I draw from the foregoing remarks may be summed up in a single sentence. I believe that Dental Science has not advanced so generally in England as in the United States, although this home truth may not be very palatable to the profession generally . . . [and] . . . until the barriers of professional jealousy and private interest are broken through . . . until a college of Dental Science is established and competent examiners appointed to test the qualifications of all aspirants, . . . Dental Surgery will not hold its proper position in England, or assume its legitimate place by the side of its parent science, Medicine. . . . By your conduct you have set a noble example to other countries. . . . I have no fears for the future prospects or the future destinies of Dental Surgery in America.[32]

Robinson was elected president of the College of Dentists of England in 1856 and worked toward upgrading English dental standards.

There were a number of significant inventions in the U.S. which spurred America to world leadership in dentistry. Two examples reveal their range and importance. Charles Goodyear, in 1855 applied vulcanized rubber as a base for artificial teeth. Soon, researchers followed with other rubber devices and prostheses. To keep the mouth dry during the long procedure of repairing teeth, Dr. C. Edmund Kells invented an automatic electric suction pump which removed saliva from the mouth.[33]

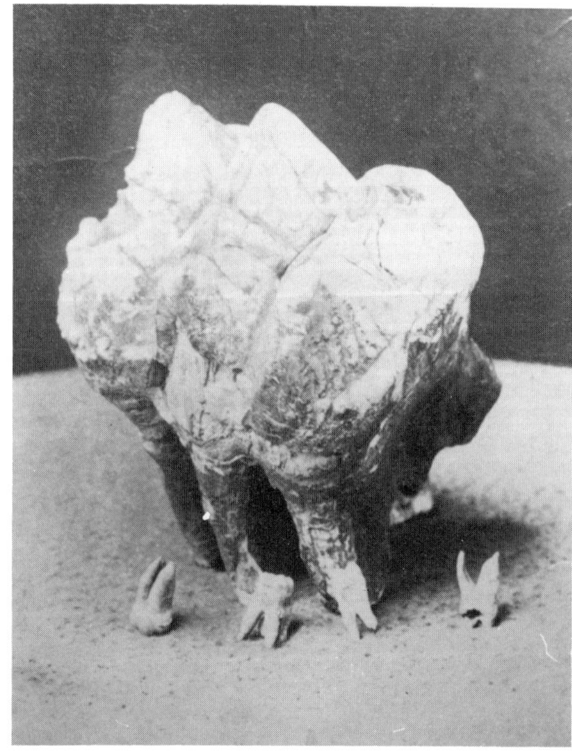

Mastodon Tooth
To get a perspective on the size of the excavated Mastodon tooth, extracted human teeth are placed beside the specimen. An unusual genre of dental interest.

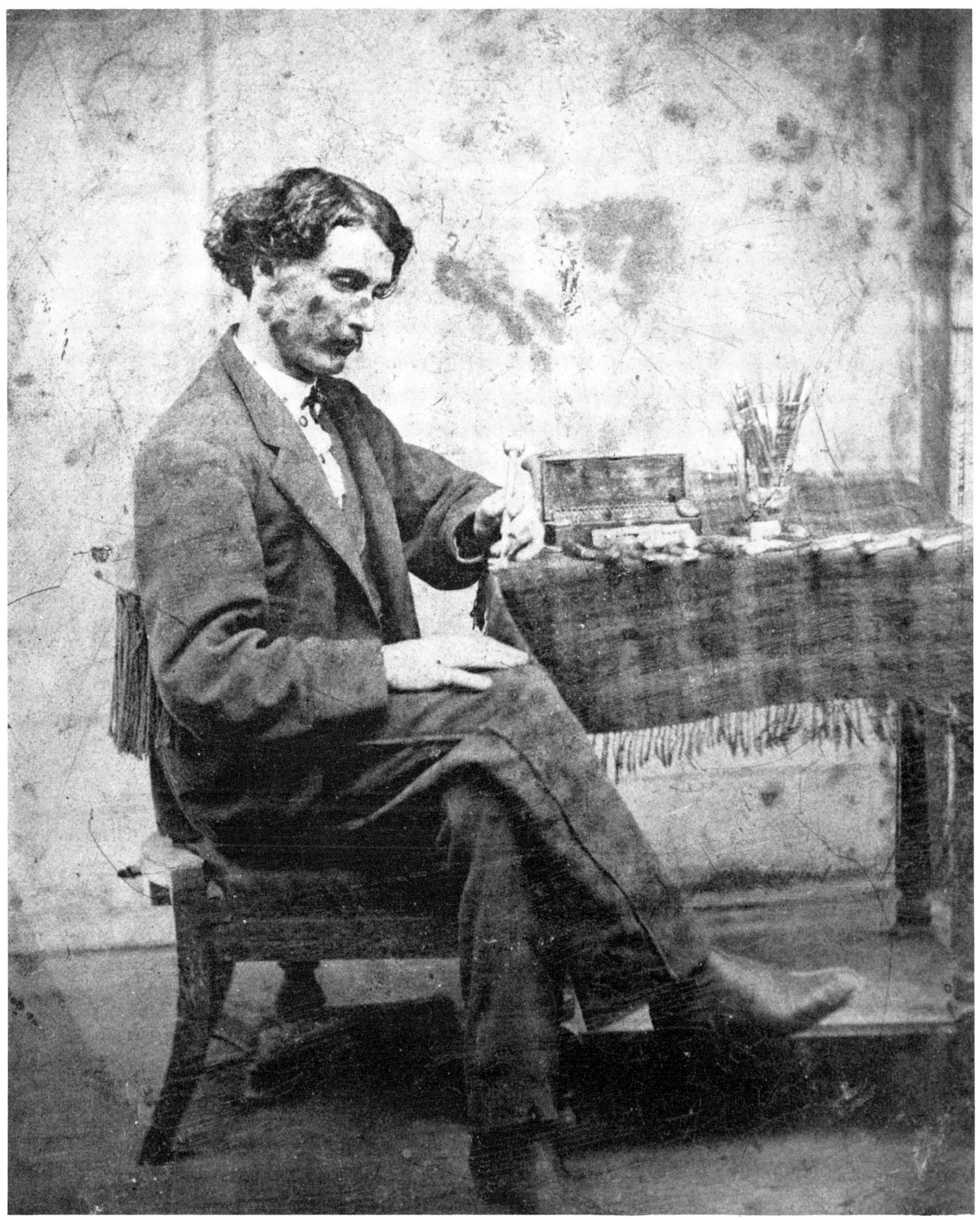

Dentist and his Electrical or Mechanical Device? Tintype 1858
This rare half-plate tintype (4½- by 5¼-inch) was taken to demonstrate this pioneer dentist's mechanical (electrical) device designed to help fill dental caries. The only known image of its type, showing a dentist applying an instrument to a tooth to promote the idea of saving teeth rather than extracting them. The dentist lays out his instruments on the table along with dental operating tools. In 1859, W.G.A. Bonwill patented a similar electric device to remove the nerve of a tooth. This is the earliest photograph of endodontics.

British Surgeon Dentist Chodwick Brown *carte de visite* 1865
English professional advertising portraiture took the normal photograph and added the practitioners respected title. There are no known European photographs of dental extraction or dentists posing with dental props from photography's earliest era, 1840-1870.

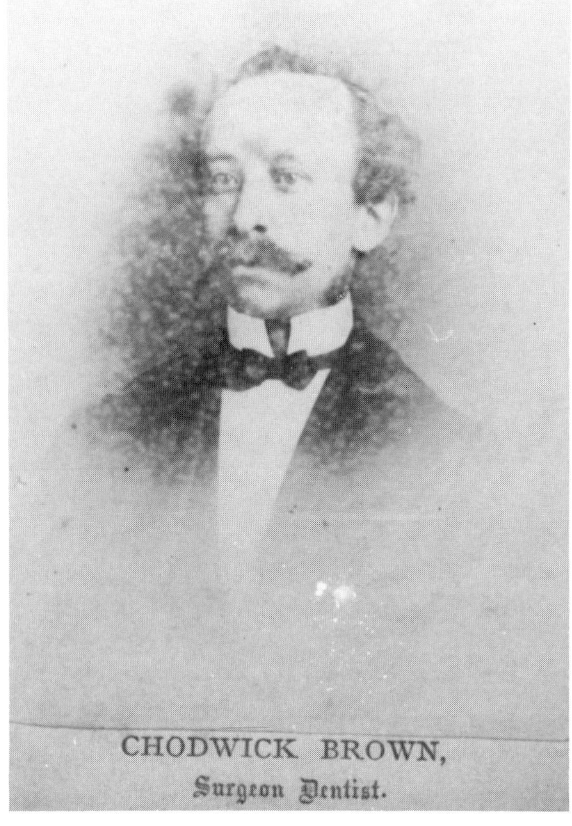

Dentist William Morton's Son Demonstrates Early X-Ray (1896)
Pioneer anesthetist William Morton's son practiced medicine, and like his father, jumped on the band wagon of medicine's new inventions. In 1896 he published the first American book on the X-ray. Here we see novice enthusiastic scientists, Dr. Morton and an electrical engineer taking an X-ray and fluoroscoping their own hands. Unbeknown to them and other early radiology pioneers, the deadly rays would ultimately cause fatal cancers.

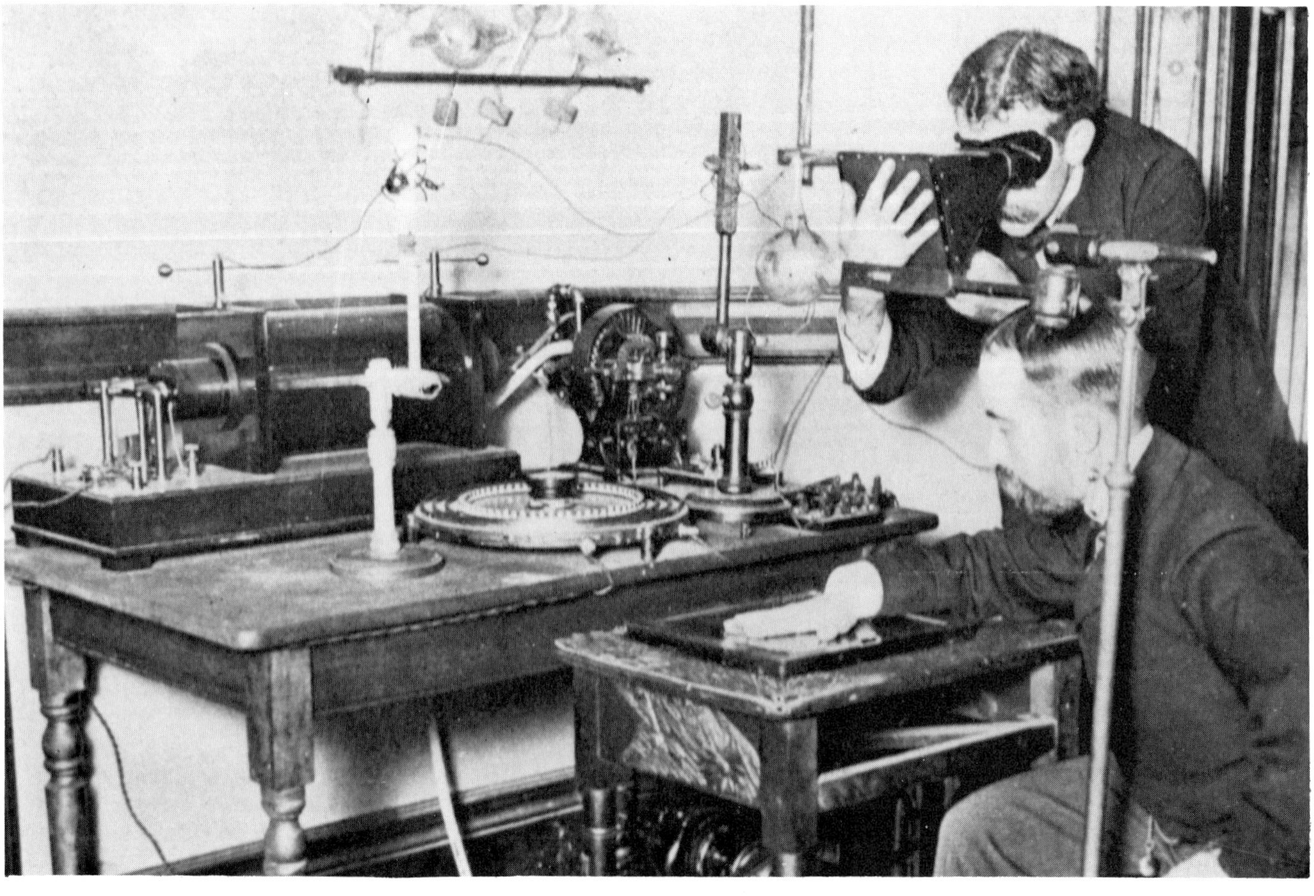

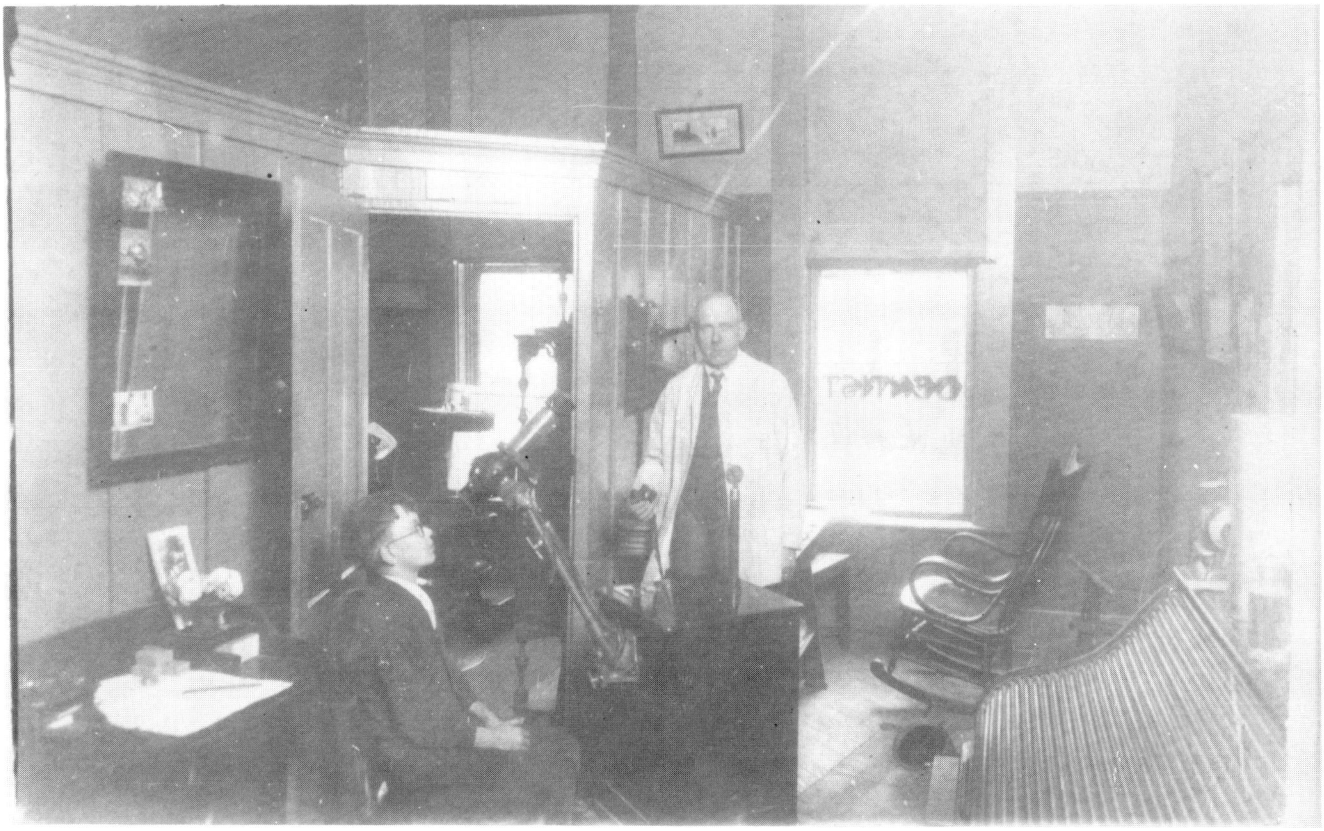

Dentist X-Raying Young Boy 1905
Showing off the latest X-ray equipment, this dentist portrays himself using the medical miracle of the age.

Typical street scene showing the Valley Hotel and incidentally the office of Dr. O.S. Carpenter DENTIST.

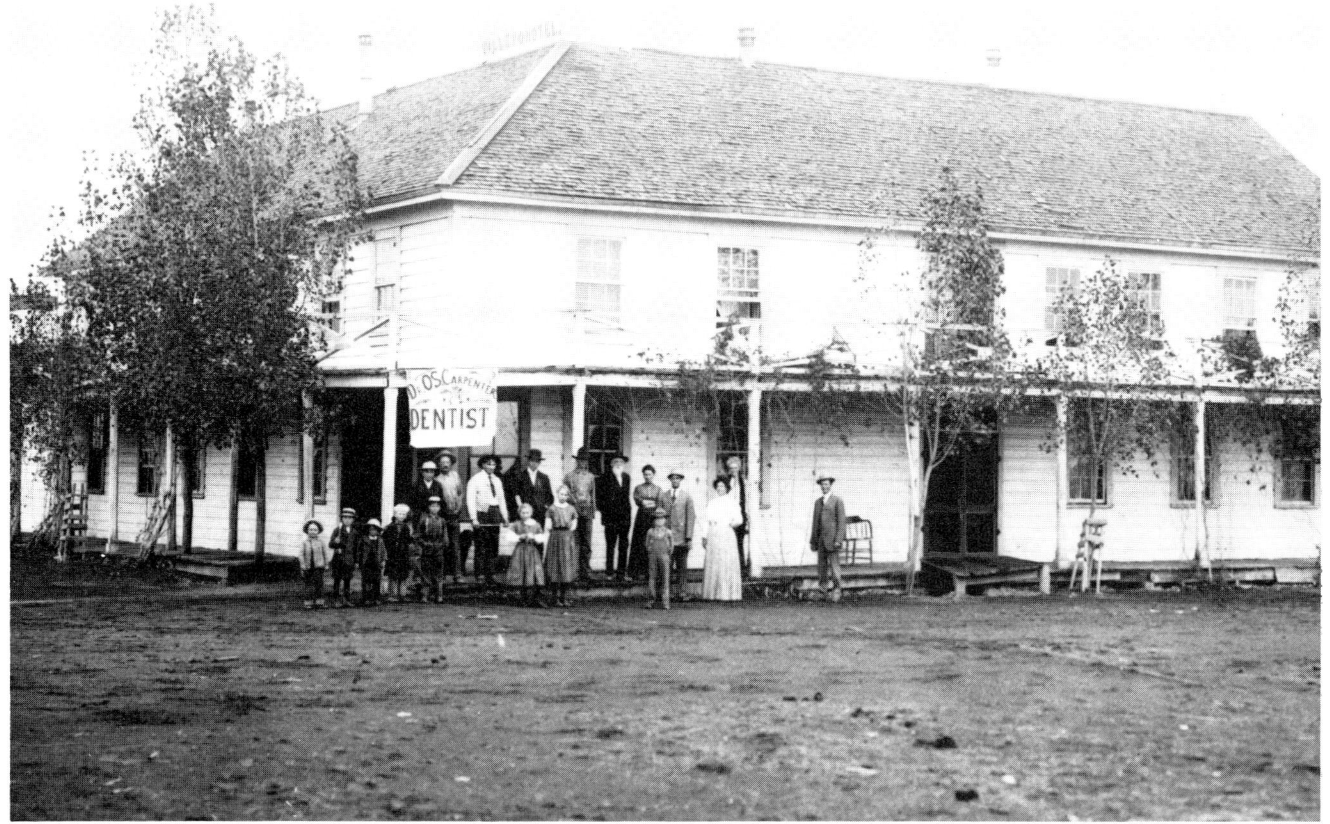

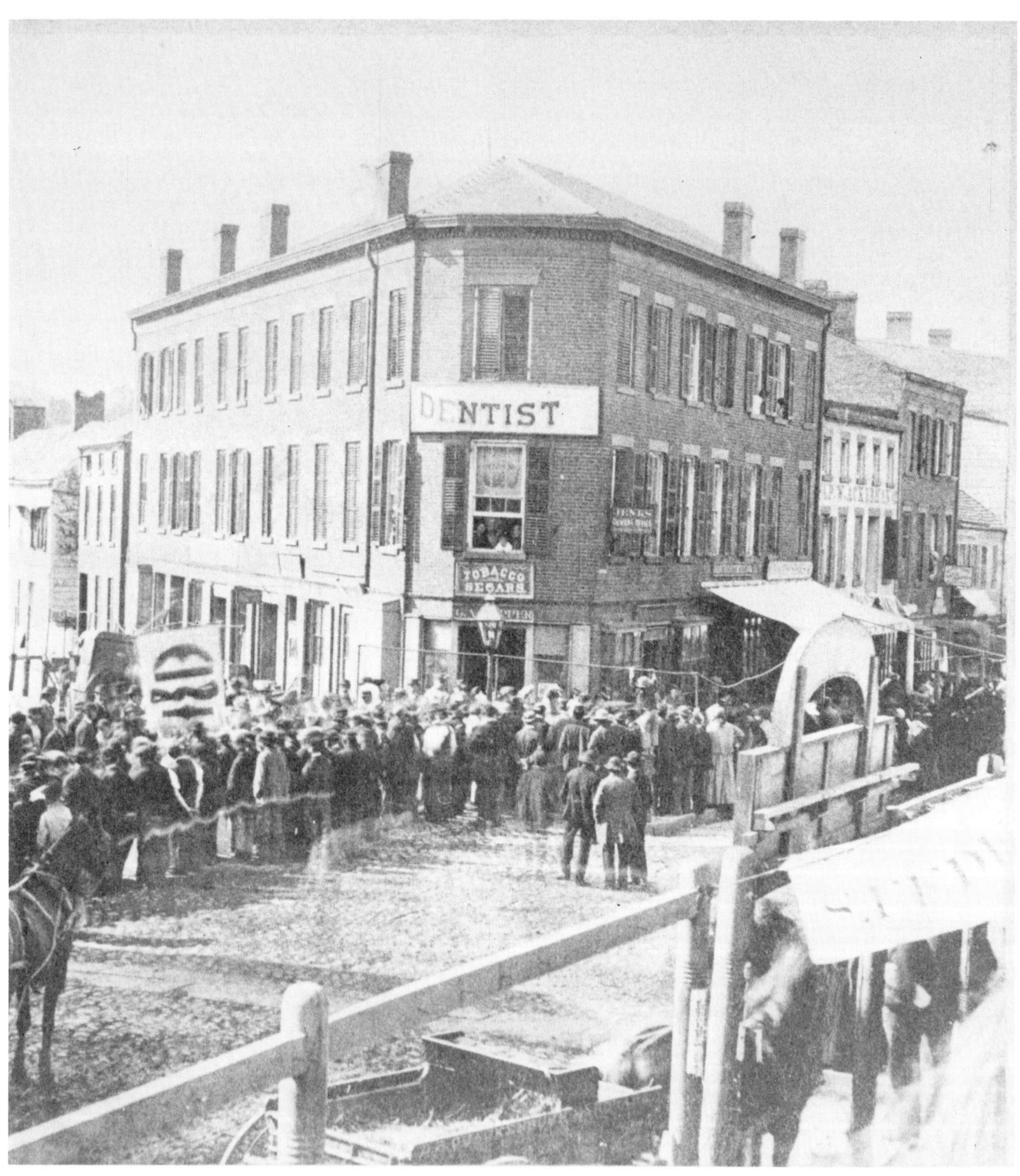

Exterior of building Dentist sign.
The photographs taken of towns and villages occasionally show exterior views of dental offices allowing us to see how dentist's practiced and their position in the local community.

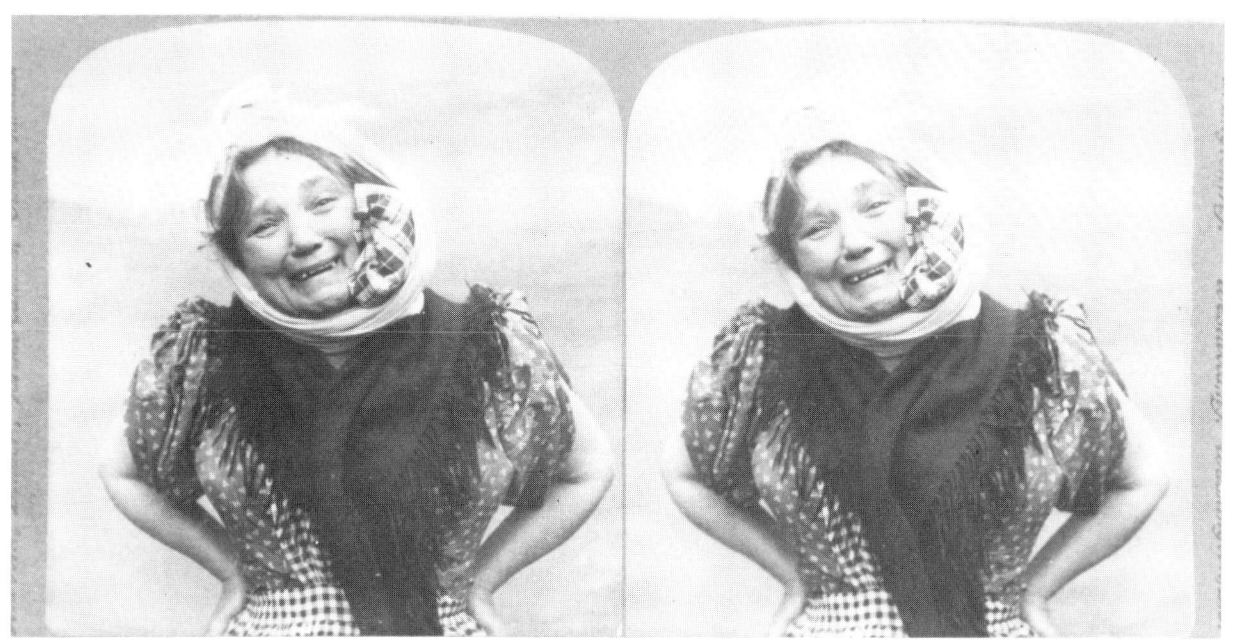

Stereo images of patients in distress were a common genre in late 19th photography. Typically the pictures show the patient with their head wrapped in a towel begging for attention.

Part of a series of photographs taken to show the medical/dental status of the Connecticut National Guard. This photo illustrates the unit's dentist at work in his office, circa 1890.

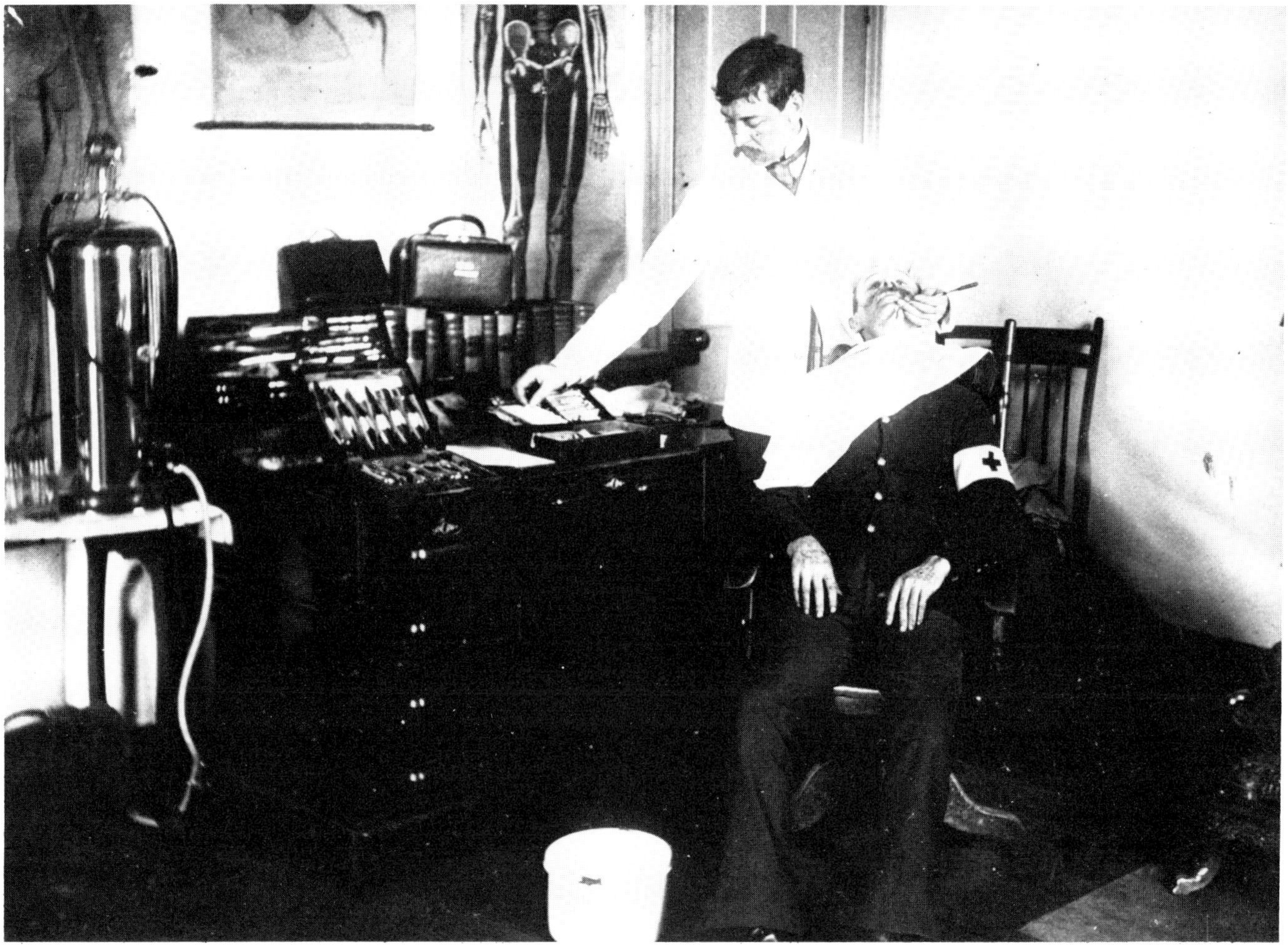

Dr RANKINS
DENTAL
PARLORS
E.J. Foley
Photo
The Rankin Reliance
B.B.C.
Edward Conroy, Capt. 1st Base. Edward Sheehan, Sec. Base. James McGarry Centre Fie
Matthew Murphy, Catcher. John Coralis, Third Base. Edward Meehan, Right Fie
William Arkman Pitcher. Alfred Burns, Short Stop. Peter Bagley, Left Fie

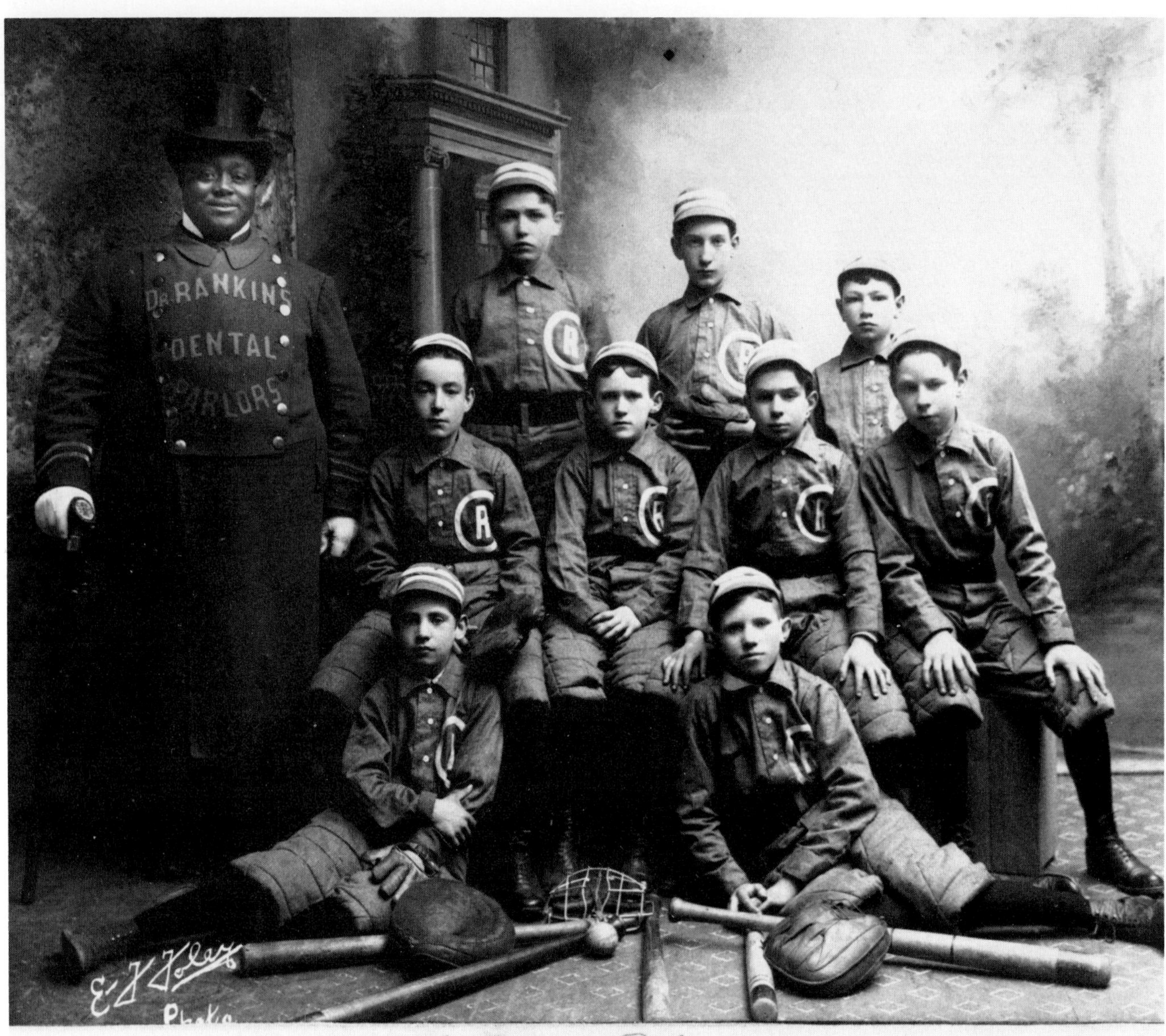

During the last decades of the 19th century baseball became the American pastime. Teams sprang up all over the United States, and most were supported by private financing. Here in this turn of the century photo we see "The Rankin Reliance," the team of Chicago entrepreneurial dentist Dr. Rankin. Not only does Dr. Rankin support the team, his fancy-dressed black man must have served as a walking advertising board for the busy dentist, who operated several dental parlors. This 8- by 10-inch photo hung in the dentist's office. Photographer E.J. Foley signed his name in the plate.

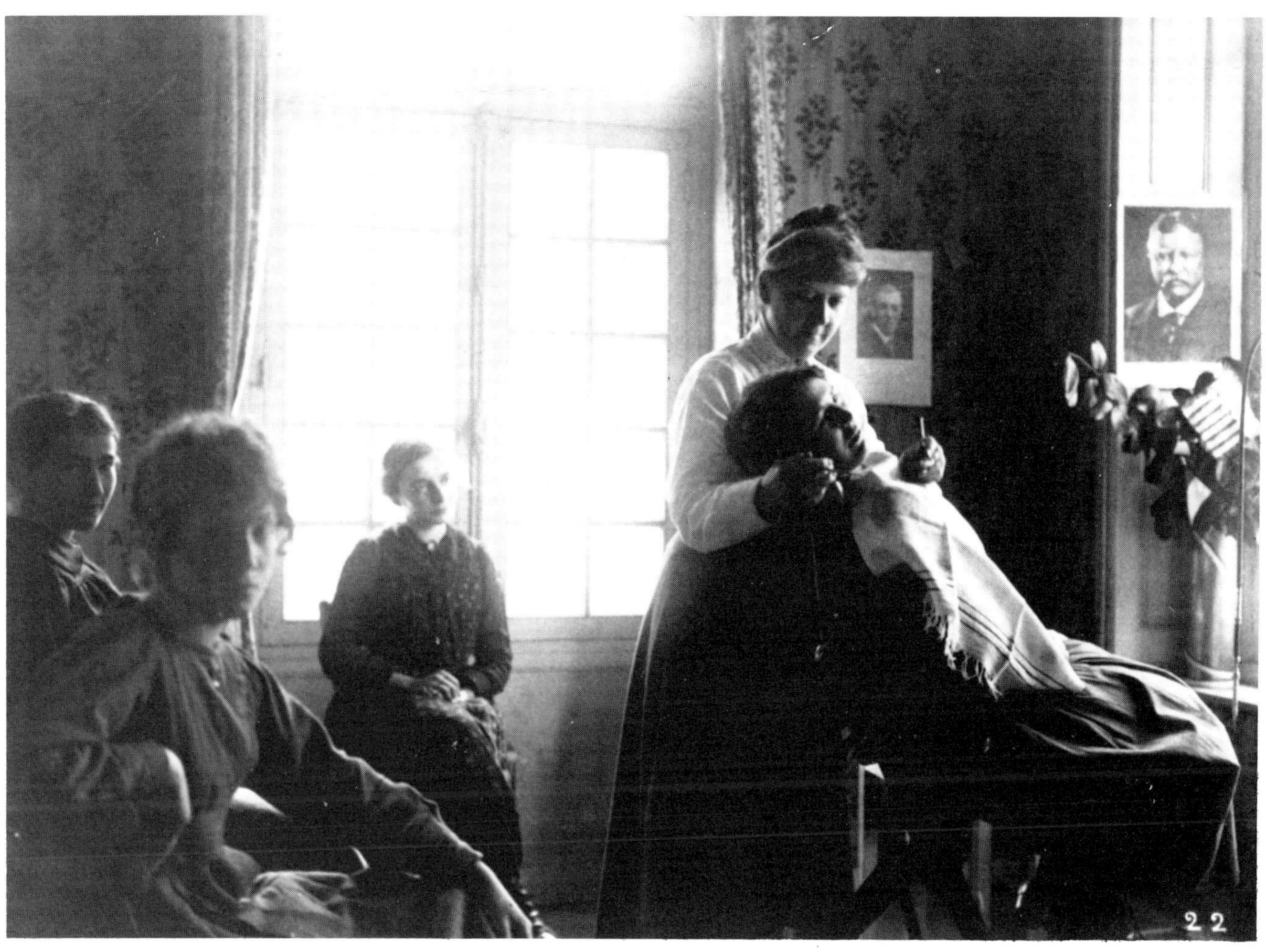

Women Dentists in WWI
Dr. Doherty at work in dental dispensary, Hospital No. 1, Luzancy, France. The American Women's Hospital was a volunteer unit of women physicians and a dentist who, prior to America's entrance into WWI, traveled to Europe to provide medical services to the wounded and the civilians of France. This photograph is part of a promotional series (#22), taken by E. Belval la Fertesous-Jouarree, to advertise the patriotic work of these noble medical volunteers. Harvard University's Medical School and several other institutions sent similar units to the allied countries.

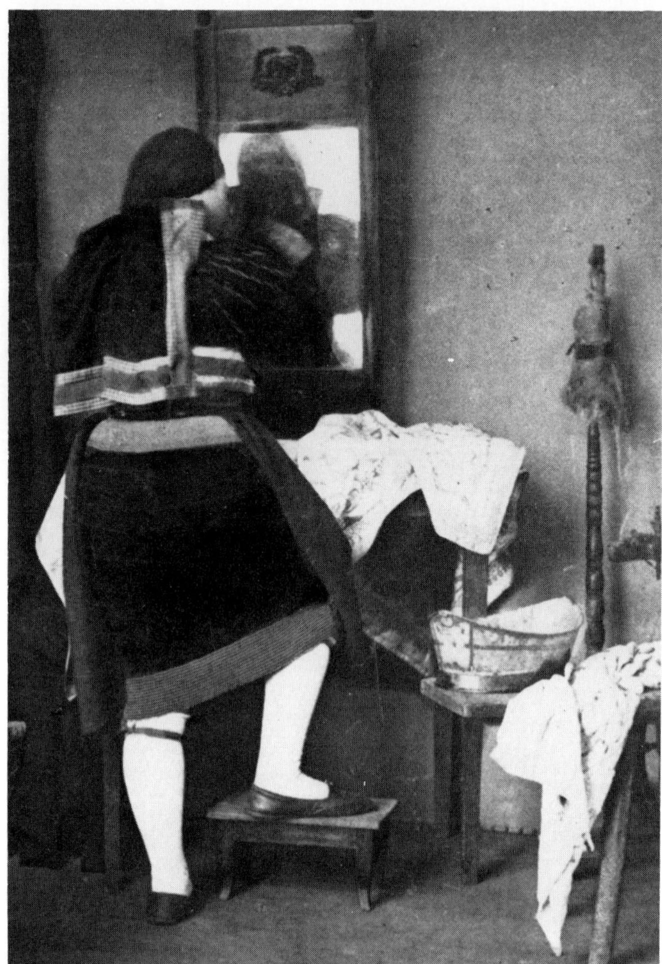

This is the only known photograph in the nineteenth century of someone brushing their teeth. Taken in Germany as part of a series on German costumes, and life it shows one aspect of "Doing ones Toilet." Berlin photographer S.P. Christman had each image hand tinted to make them more lifelike. This particular image is of a native of Sachsen-Altenburg, circa 1865.

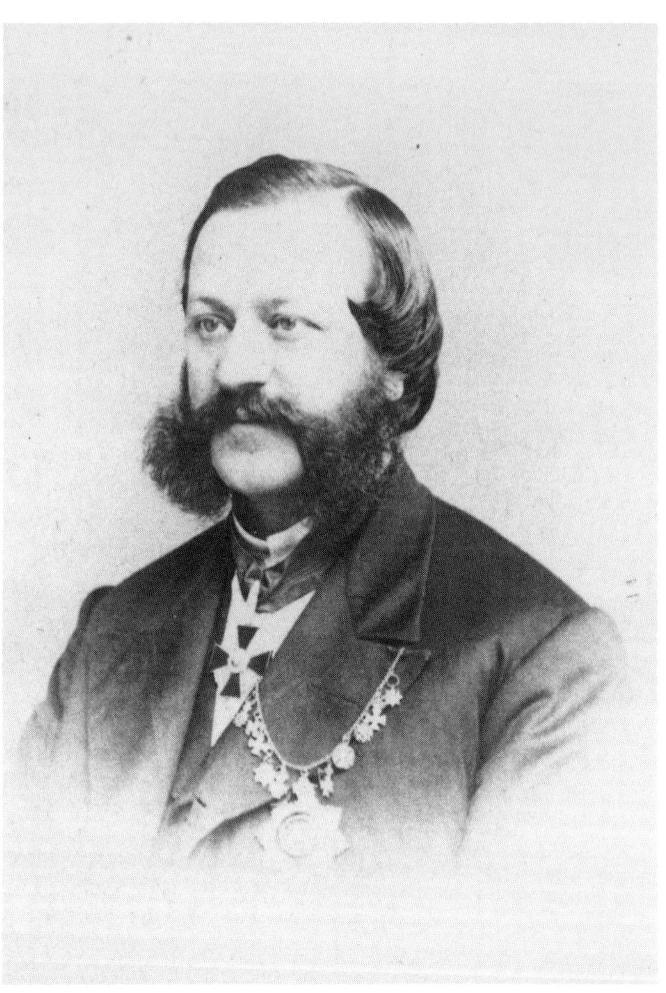

Perhaps the most famous American dentist of the 19th century was Dr. Thomas W. Evans (1823-1897). He moved to Paris in 1847, bringing American dental technology to Europe. He devised many innovative procedures during his career. His patients included notables and especially royalty, including Napoleon III of France, Czar Alexander of Russia and King Victor Emmanuel of Italy. Here we see Dr. Evans adorned with some of the international awards and orders he was presented with. This image was taken on a return visit to Philadelphia by noted photographer Frederick Gutekunst.

Studying Photographs

Studying photographs has become a modern social and cultural undertaking and a few books suggest how to begin such a program.[34] Under ideal conditions written documentation accompanies the photograph revealing who, what and where about the subject and photographer, and who preserved the photographs and why, etc. This information is rare among early photographs, so that one must scrutinize the image itself and compare it to others.

Most important in studying the photograph to identify

its era is the style of pose, clothing, dental or other equipment, and the photographic process used to take the picture. Changes in certain qualities of particular processes can be differentiated and helpful in dating images. For example, the disturbing glare from windows in interior views, called halation, was an artifact of photographs that was generally eliminated by 1895 when an inert coloring material was added to the emulsion to balance the film. Accurate dating of late 19th century office views, so popular at the time, may be made on this basis. Identification of the photographer, when possible, is extremely important as this information will give the location in which it was taken and explain some of the photograph's characteristics which were unique to the photographer. Important clues to notice in any image is the background. A calendar, or an American flag will make it possible to date the photograph because the stars in the flag were added fairly regularly in the 19th century.

Dental images transcend and supplement the written word. Early, as well as later, dental portraits are unusual in their frequent inclusion of a patient. In addition to the changing image of the dentist in photographs, the image of the patient is also transformed. Visual representation of what a patient expected and how he reacted is an important aspect of dental photography. In looking at the pictures in this book there are obvious changes in patient demeanor, composure and attitude. Patients change from appearing physically restrained and fearful to looking peaceful and cooperative. Although there are some exceptions, in general, we observe that the patient is physically restrained and fearful from 1840-1870, facing a window anonymously from 1890-1920, and cooperating calmly with the dentist beginning in the 1930s.

Dental images offer other critical information such as the introduction, role and type of assistants employed in the dental office, and the origin, kind, and use of equipment and instruments. All of these events contributed to the environment to which the patient responded. Photographs taught people how to behave with the practitioner.

The dental extraction genre photograph had its own specific occupational photographic convention.[35] In analyzing early medical views it was noted that these photographs are depicted with a recognizable background. None of the early dental extraction views are depicted with a recognizable background; it is plain. The usual studio format was not used. There is nothing in the picture but the dentist, his tools and the patient. This pose had to be a planned arrangement. The center of attention in all these images is the dentist and his patient. It is a very personal, direct and dynamic visual experience. Distracting tables, rugs, painted backdrops, etc., all of which appear in other occupational portraits of the era, even medical, are not present.

Historic Photographs Become Valuable

In 1938, a century after the discovery of the daguerreotype, there were only a few recognized collectors in America of these images.[36] It was not until the early 1970s that photography was generally appreciated and recognized as providing an important historic, social and cultural document, as well as being an art. Serious collecting and study began in the 1970s resulting in major accumulations in specialty areas of interest such as medicine, black American, folk art, erotica and other images. Those photographs previously discarded were snatched up by collectors. Today there are hundreds of daguerreotype collectors and as many institutions that covet early photographs. The result of this interest and subsequent increased value of early photographs has been the recovery and preservation of the early dental image.

Written descriptions of an event photographed, while important, are obviously influenced by the conventions and concerns of the time. Original photographs are now recognized as unique historic documents which may be studied, and then, re-studied in the future; constantly shedding new light and providing other possibilities for interpretation of past events. Included in the re-evaluation of these images is a discussion of whether the photograph is a perfect picture of reality. The intentions of the photographer, attitudes toward the client, beliefs and stereotypes of the period all enter into the composition, character and details revealed in a photograph. Framing and camera angle are among the techniques which the photographer uses to interject his feelings toward the people and objects photographed.[37] Eric Margolis cautions students of photographic images that

> "There is much to see in these pictures beyond the details of the actual image. Understanding depends on 'hidden' meanings, which only become available when the viewer has access to background information that makes it possible to read the pictures with an increasingly complex and deep recognition. Photos require context to fulfill their potential to inform—every picture does not tell a story.
>
> Photographs can only provide a skeletal image for our imaginations to fill out. These imaginations are professional—sociological, historical, anthropological—and they are informed by other data as well.[38]

The next chapters, also illustrated by contemporary photographs, reveal other aspects of the American dentist's struggle for excellence in a society absorbing numerous challenges from fluctuating ethnic, ethical, social, financial, health care and other systems. The photograph not only helps to tell the story of the American dentist, but compels us to ask other questions, thus extending the historical process and enriching our awareness of the growth of an American professional.[39]

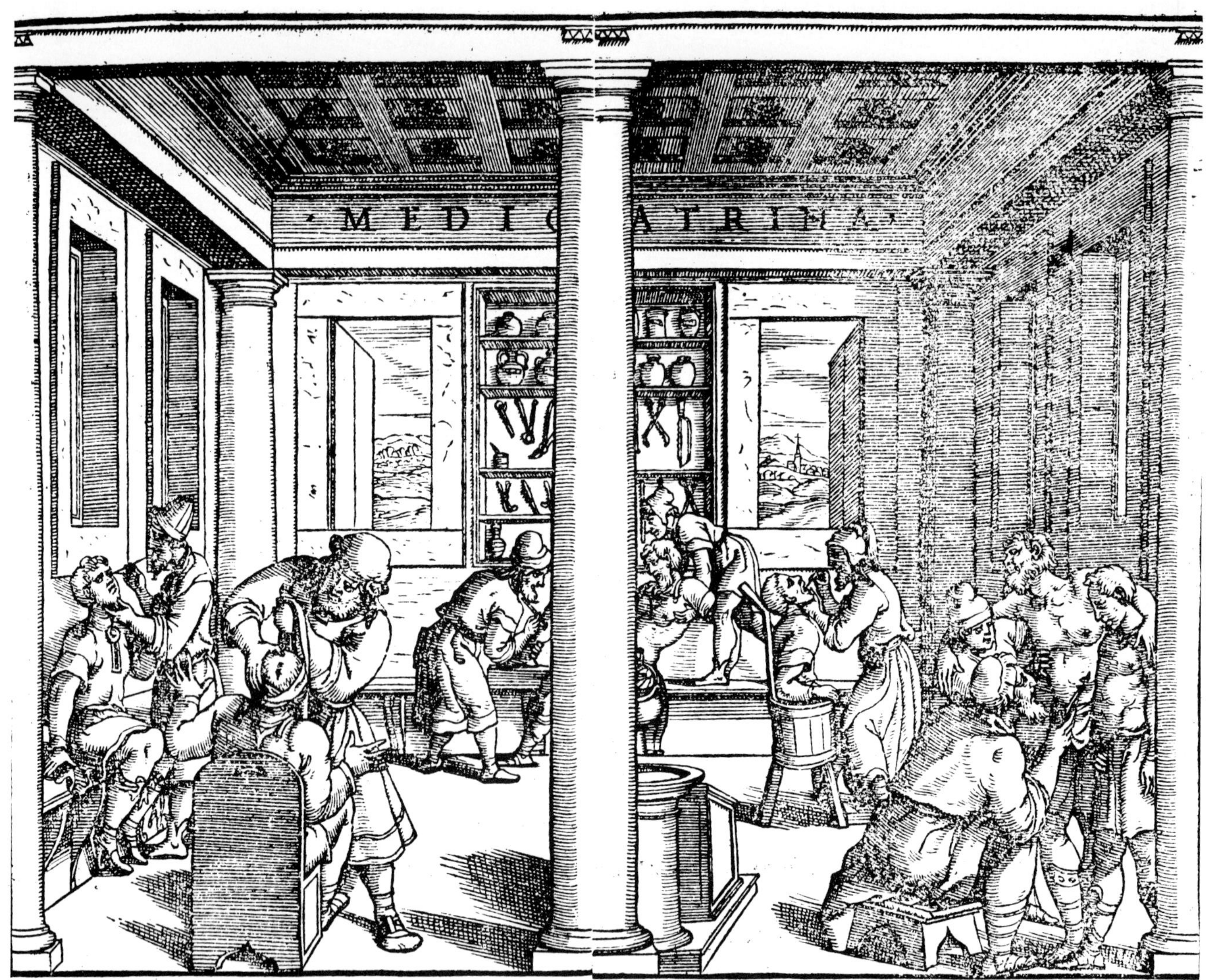

GALENI IN LIBRVM HIPPOCRATIS

Clinic, woodcut illustration from Galen, *Opera Omnia*, Venice, 1550. Dentistry was part of medical practice usually performed by the surgeon. The dental patient, in the center and to the right of the column, sits in a chair with a tilted headrest. Dentistry separated from medicine in the U.S. after the first dental school was established in 1839-40 in Baltimore, Maryland. From National Library of Medicine, Neg. No. 67-238.

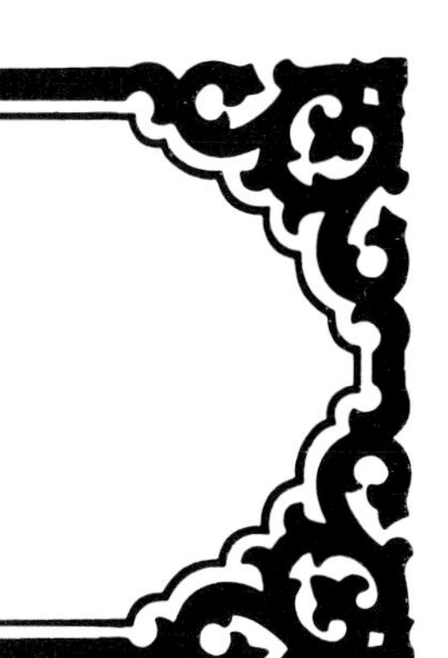

CHAPTER ONE

The Rise of the Dental Office

Eighteenth Century Background

The American dentist is the culmination of converging social, cultural, technological and medical factors in the 19th century. The basis for his craft was laid in the previous century when the instruments and techniques were imported from Europe, especially France, the cradle of modern dentistry. Dental instruments and techniques were refined and adopted from tools and procedures used by mechanics, watch makers, jewelers, enamelers and other craftsmen. The impetus to improve dental practice stemmed from two related events: the need to treat young sailors with debilitating dental disease and the exposure of a talented surgeon to naval dentistry early in his career. Confronted with many patients suffering from the deficiency disease, scurvy, the naval surgeon was forced to provide relief for extensive dental problems. French naval surgeons responded innovatively to the many seamen who contracted scurvy and other dental diseases. Foul breath, soft gums and toothache were symptoms of scurvy to which seamen fell victim after long voyages subsisting on a deficient diet. To prepare surgeons for treating the expected oral disease, as early as 1736, dentistry was included in the curriculum of the naval hygiene school at Rochefort, France.[1] France became a center for advanced dental techniques.

A leader among French dentists, whose career was launched in the navy, was Pierre Fauchard[2] (1678-1761). Guided into dentistry by the surgeon, Maj. Alexandre Poteleret, Fauchard soon introduced a new treatment for scurvy weakened teeth. He recommended scraping the teeth and cleaning the gums to treat the effects of this disease known as pyorrhea alveolaris. His useful treatment led to the name Fauchard's disease.[3]

Fauchard's text on dentistry, published in 1728, was the first to redefine significant issues which would become the art and technique of modern dentistry. Although the text was derivative, the book's title, *Le Chirurgien Dentiste*, encapsulated Fauchard's understanding of the expanding role of the dentist. Fauchard was the first to call himself a surgeon-dentist after he entered private practice in 1696 in Angers, France. Among his suggestions for improving dentistry, which would become the nucleus of dental care designed to save teeth, was advice about supporting the patient's body during treatment. He recommended an armchair of a size that the patient could grip and be able to place his feet on the floor to steady the body during the dental procedure. His chair was designed with a high back covered with horsehair and adjusted with pillows to keep the patient's head stationary and in the proper position for the dentist to see and reach the teeth.[4] Those patients too ill to sit up were to be treated in bed. Fauchard's suggestions came in a period before the dental chair existed, when standing, sitting or lying on the floor were accepted positions for a patient receiving dental treatment. To extract painful, loose or rotting teeth these extemporaneous positions may have sufficed, whereas to drill, fill, clean, polish and insert teeth a more stable, comfortable position was needed for both dentist and patient.

French and British surgeons, who generally served for three years in the colonies, brought Fauchard's techniques and their own modifications to America.[5] Surgeons continued to practice dentistry until the end of the century when dentistry became a specialty practiced by surgeon-dentists.

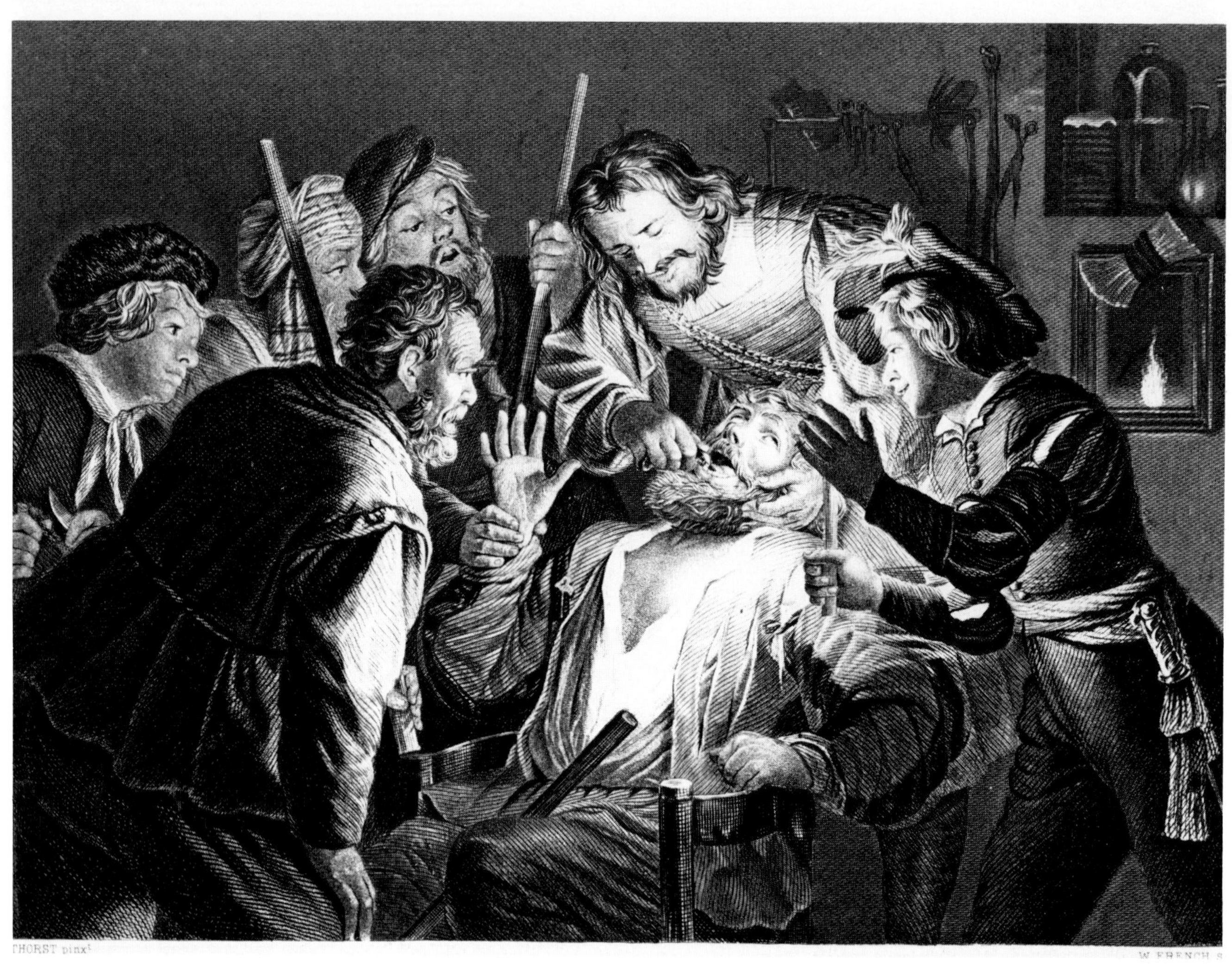

The Toothdrawer. Engraving by W. French after painting by Gerald Honthorst, 1622. The first representation of dental treatment by candlelight. Many poignant scenes of tooth extractions were painted over the last three centuries and many of them have been collected and published by Curt Proskauer, *Iconographia Odontologica*, 1927. (NLM Neg. No. 59-238)

CHAPTER TWO

Itinerant Dentistry

Preceding the surgeon-dentist and co-existing with him were those who extracted teeth almost exclusively. The most graphic descriptions of the specialized dentist or tooth-drawer in action are conveyed by paintings, sketches, drawings, cartoons and satirical illustrations. The most dramatic and unusual representations of the dentist have been copied and published. The images have generally been allowed to convey their own messages, which are among the profound human emotions centered on pain, compassion, curiosity, malice and ingenuity in overcoming adversity. Only a few are illustrated in our book, because many paintings, drawings, etc., were reproduced and published in several editions of Curt Proskauer's classic book *Iconographia Odontologica* and an interesting collection of early and contemporary dental art by J.J. Pindborg and L. Marvitz.[6] Several recurring motifs appear in these paintings. These are a string of teeth suspended near or on the tooth-puller, barely sketched in dental instruments and a bench or minimally supportive chair, which forces the dentist to hold the patient with one arm locked under his armpit.

One example of the painter's powerful insight into dental illness and treatment is represented by the Dutch painter, Jan Victors' "The Toothdrawer." Victors (1620-1676) was among those who vividly recorded the itinerant dentist's visit to a small town. The scene depicts the patient standing to have his tooth removed while another seated patient holds her swollen jaw. Extracting painful and rotting teeth could be quickly completed in a temporary "office" placed in front of shops. Spectators of all ages observe the patient, the dentist, and the table set with an open leather case, a bowl, a number of small bottles and several instruments laid upon a colorful table cloth. The table is shaded with an umbrella and adorned with a monkey who was brought along by the dentist to amuse the audience.

Throughout the 18th and 19th centuries, colonists were served by English and French surgeon-dentists who traveled to major cities where they carried out sophisticated procedures to clean, remove and replace teeth with artificial or human transplants. American dentists[7] followed their leadership in serving patients as itinerant dentists throughout the century because they could not afford to settle in one town and dental technology did not demand a permanent location. Itinerants tended patients in various settings: the home, factory, farm, hotel, coffeehouse, a borrowed physician's office, market place, village fair, bazaar or any place where a patient was stricken with a toothache. Newspapers[8] reveal that these American and foreign itinerants were adaptable and eager to please. They announced their arrival in town and invited patients to their hotels or offered to come to the patient's home, thus making the dental procedure private, when previously it had been a public demonstration. Oliver Holmes, surgeon-dentist from Baltimore, announced in the St. Louis paper, the *Missouri Gazette*, of April 26, 1820 that he would "wait upon patients in his home."[9] Among his services he included cleaning, separating, polishing and mending teeth with gold and foil, extracting those unable to be fixed, and supplying artificial teeth which he constructed. George S. Greene announced in *The Beacon* of St. Louis of 1830 that he would accept patients at the Major Hopkins Hotel and "wait on ladies in their residence when required."[10] For those unable to pay for his services he offered to treat them without charge between 6 a.m. and 8 a.m. daily.

Dentists also cooperated with patients unable to receive their services when they were out of town by suggesting ways in which they could preserve their teeth. S. Hardyear, the first traveling dentist in Cleveland, in 1826, explained that anyone could use a penknife to remove tartar from the teeth and keep the the teeth clean with charcoal made from burned bread. He advised that the toothbrush be placed perpendicular to the teeth and the gums.[11]

Enterprising dentists seized the opportunity to be of assistance whenever a demand occurred. A Michigan dentist reported in the 1820s that he treated the tooth of one patient in a tavern. He explained several of his methods:

"I made a dental operating chair by standing on one foot and placing the other foot in a chair back of the person and resting his head against my knee to steady it while I cleaned and filled his teeth, and if I visited the house to work for the women folks I sat down on a low cushion and had the persons sit on the floor and place their heads against my left arm for a headrest while I operated on their teeth. Sometimes my lady patients would remark that this was 'a very awkward and singular position to be placed in' to have their teeth fixed, but as we had no other conveniences it was made to answer the purpose of the dental chair."[12] The patient, "to a large extent, deprived of the power of movement, played a comparatively undistinguished part in the ensuing drama."[13]

Equally impressive and authentic representations of permanent dental offices are depicted in paintings, drawings, and after 1890, most often recorded in photographs. These scenes reveal which equipment a dentist selected, and then, arranged to serve patients, and sometimes, the reactions of the patient to dental treatment. The shape and ambiance of an early dental office appears in a richly detailed painting by Edouard Pingret of the office of the Parisian dentist Georges Fattett, who practiced during the mid-19th century.[14] The picture shows an enclosed cabinet filled with dentures and appliances neatly arranged on seven shelves, a cushioned, high-backed chair, a spittoon and instrument table. The table contains a magnifying lens, forceps, a dental key and dentures. The dentist is about to insert a set of teeth into his patient's mouth. A black dog and two dark-skinned attendants observe the action. Animal parts including preserved reptiles, elephant tusks, skins, teeth, etc., are on display in the room as was the custom in this period, especially in pharmacies, for these organic substances were a source of various drugs.

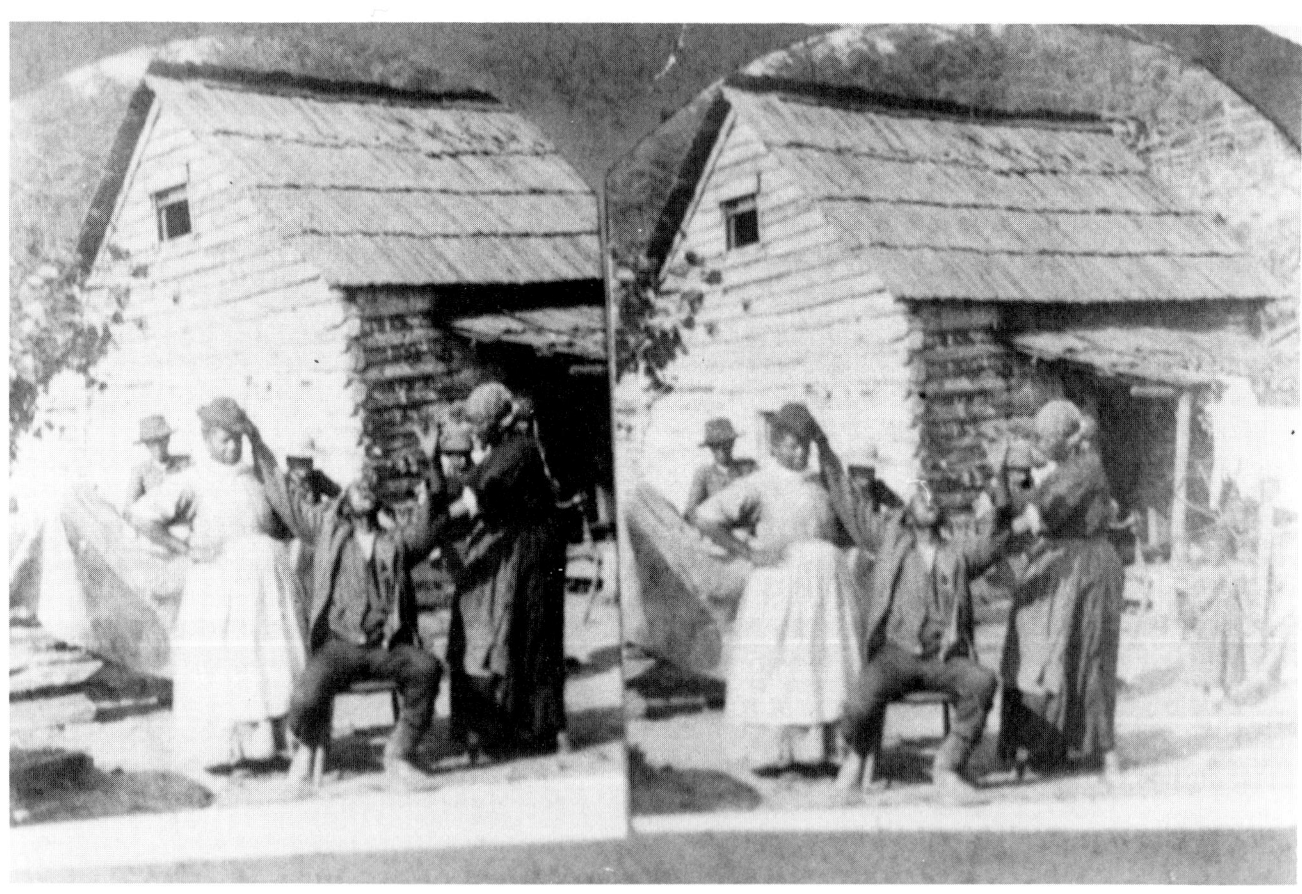

Dentistry was practiced by itinerants, apprentices and graduate dentists of both sexes, but primarily males, through the end of the 19th century. A rare photograph of a black woman in practice is this one of "Aunt Sophia," who ministered to miners in the Rorer Iron Mines of Virginia in 1890. These two illustrations, from stereopticons, show her about to remove a tooth while her daughter holds the patient's head steady. From Library of Congress.

CHAPTER THREE

Who Became Dentists in America

By 1825 the number of dentists in America was approximately 100, and by 1840, the number had grown to 1,200, although they were commonly called tooth-drawers or by related terms, rather than dentists. The first dental school in the U.S. was founded in 1840, however, only a few students graduated each year from this and several other private and university affiliated dental schools, so that most American dentists, until the last decade of the 19th century, were not dental school graduates, but graduate apprentices, physicians or poly-craftsmen,[15] who plied other trades and professions simultaneously. The dentists who settled in an area are listed in city directories. Thus we learn that Martin Lawrence Cardell of Detroit, in 1837, was a "Surgeon Dentist . . . permanently fixed in Desnoyers' new building."[16]

By 1840, the ethnic diversity of dentists was not limited to those who had migrated to the country by choice. There were approximately 120 black dentists. Most black dentists learned their techniques as apprentices and laboratory assistants to white dentists. As assistants to some of the most prominent white dentists, blacks were involved in the delivery of dental care into the 20th century.[17] One "gentlemanly Ethiopian" assisted the renowned New York dentist M.L. Rhein in his elaborate Victorian office of the 1890s.[18]

Black people were believed to possess generally good dental health, which disappeared in later generations, after adopting a different American diet. Blacks, who needed dental care, were refused treatment by most white dentists or were treated out of sight of other patients.[19] Preferential treatment for white patients, sometimes had advantages for the black. Dentists, who bought sound teeth from those willing to have them extracted, to use in transplantations into their wealthier patients, usually refused to buy teeth from slaves.[20] Lacking dental care from white dentists, opportunities were created for unusual black dentists to practice. An account of one of the earliest of these practitioners reveals that dentistry took many forms in the colonial period. Samuel Mordecai of Richmond, Virginia, a patient, in 1765 described his dentist, Pere Hawkins as: a tall, raw-boned, very black Negro, who rode a raw-boned black horse, for his practice was too extensive to be managed on foot, and he carried all his instruments, consisting of two or three pullikins, in his pocket. His dexterity was such that he has been known to be stopped in the street by one of his distressed brethren... and to relieve him of the offending tooth, gratuitously, without dismounting from his horse. His strength of wrist was such, that he would almost infallibly extract, or break a tooth, whether the right or wrong one."[21]

The dentist seated on a horse was the subject of painters who lived before and after Hawkins practiced. A career as a dentist brought freedom to one black man. Cesar, a slave, was freed in 1792 after performing medical and dental "cures." The Assembly of South Carolina voted the money to purchase his freedom and provide him with an annuity of $100.[22]

Expectations were optimistic that a black person could obtain a proper dental education. Robert T. Freeman, a black, was among the first six graduates to obtain a doctoral degree in 1869 from the Harvard Dental School, the first dental school to be a part of a university. Denied entry into independent dental schools, Freeman applied to Harvard Dental College in 1867.[23] In 1881 the Howard University College of Dentistry in the District of Columbia was founded and remains a major institution for educating black dentists. In the first class, six students enrolled and the first dentist graduated in 1885 with a D.D.S. In 1900 graduates organized the Robert Freeman Dental Society in Washington, D.C. which became a constituent society of the National Dental Association. In 1910 when there were over 30,000 American dentists, only 478 of them were black and by 1930, the number had increased to a mere 1,773.[24]

In the 19th century women rarely practiced dentistry unless their husbands, fathers or brothers taught them to assist with their patients. Occasionally, upon the death of their tutors, women, who had learned and enjoyed dentistry, carried on the dental practices they inherited.

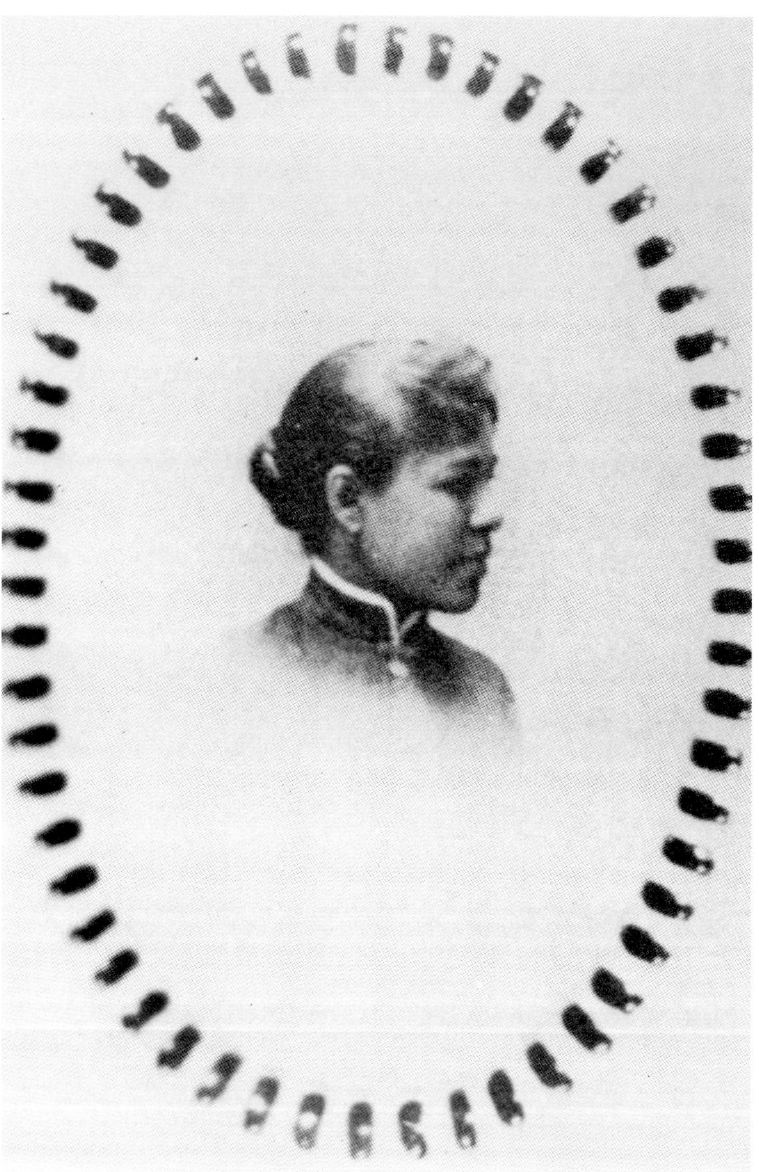

Ida Gray, who graduated in 1890 from the University of Michigan School of Dentistry, was the first black woman to receive a dental degree. In 1869 the first black male, Robert Tanner Freeman, received a degree from Harvard University. From University of Michigan School of Dentistry *Alumni Bulletin*, 1977-78, pg. 51. Smithsonian Institution, Neg. No. 88-9886-28.

CHAPTER FOUR

Early Dental Equipment

Itinerant dentists usually carried a tin or leather box containing a variety of extracting instruments including a pullikin or pelican, a turnkey and forceps, as well as excavators, probes, and a piece of bone out of which to carve teeth. The itinerant dentist placed his instruments on any convenient table, chair or barrel while he worked on the patient. Among the most common instruments was the pelican that Ambroise Paré (1510-1590), French surgeon, had recommended to remove a tooth that was firmly entrenched. The bolster of the pelican placed against the gum enabled the dentist to force the tooth out sideways. Then, with another instrument, the elevator, he lifted out the root.[25] Since 1740 the turnkey was accepted as the more efficient instrument for extracting less resistant teeth. Fitted with a claw it resembled "a ratchet wrench used by mechanics to attach and remove nuts and bolts."[26] By applying the key to the patient's tooth while he lay on the floor with his head between the knees of the operator, the tooth could be extracted more quickly than with a pelican. If incorrectly applied the turnkey could break away part of the jaw bone, and therefore, was not recommended by a dentist like Fauchard.[27]

Barber surgeon set containing a dental key and two forceps in a cloth case. These dental instruments were part of an early 19th century barber surgeon's kit. From Smithsonian Institution, Neg. No. 43-4221.

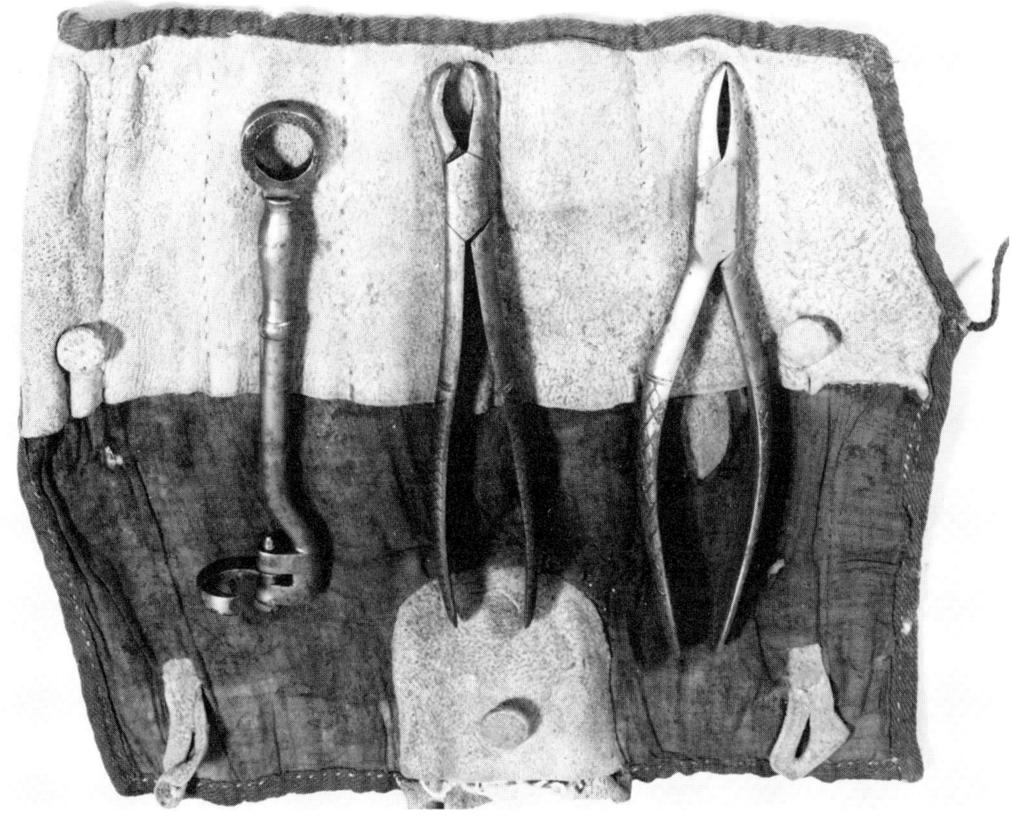

Dentists often made their own instruments such as the Michigan dentist who made "small excavators, pluggers and burrs out of shoemakers' awls."[28] Dental students were expected to fashion their own instruments until the last quarter of the 19th century. Dental instruments adapted from other tools were effective when applied skillfully. The anatomist, Astley Cooper, witnessed one instance. After Cooper tried unsuccessfully to remove his patient's tooth, Josiah Flagg Jr., captured during the War of 1812 and brought to London where he became Cooper's assistant, used his jeweler's tool to pry out the tooth. It "flew across the room," to Cooper's astonishment.[29]

The more expert itinerant dentist made "teeth for old ladies . . . from calves' teeth and the teeth of sheep fastened on a piece of thick leather and worn under the upper and lower lips."[30] These teeth were usually worn for their appearance and were taken out before eating. Where partial sections were needed they were carved from bone and tied in place with a ligature attached to the back teeth. Ivory was salvaged from many sources including piano keys, to make teeth, such as those made for the mother of Ralph Waldo Emerson. Patients occasionally made their own teeth. One lady, in an emergency, carved her teeth out of a baga turnip. She wore her "turnip plate" to a party with success, but returned to her dentist for a more permanent denture.[31]

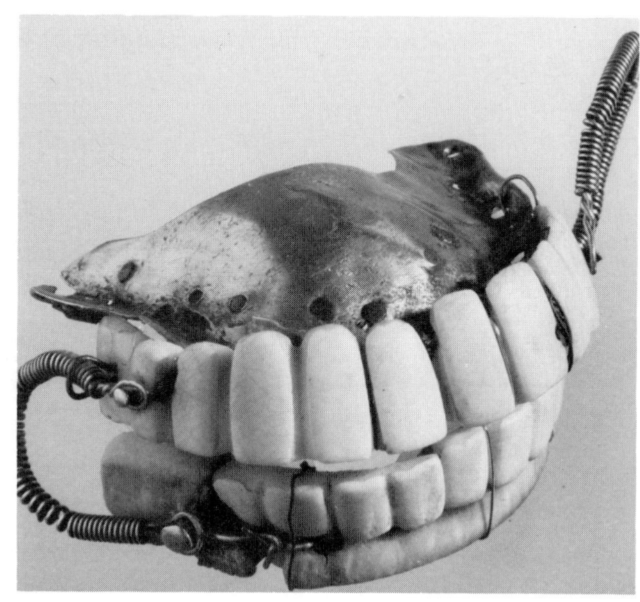

Set of George Washington's teeth made by John Greenwood and loaned by the University of Maryland School of Dentistry to the Smithsonian Institution in 1964. The set remained on exhibit until 1983 when the upper half of the denture was taken and has not been located. These teeth are made of ivory. The upper plate was made of gold and the springs are brass. From Smithsonian Institution, Neg. No. 75-3665.

Hand tools designed by Horace Hayden, founder of the first dental school in the world in Baltimore, Maryland (1839-40). These tools are on exhibition in the National Museum of American History (NMAH). From Smithsonian Institution, Neg. No. 73-12794.

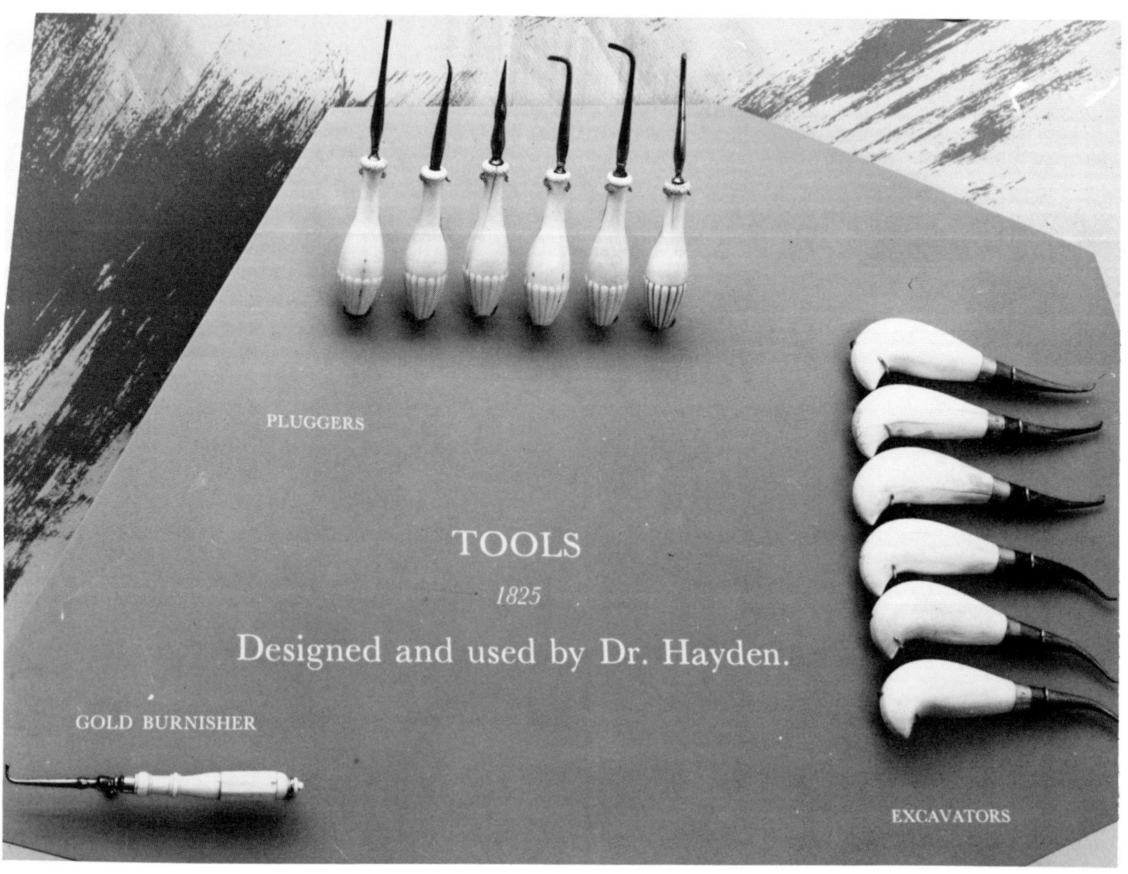

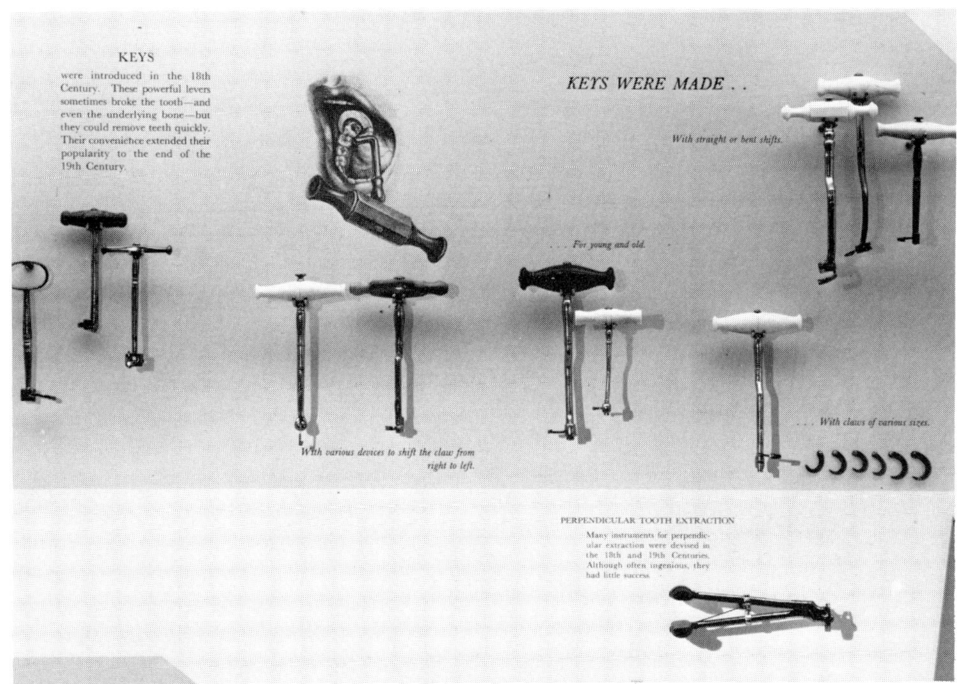

Dental keys on exhibit in NMAH. Keys were introduced in the 18th century and could be used to quickly remove a tooth in the period before anesthetics were available. This convenience, in spite of the disadvantage of breaking the tooth or jaw bone, extended their use until the late 19th century. Keys were made with straight, or curved and bent shafts, for children and adult teeth, and with various size claws. From Smithsonian Institution, Neg. No. 64741.

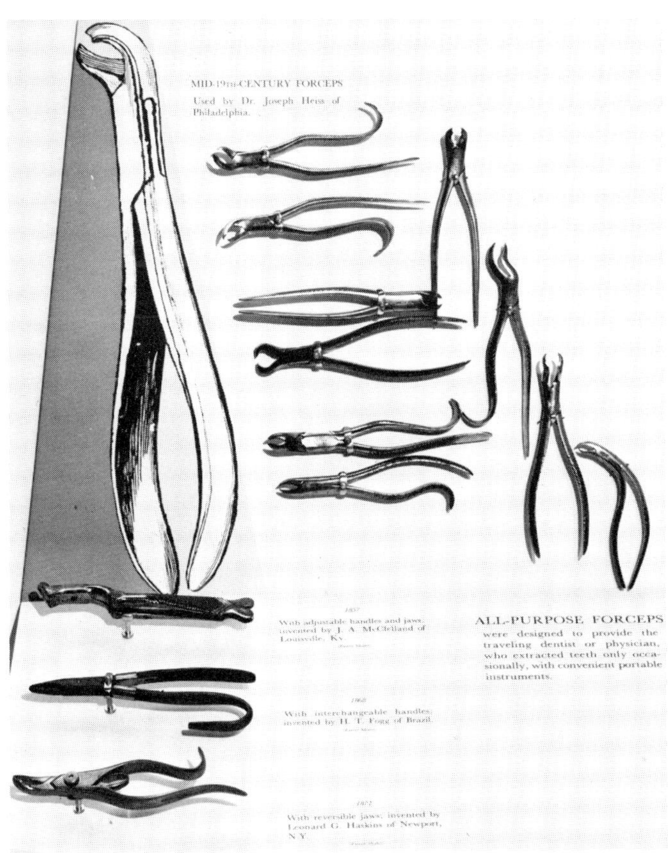

Forceps replaced both keys and pelicans, and remain the instrument used to extract teeth. Forceps were designed specifically to extract teeth in each part of the jaw and to accommodate different sizes in mouth cavities. From Smithsonian Institution, Neg. No. 64735.

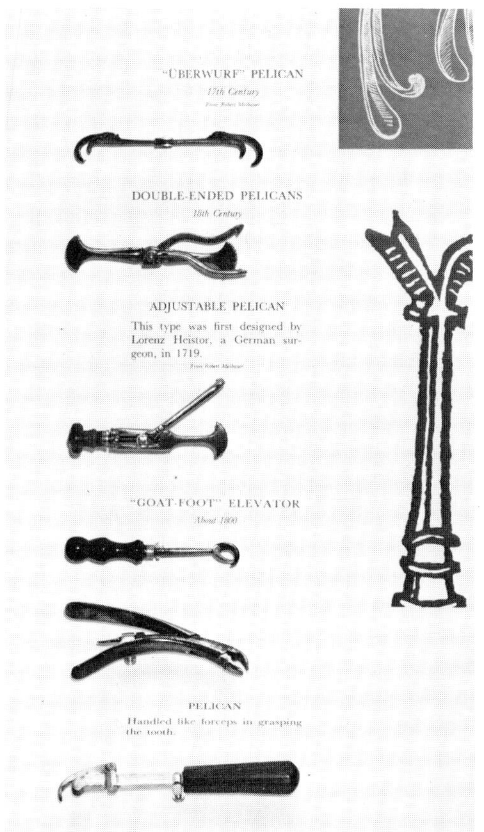

Pelicans, also on exhibit in NMAH, were promoted early by the father of modern surgery, the Frenchman, Ambroise Paré. (See Richard Glenner's, *The Dental Office,* p. 113 for a comparison of pelican and keys.) From Smithsonian Institution, Neg. No. 64740.

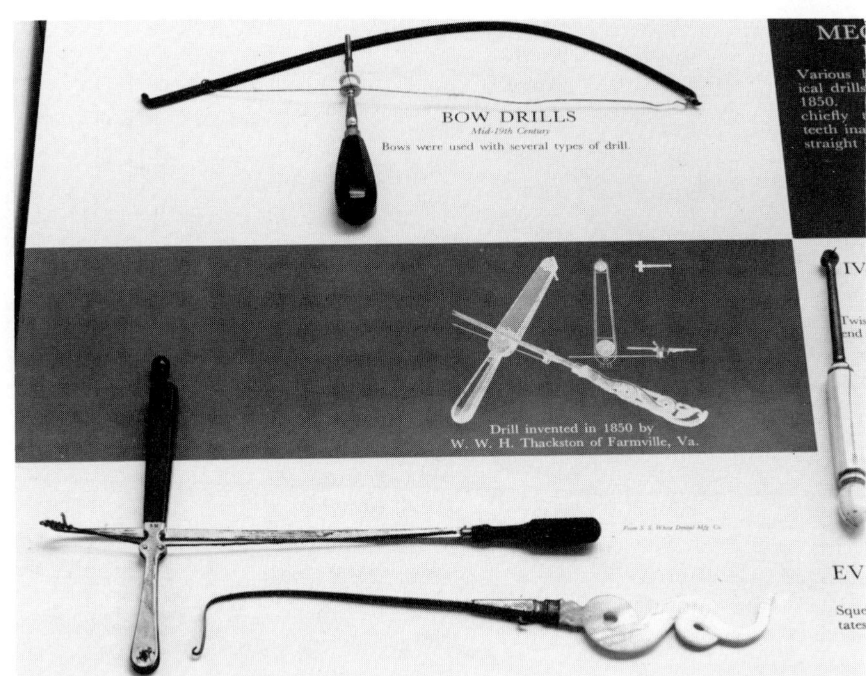

Drills were used to remove decay from a tooth before filling it with a metallic "stopping" to prevent further decay and permit use of the tooth. The earliest drills were hand-turned and called bow drills from their obvious arrangement. From Smithsonian Institution, Neg. No. 64738.

This photograph of an exhibit case shows models of engines used to power hand drills, four of them lined up on the left of the large foot-pedal drill. From top to bottom: Harrington's key and drill (1864); from Kalamazoo, Michigan, George F. Green's pneumatic drill of 1866; and Green's electric drill. The foot-pedal drill was invented by J.B. Morrison of St. Louis in 1871. Electric motors replaced the foot-pedal in the early 20th century, although when electricity was not available, as on a battlefield, the foot-pedal drill had its use well into the century. From Smithsonian Institution, Neg. No. 64739.

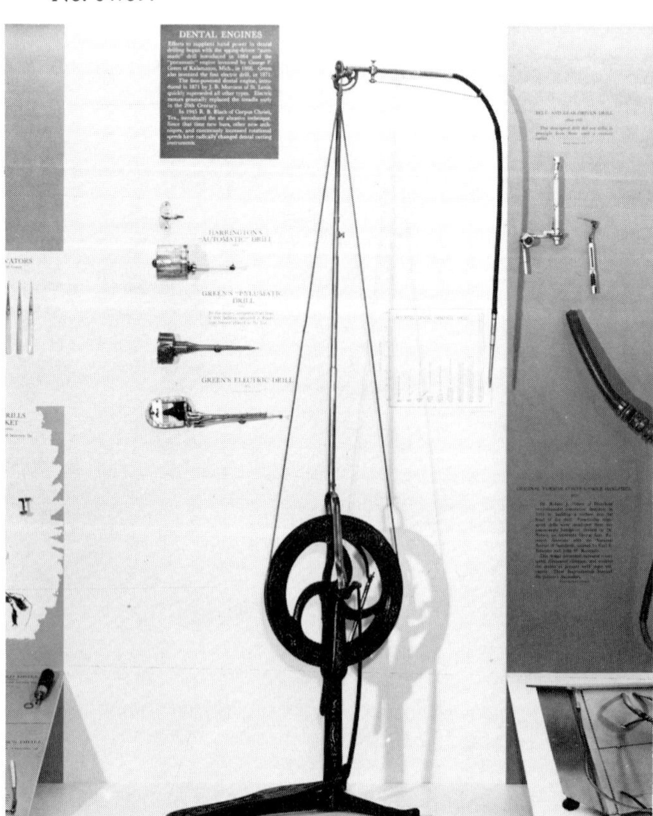

Enlargement of foot-pedal drill.

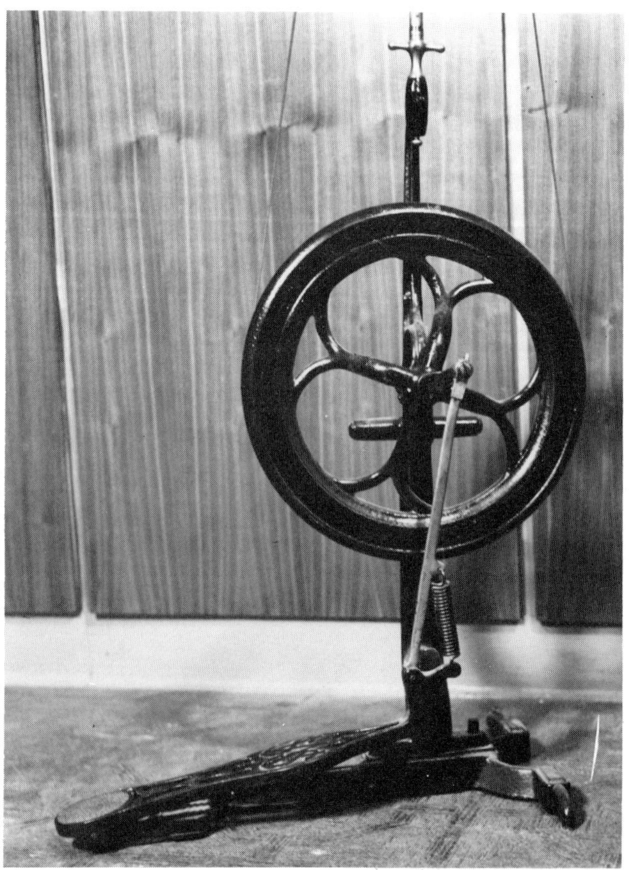

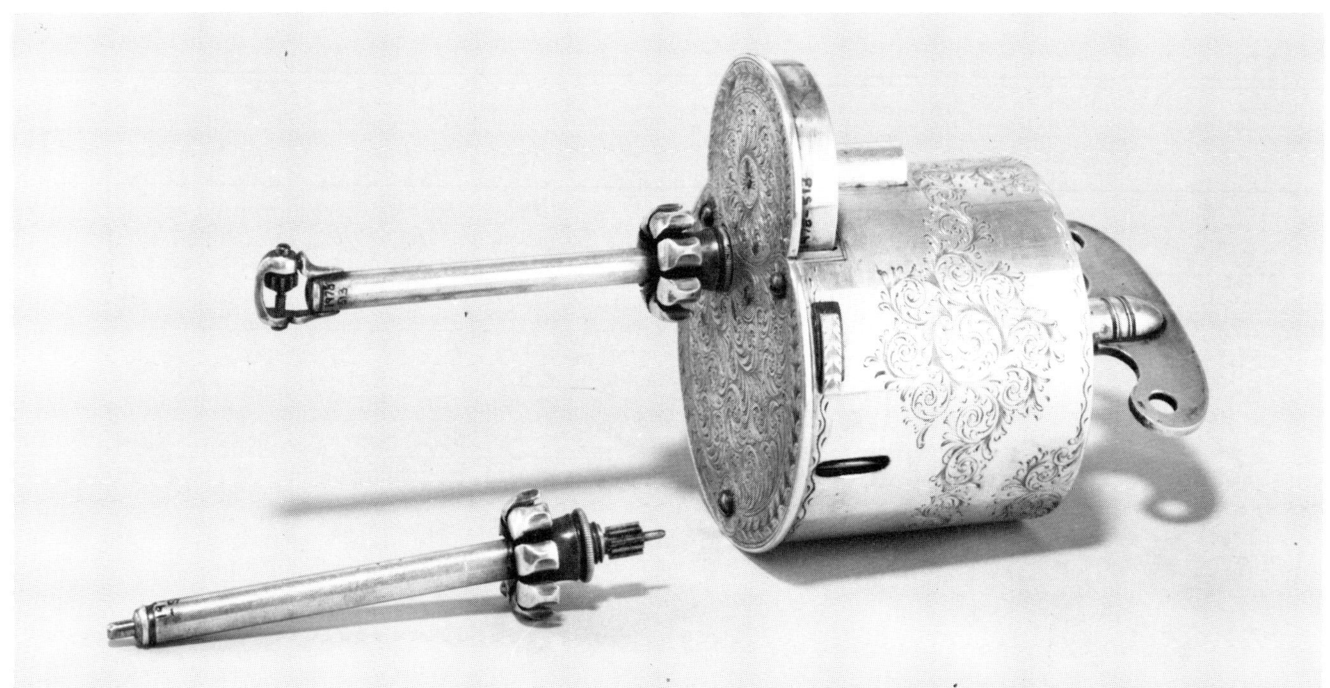

The first motor-driven dental engine was patented in England by George Fellows Harrington in 1864. It was operated by spring clockwork and was provided with a key for winding up the spring. It is believed to be the oldest motor-driven dental engine. This drill ran for two minutes, and could easily be applied with one hand. Its construction was similar to a child's toy of today. From London Science Museum, Neg. No. 751/80.

Electric panel or switchboard advertised in 1911 by Marshall-O'Brien-Worthen Company showing the different pieces of equipment which could be wired into the panel. The company under the name O'Brien Worthen had offices in St. Louis, Missouri; Des Moines, Iowa; and a number of other midwestern cities. Equipment that could be linked to the panel beginning with the upper right and moving around the panel clockwise includes a fan, sterilizer, light for the mouth, hand-piece, drill, mirror, set of hand-pieces, water heater, and heater.

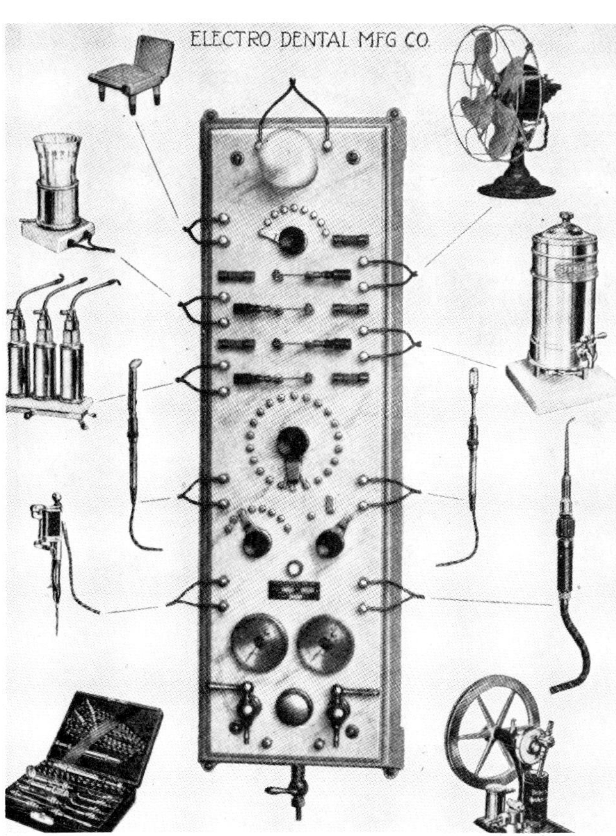

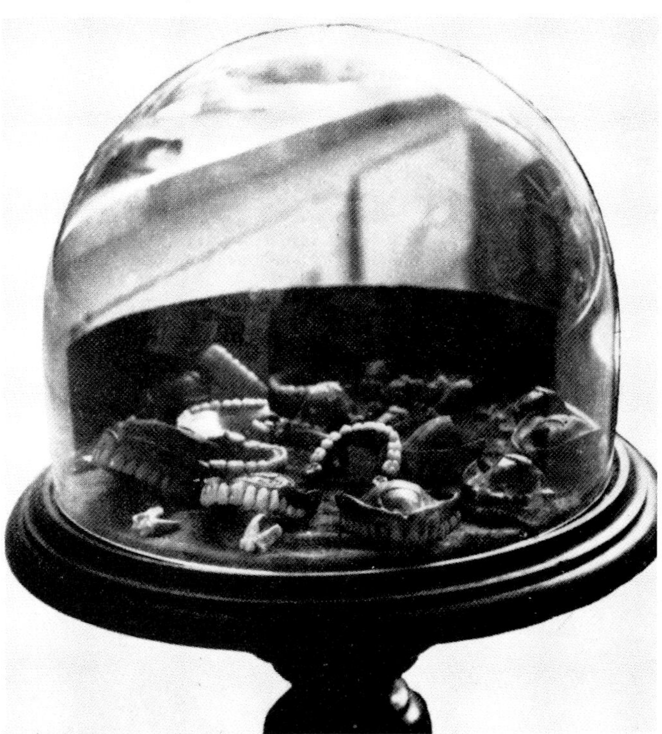

Dental parlor stand of Dr. Herman R. Eavey. Displays of artificial dentures were part of the dental office in the late 19th century.

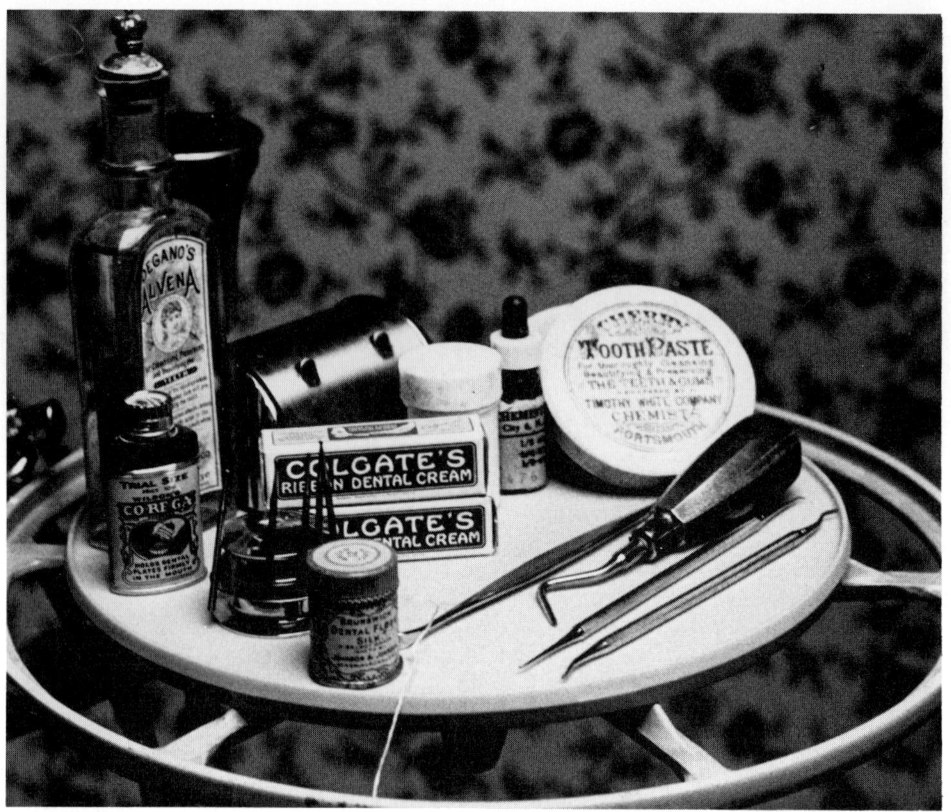

Assortment of tooth cleansers arranged on a dental tray. These items were available at the turn of the century. The instruments were used to scrape teeth and remove tartar from the teeth.

Several dental products photographed by the Lincoln Dental Supply Company. Of special interest are the two ceramic bottles labeled mercury, which was used in making silver amalgam filling material. The brick-shaped item to the right is a flask used to mold artificial dentures. From Lincoln Dental Supply Company, Philadelphia, Pennsylvania.

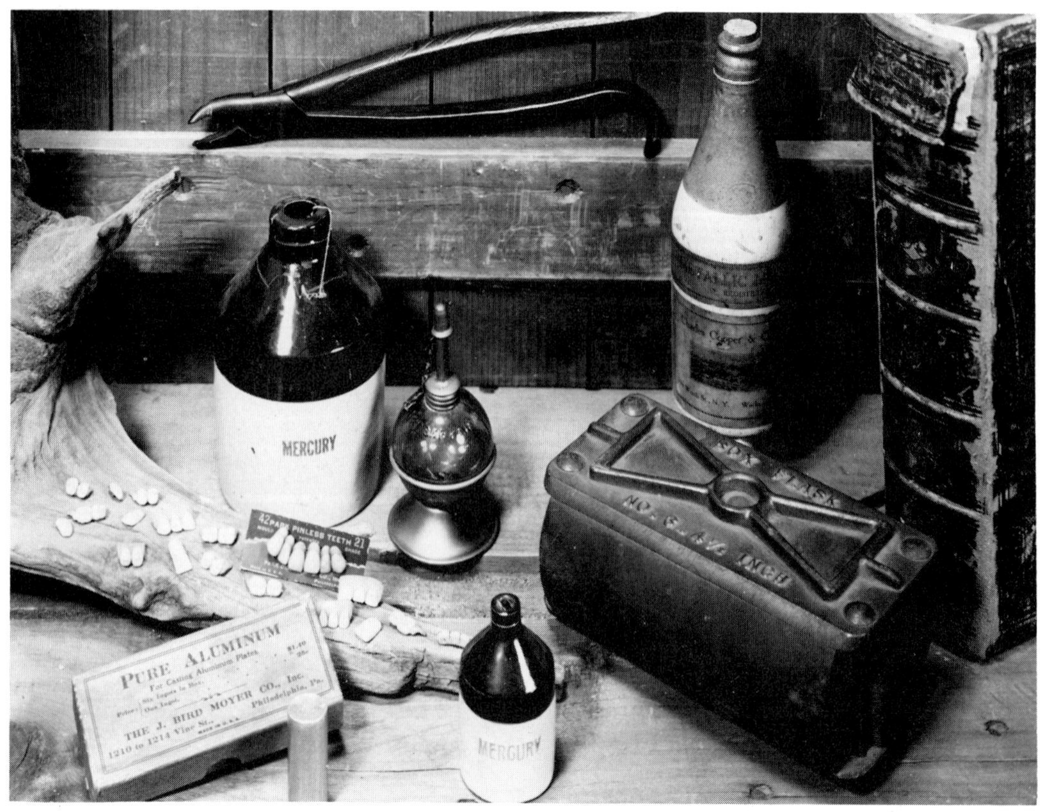

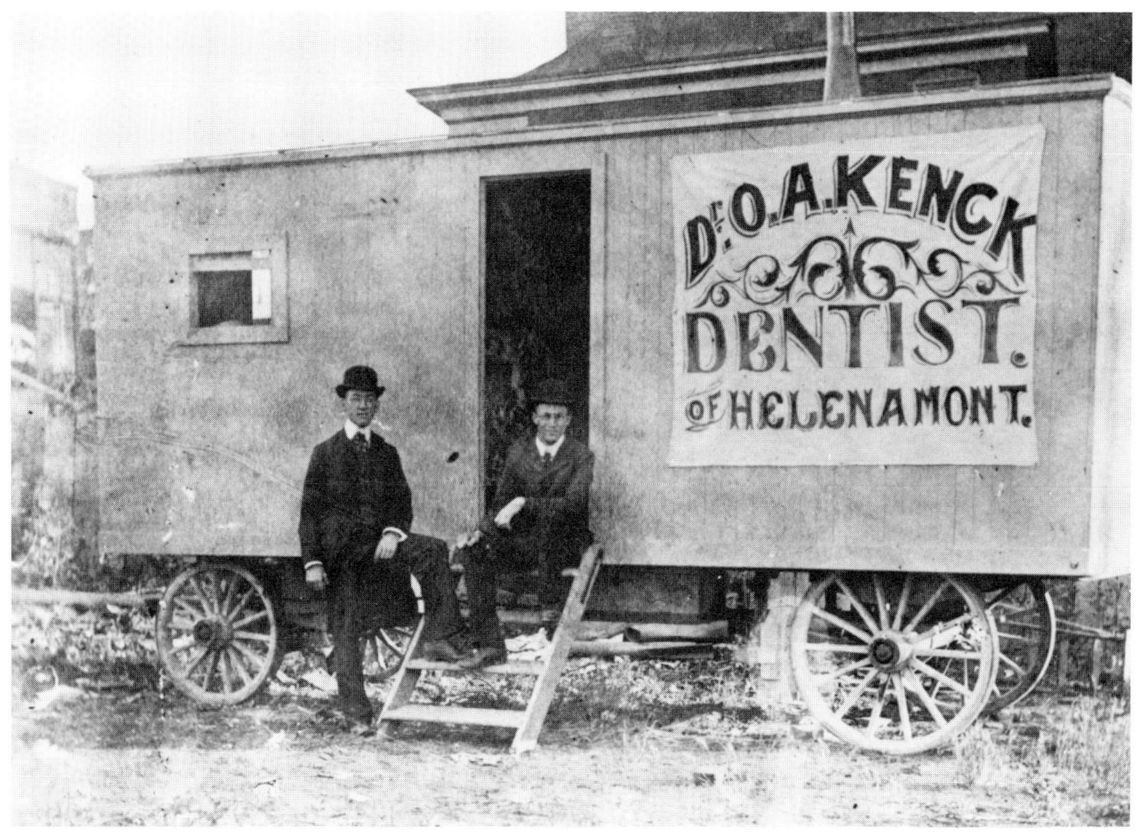

The dental office on wheels of itinerant dentist, Dr. O.A. Kenck, of Helena, Montana, circa 1899-1900. From Montana Historical Society, Helena, Montana.

Itinerant dentist, Dr. O.A. Kenck of Helena, Montana, in his office on wheels, circa 1899-1900. From Montana Historical Society, Helena, Montana.

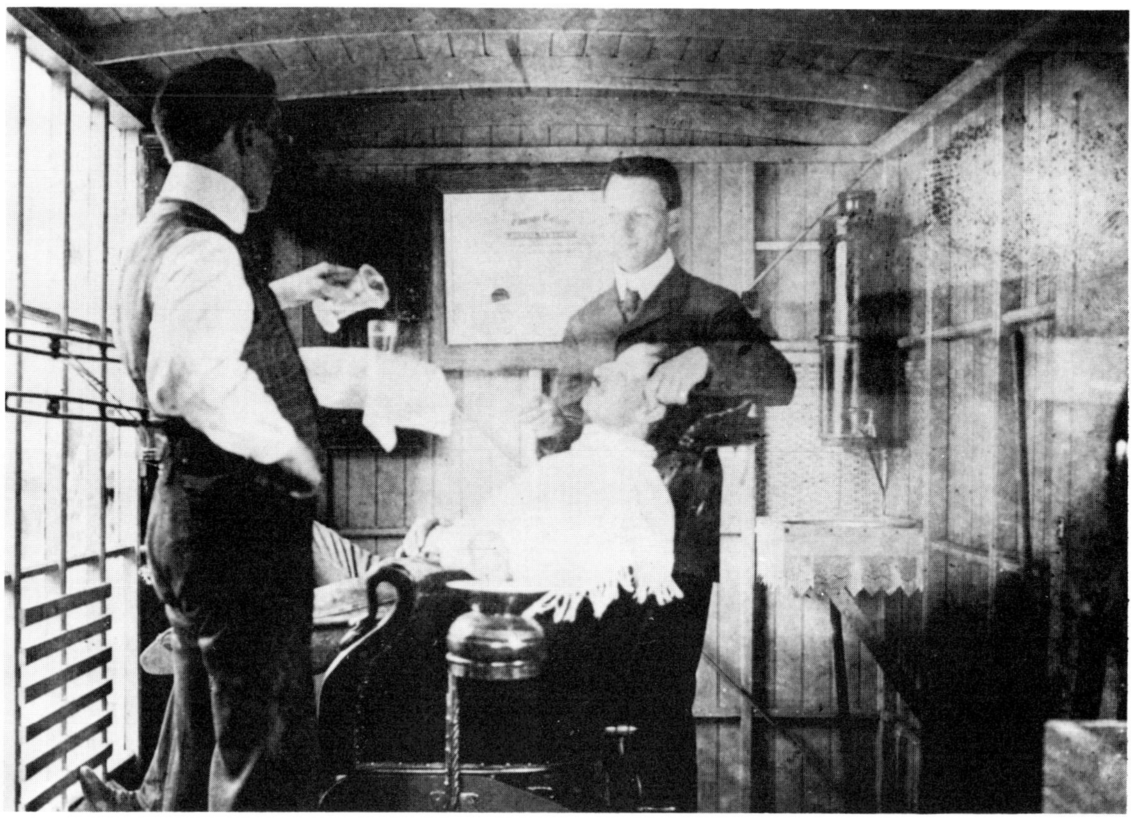

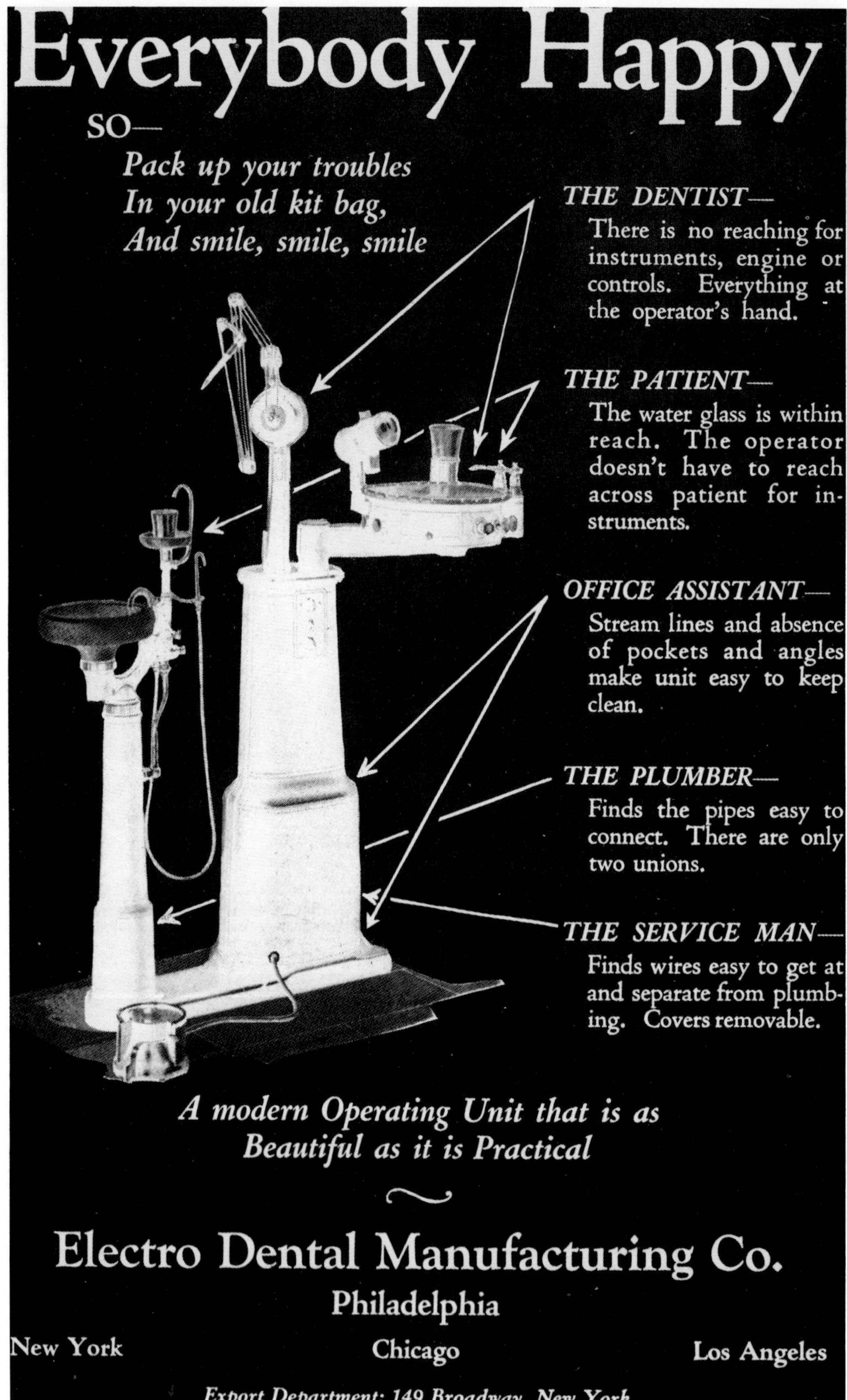

Dental unit as advertised in the early 1920s.

CHAPTER FIVE

Early Dental Chairs and Offices

In 1790 the dentist, Josiah Foster Flagg Jr., who as we noted before used the jeweler's instrument so well, designed the first special chair for dentistry in America by attaching a headrest to a Windsor-style armchair. The chair became the emblem, as well as, an essential piece of furniture for the patient and dentist. Flagg's dental chair has become an icon of the history of dentistry where it resides in the Temple University School of Dentistry Museum. Upon occasion itinerant dentists carried a chair with them on their journeys to patients. One of these is depicted in a recent painting by Hedda of the period, circa 1800. The dentist drives a horse and wagon in which are seated his family, and behind them, a Flagg dental chair.[32] For traveling dentists, who did not wish to transport a complete chair, Samuel Stockton White, an American dental manufacturer, began in 1848[33] to sell headrests, the most essential part of the chair, from the dentist's viewpoint. The headrest could be attached to any chair with a back and used to cradle the head and neck in a convenient position for the dentist to see and work on the teeth. Comfort for both patient and dentist was difficult to obtain and remains a selling point in new designs for dental equipment. The dental chair became, by the last quarter of the 19th century, the stationary focus of a space called the dental office and was surrounded by foot-pedaled drills, multi-drawer cabinets for storing an array of hand instruments and supplies, a spittoon, gas and electric lamps, anesthesia devices and other specialized equipment.

The decor of dental offices often reflects the dentist's personality, as well as his technical proficiency. None more so than Martin van Butchell, an eccentric and flamboyant British dental practitioner, who operated out of an office on Mount Street near Berkeley Square in London between 1770-1814. He arranged his office to include one macabre display—the embalmed body of his first wife, which remained on view for 30 years. Since then her mummy has been preserved by the museum of the Royal College of Surgeons to which her body was willed. Butchell learned about the embalming technique from his friend William Hunter, "The Father of Modern Surgery," who also advised him on the treatment of dental disorders.[34] His office symbolizes the tolerance for harsh, uncomfortable and uninviting offices in this period. Throughout the 19th century and the next, changes in the appearance of the dental office indicate a desire to transform the office into a planned, less stressful environment for the patient. To accomplish this end, dentists employed a range of schemes dictated by their technical needs, their hobbies and in response to their patients' sensitivities.

James Snell, member of the Royal College of Surgeons, whose volume on the teeth was printed in London and Philadelphia in 1832, was the first to describe and illustrate in detail the qualities of a specially designed dental chair. He noted the unnecessary discomfort for the patient due to sitting in an improper chair and recommended a specially tailored chair, admitting that its appearance might frighten the patient at first sight, but would provide a much less uncomfortable experience while having his/her teeth cared for. The chair he had used for years was constructed of a heavy wooden framework, with its feet firmly fastened to the floor, a broad seat and a back four feet in height. Snell's method of operating on the upper teeth required that the chair and patient be raised above his head.[35]

Attached to Snell's chair was a mirror and a stand to hold instruments, thus the basis for the dental chair and unit was laid, to be refined and improved over the next century and a half.[36] In other instances, a stand with hot and cold water was placed near the chair containing, in addition to instruments, several bottles of fluids such as creosote, oil of cloves and tincture of myrrh. The instruments used varied from the simple to the elegant and are reported to have included an ivory-handled corkscrew or dental key, gum lancet, elevator, tenaculum with cotton-wool and lint, excavators and pluggers with elegantly carved mother-of-pearl handles, scaling instruments and small books of gold leaves and tin foil to replace decayed tooth structure that had been removed from the teeth.[37]

Directing sufficient light into the mouth is one of the

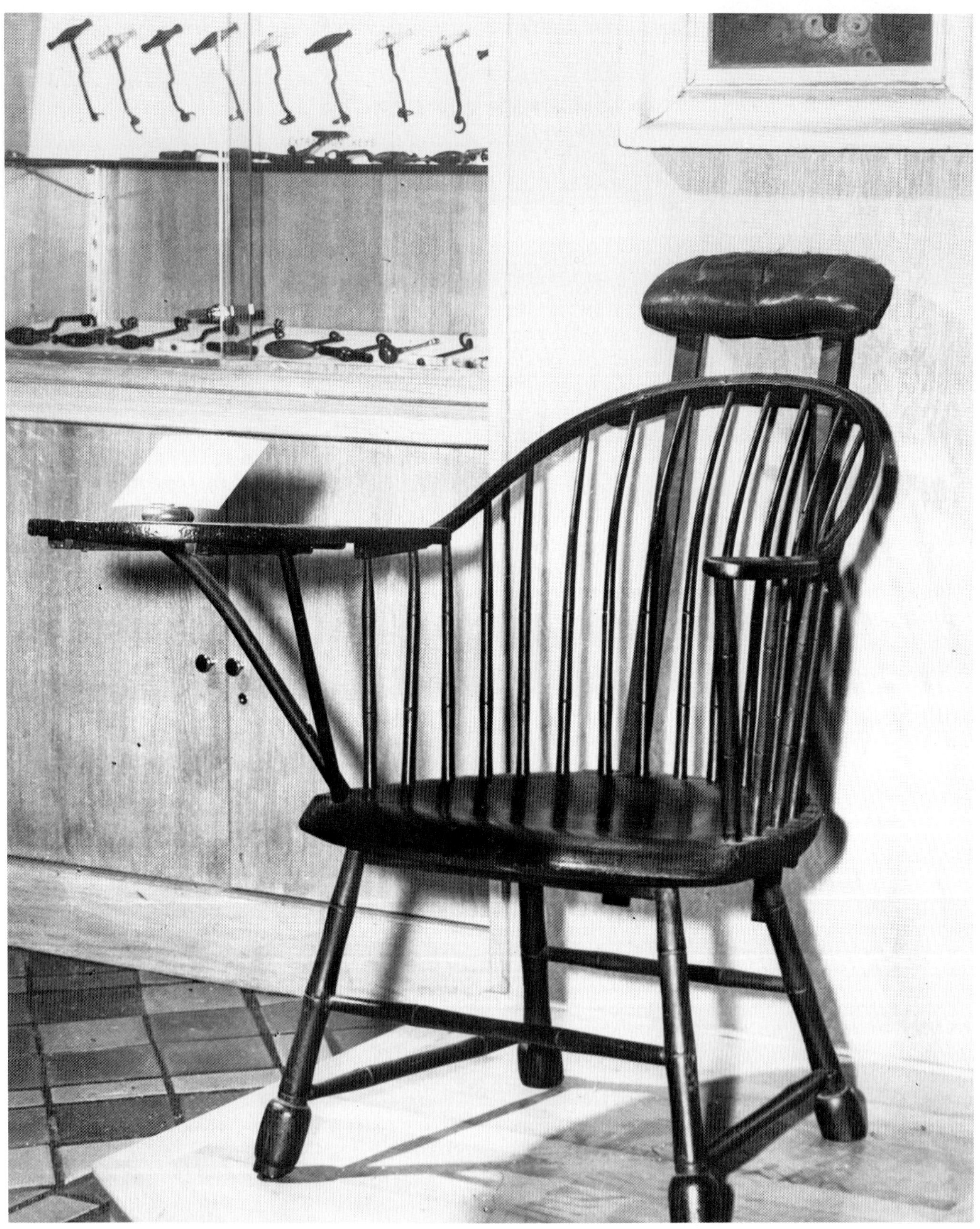

Josiah Flagg chair, earliest American dental chair from 1790-1812. Flagg converted a Windsor-type chair, by inserting an adjustable headrest made of horsehair and leather, and drawers for instruments were placed under the right armrest and under the seat. From Temple University School of Dentistry.

most important requirements in a dental office which, before the period of electricity and specially designed lamps, taxed the ingenuity of the dentist. An account of a British office in 1830[38] reveals that the most satisfactory light was obtained by placing the chair in front of a large window, a practice that would continue for another century. The type of daylight—whether soft or bright sun, shadow, etc., made a difference, so that offices were selected and arranged to face in the most advantageous direction for the region to take advantage of natural light. For those who used artificial light, Snell was the first to suggest that a lamp be attached to the dental chair so that the patient would not be burdened with holding a candle. He commented: ". . . for the patient to hold [the candle] in his left hand . . . is in all cases a clumsy expedient, and nothing can be conceived more awkward than to request a lady to perform such an office, especially when she is agitated by the anticipation of pain."[39]

Snell's design for a dental chair gradually led to other designs and their commercial production. The first American patent for a dental chair, which was never produced, was granted to M.W. Hanchett in 1848. Its seat could be raised and lowered like a piano stool. A similar chair, patented in 1855, was the unstable Perkins chair. The seat was supported on a ball and socket which could be moved into any position, but could also be tipped over with the patient in the chair.[40]

The evolution of chairs followed the establishment of dental offices. Before the Civil War permanent dental offices were uncommon in the U.S. One office reputed to have been in use in 1822 was on display in the museum of the Harvard Dental School in 1925.[41] The office had been used by John Randall, who practiced medicine and dentistry for 40 years in Boston, beginning in 1802, after he graduated from Harvard College. The office on exhibit measured 7 feet by 8 feet and contained a Windsor chair for the patient, but little else, that later, would become essential in the dental office.

An office, representative of the next generation of dentistry, when ether first was applied as an anesthetic (1840s), was described half a century later by Dr. J.L. Asay of San Jose, California. He recalled that it was common to remain silent about the furnishings and supplies of the dental office and laboratory. Guarding the laboratory or "work-shop" and instructing his apprentice not to discuss the methods and practices carried out by him, the dentist worked alone and without the support of professional colleagues. One room was divided into an office and laboratory. Without an artificial source of light, a rocking chair was placed on a platform in front of a window, so the dentist could move the patient by tilting the chair to get more light into the mouth. Nearby stood a wash basin, which served as a cuspidor, on a covered stool. On a table the instruments, towels and napkins were laid out. The instruments were described as a half-dozen crude forceps, an extracting key and four or five smooth-pointed pluggers. The excavators, chisels and drills were forged and tempered by the dentist or a local metal craftsman. Pearl- or ivory-handled instruments could be purchased in France or England, and from Chevalier of New York City after 1850. These items served as elegant display instruments in the American dentist's office, when not in use on the patient.[42]

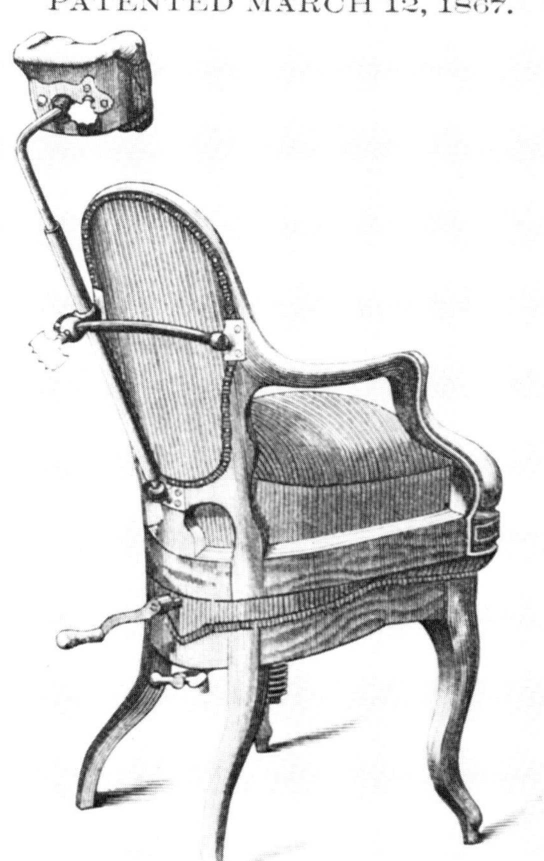

O.C. White's headrest attached to chair. It was patented on March 12, 1867. This drawing is from the 1876 catalog of S.S. White.

By midcentury there were notable exceptions to the simply equipped American dental office. Carl Ludwig Fleischman, a German, who toured the U.S. in 1850, observed and described many crafts, trades and occupations in a publication which appeared two years later in Stuttgart. Recently translated, this book provides a favorable view of dental practice before the Civil War and indicates that office practice was beginning to augment or replace the variable locales of itinerant dentistry. Fleischman was impressed with the best American dentist's equipment. He commented:

> If one visits one of the more respected dentists here, one finds reception rooms tastefully furnished, the surgery provided with elegant armchairs and other mechanical furniture in order to put the patient into the right position for an operation, and then beautiful cabinets with all kinds of instruments, so neat and shiny that one feels inclined to have the dentist use them in one's mouth.[44]

Fleischman further complimented dental practice in this period when he added that

> the dentist's main activity is the drilling and filling of bad teeth, insertions of artificial teeth or entire dentures, and similar services which maintain or replace teeth. It must be acknowledged that America is very far advanced in the field of dentistry. The dentists here have nothing in common with the tooth breakers of the Old World, who indeed tear out their patient's teeth with an old rusty hook.[44]

Some of Fleischman's comments may reflect the enthusiasm and tact of a foreign visitor, however his conclusion that the best American dentistry was superior to European dental practices is borne out by the prizes and medals which American dental inventors and manufacturers of dental equipment began to receive in national and international competitions and exhibitions beginning at this time. Even dentists, who had the least expectation for a good education, like the black dentist John S. Rock, were among those who received a silver medal in 1851 for making artificial teeth. These prize winning teeth were exhibited at the Franklin Institute in Philadelphia.[45]

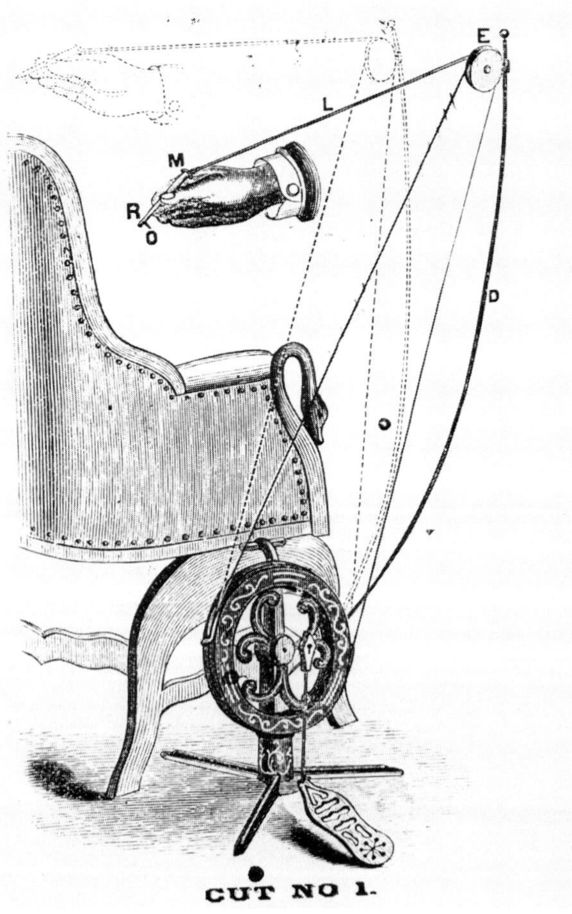

Dr. A.W. Todd's dental drill (1876) in position beside an Archer dental chair. The drill reached 500 rpm.

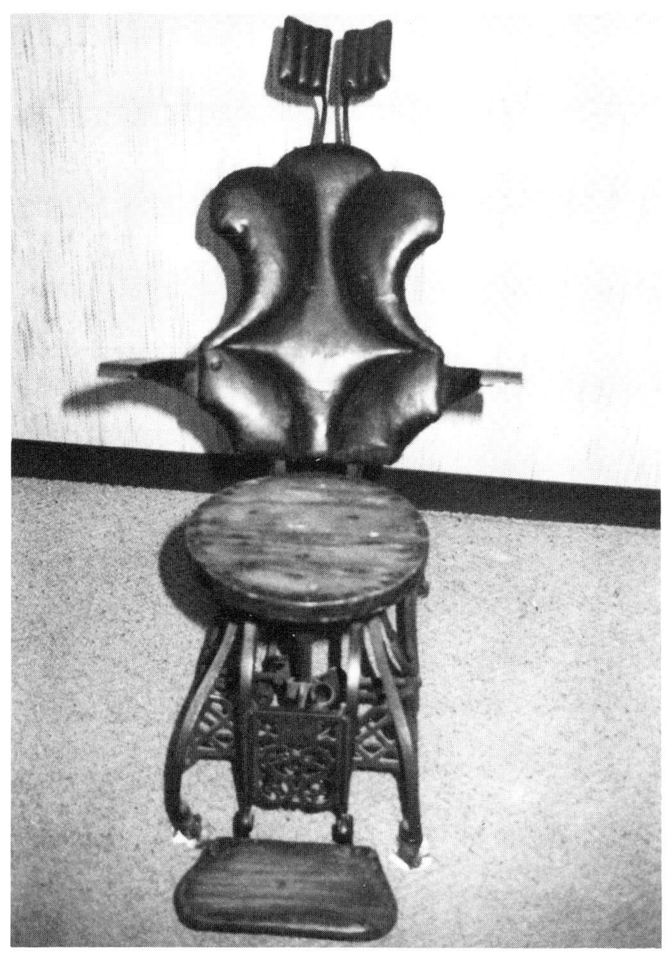

Interesting 19th century chair which was portable, containing a round wooden seat, leather back and headrest, and metal support.

Morrison chairs at the Chicago College of Dental Surgery Clinic, published in 1968 in the Loyola College of Dentistry alumni magazine, *The Bur*. The Chicago College merged with the Loyola University in the 1920s.

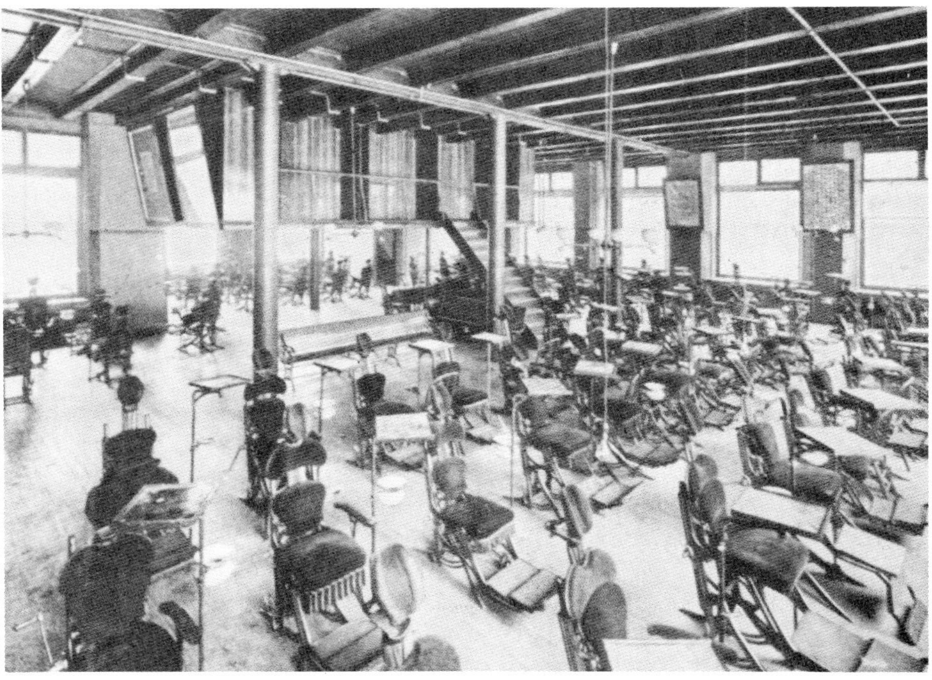

Ritter pump dental chair of 1919. From Ritter Dental Manufacturing Company, Rochester, New York.

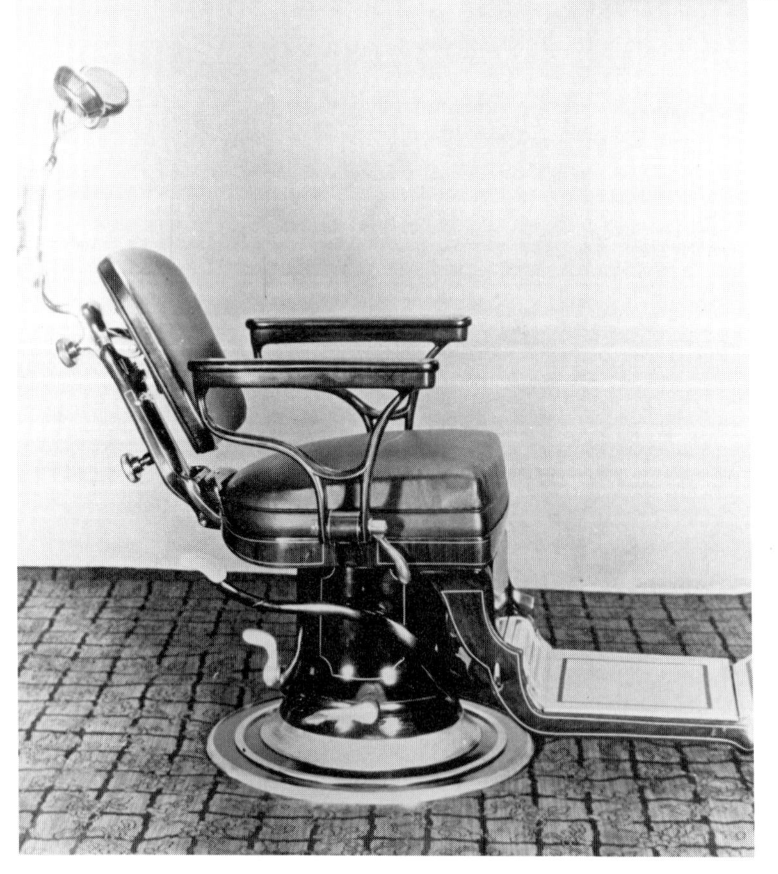

The Harvard dental chair in 1930. From Weber Dental Manufacturing Company, Canton, Ohio.

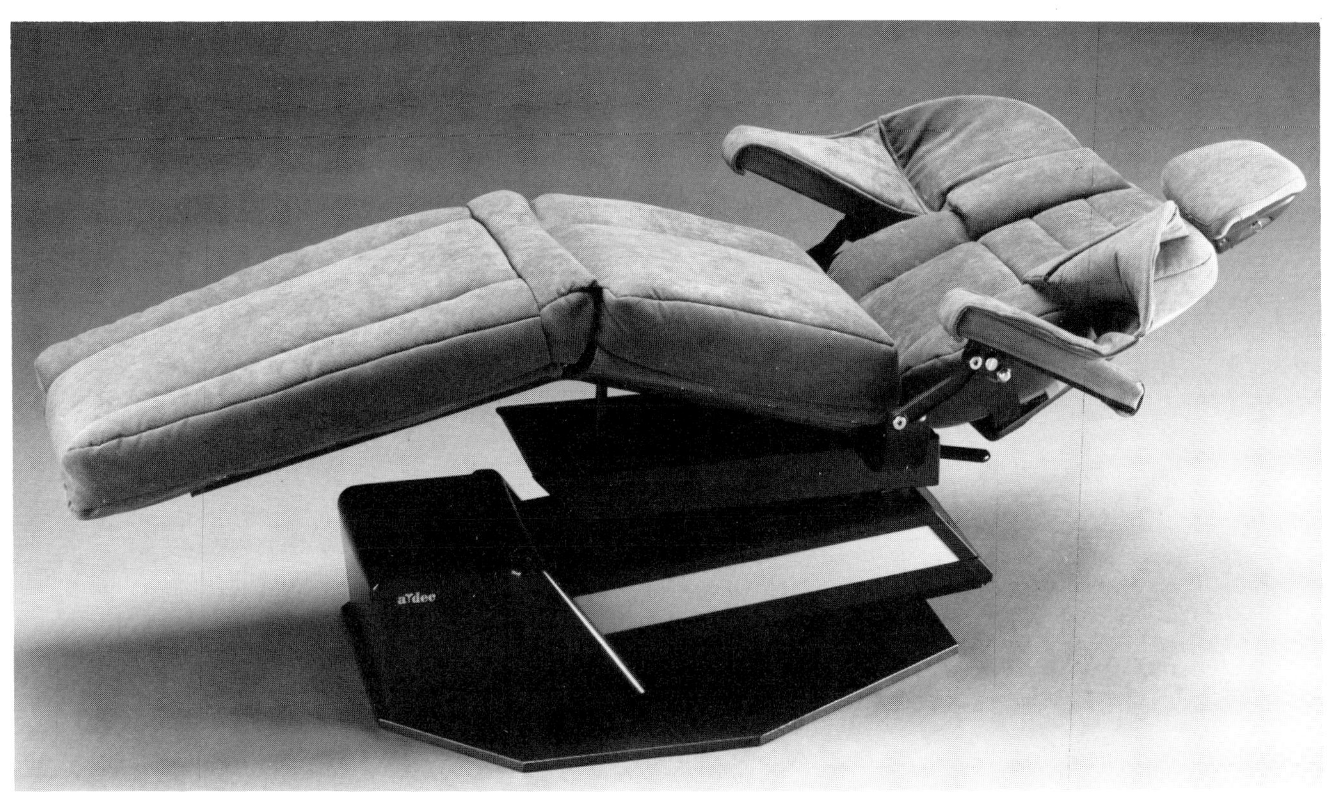

Priority Plus Chair of 1986 by ADEC of Newberg, Oregon.

Uni-Chair unit with cuspidor, 1975. From ADEC, Newberg, Oregon, the leading supplier of dental chairs at this time.

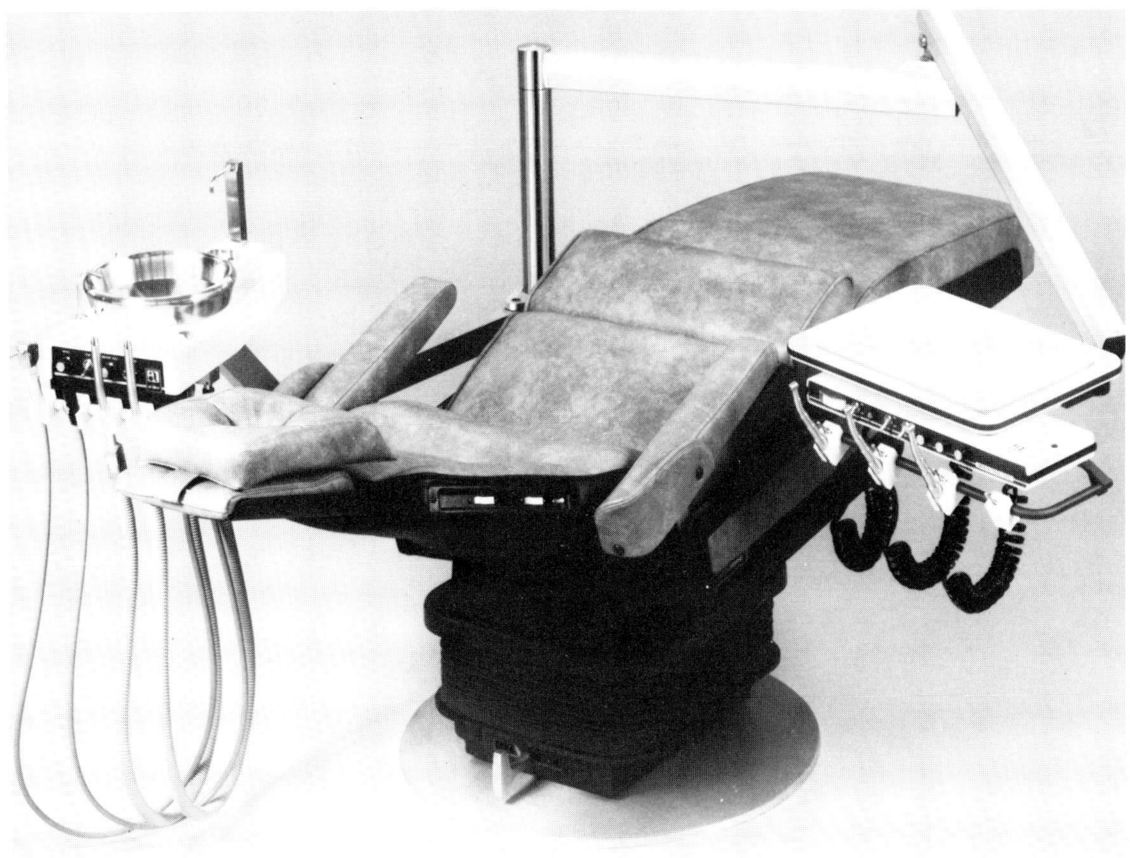

CASE FOR THE DENTAL ENGINE

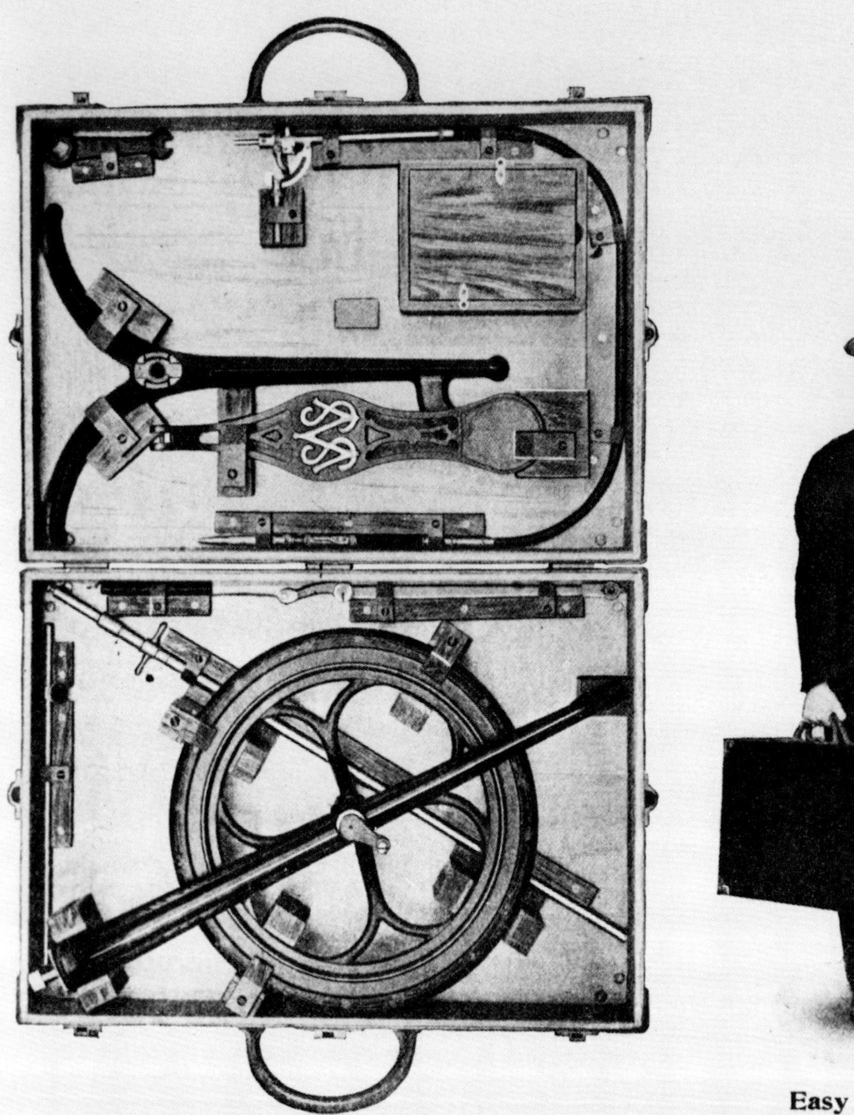

The Case Packed

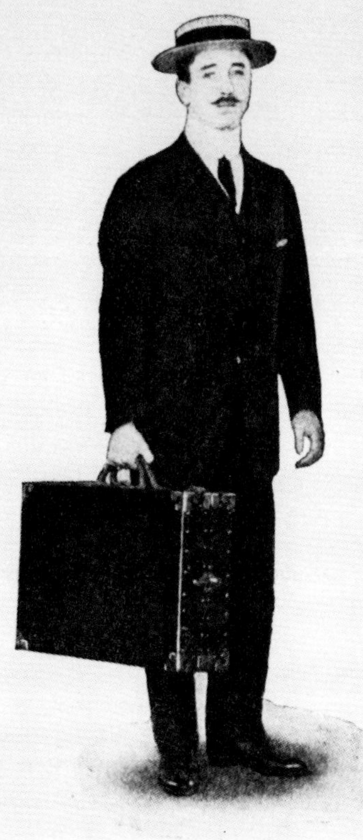

Easy to Carry

The transportation of his engine is a serious problem for the traveling dentist, more especially in mountainous regions, where practically all freight is carried by "packing" it on mules. The problem is solved by the portable case shown herewith, which was devised for and is largely used by the dental surgeons connected with the United States Army, whose duties require frequent and sometimes hurried removals from one station to another.

This case opens like a suit case, and the two sides are provided with blocks and stays fitted to take and hold securely the various parts of the S. S. White Cable or Belt Engine. A compartment in one side serves to hold equipment.

The case can be unpacked and the Engine set up, with ease, in five (5) minutes. Taking the engine apart and packing it requires no longer time.

Strongly made, Leatheroid covered, with double handles, lock and catch locks, and metal corners; will stand hard usage. Size over all, 22¼ x 15½ x 6½ inches. Weight of engine packed in case, exclusive of equipment, about 40 pounds.

In ordering indicate whether for Cable or Belt Engine.

Price, Case, for either Engine **$18.00**

S.S. White portable foot-pedal dental drill used by itinerant dentists and advertised in the 1915 catalog of the company.

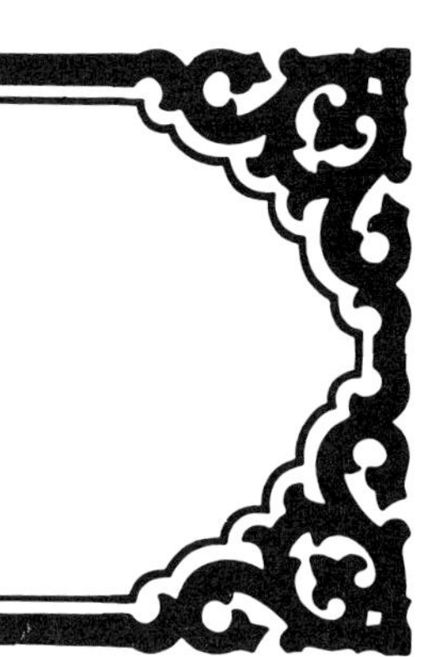

CHAPTER SIX

Greene Vardiman Black and Dental Innovation

An outstanding American dentist, whose career has been well documented by historians,[46] provides an example of how the talented and energetic dentist approached and improved his practice. Greene Vardiman Black (1836-1915), a leading reformer of American dentistry, began to practice in the period just before the Civil War. Black's dental education remained informal, but intensive throughout his life. Under his brother, Thomas' guidance, he studied medicine. In the course of his studies he met the dentist, J.C. Speer. After a few weeks of apprenticeship with him, Black went into dental practice in 1857 in a small office outfitted with a Flagg chair. Black also canvassed the area for patients by journeying to people who lived nearby. His first office in Winchester, Illinois, the place of his birth, closed when the Civil War erupted. Black and three of his brothers joined the Union Army. He was injured and discharged in 1862. His second office was set up a year later in conjunction with a partner, Dr. Cox, in nearby Jacksonville, Illinois. Cox left Jacksonville within a year. About a decade later Black built an addition to his home in a building near his first office and practiced until 1897 when he became dean of the Northwestern University Dental School.

He introduced equipment which resulted in fundamental changes in dental technology. Black, like other dentists of the period, was compelled to design a dental cabinet to store, and keep organized, the growing assortment of dental implements, in addition to an expanding selection of dentures and drugs. Individually conceived, and often, portable cabinets, preceded mass produced and more elaborate chests, which were finished in fine wood and decorative carvings used to make fine furniture. These cabinets contained numerous, and uniquely shaped spaces that offered access to suit the special uses of the dentist.

Another design of Black's made him the inventor of the foot engine, which was the first to have the shaft of the hand-piece directly driven by the cord from the driving wheel. These engines, which freed the dentist's hands from running the hand-piece, were manufactured on the third floor of Black's office building. Although the hands were not required to power the engine, one foot had to continuously pump the foot pedal to keep the hand-piece in motion, a function that soon tired the dentist, who was forced to stand on the other foot.

An active member of the St. Louis Dental Society, until he moved to Chicago in 1891, Black introduced his foot engine to his colleagues in that city. W. DeCrow, a member of the Illinois State Dental Association since 1869, claimed in 1896 to have bought the first engine sold by Black after it was exhibited before dental society meetings in St. Louis in 1872, 1873 and 1874.[47]

Missouri dentists were keen inventors in this period, which may have attracted Black to their meetings. Another famous inventor of dental equipment living in St. Louis at the time was James B. Morrison. He learned fine craftsmanship as a boy in Springfield, Illinois and produced precision gold dentures in dental school which won first prize in 1852. He patented the first popular American dental chair on September 29, 1868, which remained in demand even after it was superseded by the hydraulic chair. By an unobtrusive lever device, the chair was adjustable in all directions.[48] Improvements in the dental office at this time, especially the chair, drew praise from America's leading medical spokesman, Oliver Wendell Holmes. He praised the new dental chair in 1872 when he addressed the Harvard Dental School. Of the newly invented Morrison adjustable chair he said "one of those magic chairs, which fill alike the giant and the dwarf, which would accommodate the visitors of Procrustes and suit itself to all the transformations of Proteus."[49]

The Morrison chair was the first dental chair to permit the dentist to change the height of the chair and the patient in it by means of a crank, and therefore, permit the dentist to choose between standing or sitting while operating on a patient.[50] Vertical movement of the chair not only permitted a wider latitude in reaching and seeing into the patient's mouth, but permitted the dentist to "talk down" to the patient, thereby enforcing a psychological advantage in the dentist-patient relationship.[51] Use of the dental chair to subjugate and intimidate the patient served to strengthen the image and power of the dentist before he could rely on his status as a professional with unusual skills to win the goodwill and respect of the patient.

Black may not have concurred with Holmes' assessment of the Morrison chair since he purchased a chair made by R.W. Archer of Rochester, New York. Archer produced several chairs resembling barber chairs in the 1860s and 70s, of which the most spectacular was No. 2, that was "made with flaring arms, [each decorated with a] carved imitation of a swan's neck and head, [and a] seat wide enough for the convenience of any patient."[52] This chair was constructed of black walnut and upholstered in green or crimson plush and trimmed with porcelain, gilt- or silver-headed nails. Until the age of sterility, these handsome chairs were the norm in a well-equipped dental office and have since become prize collector's pieces.

Black's talents resulted in other inventions. He built his own operating tray, work bench and stool, and to facilitate his multitudinous research projects, he designed a number of specialized tools. These included a manudynamometer for testing finger pressure, a tupfodynamometer for measuring the force of mallet blows to put in a gold filling, a phagodynamometer for measuring the force required to chew various foods, and a gnathodynamometer for measuring the strength of the bite. Black discovered the usefulness of the microscope after a German physician immigrated to his town. To improve his microscopical skills and study the latest discoveries in cell pathology he learned to read German.[53]

The foot engine, Archer chair, two brass microscopes and a cabinet from Dr. Black's office, which he used in 1885, have been on display in the Smithsonian Institution since 1955, and in the National Museum of American History since 1964. Originally his office was displayed at Northwestern University in a setting which more accurately resembled his last office in Jacksonville.

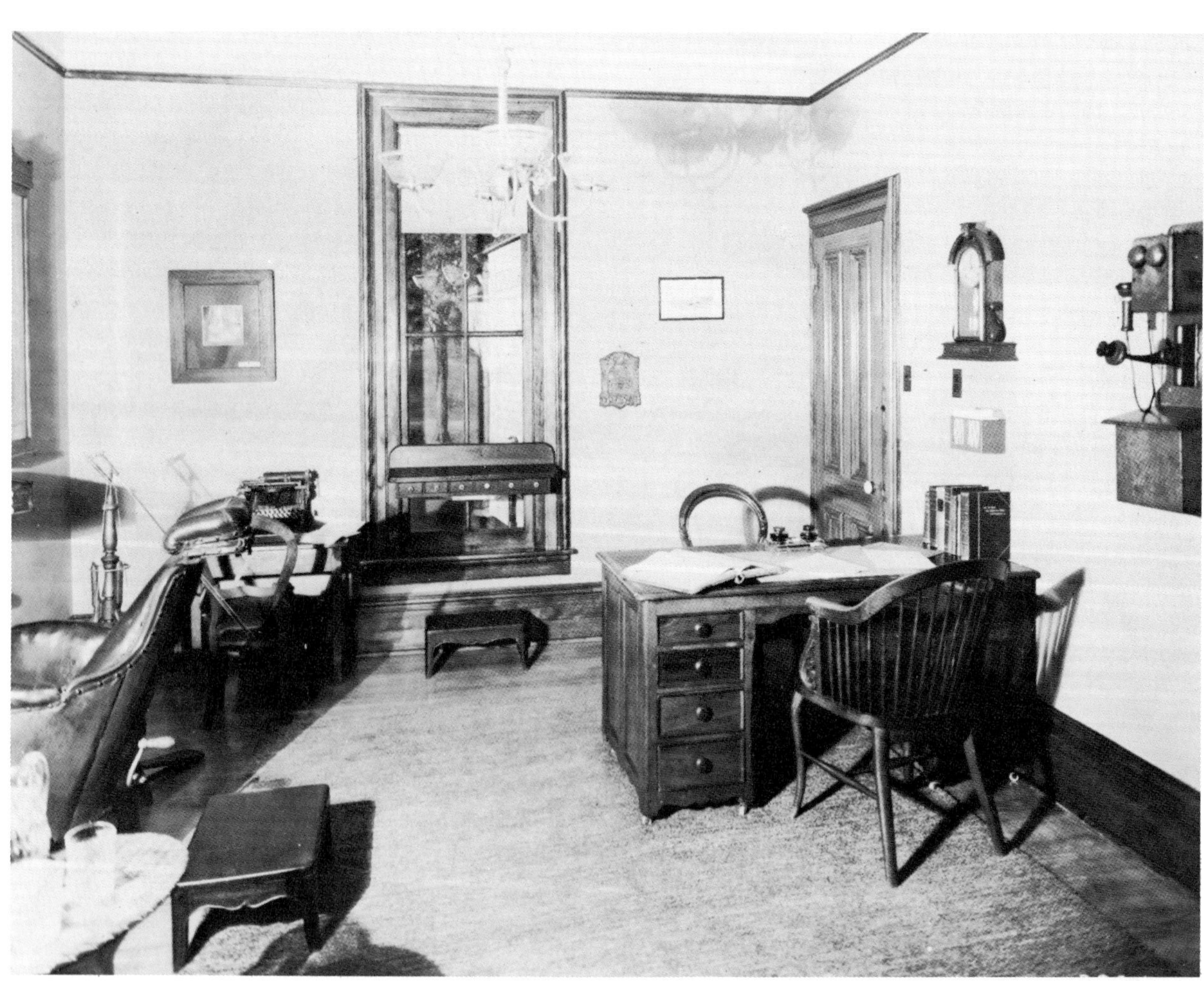

Reconstructed dental office of Greene Vardiman Black on display at the Northwestern University Dental School until 1955. The room is an exact replica. The doors and part of the wood trim were removed from Black's Jacksonville, Illinois office for this display. The views from the windows are reproduced on canvas. Black opened an office in Jacksonville in 1864 where he practiced until 1897. This operating room was used by Black from 1875 until 1897. His laboratory was next door. The typewriter was one of the first models of the "Caligraph." All of the furniture was made of walnut wood. From Northwestern University Dental School.

CHAPTER SEVEN

The Shaping of the Commercially Supplied Dental Office

In the ensuing decades dentistry changed from a largely tooth removing to a tooth preserving and beautifying practice. In the pursuit of methods to remove decay, save teeth and heal diseased gums, dental equipment and techniques exploded and the dental office grew into a suite of rooms to accommodate all this equipment and furniture, as well as, the dentist and his assistants. The shape and extent of the office responded to the special technical needs of the dentist and the aesthetic requirements of dentist and patient.

Over the past century and a quarter the American dentist's office environment evolved within the context of room designs familiar to middle- and upper-class society. The dentist's office expanded to include separate rooms for patients to wait, pay their bills and receive special instruction in tooth care. The materials and structures used in the home were installed in the waiting room and rest room that was separated from the dental operatory, where the patient was treated. Making the waiting room comfortable provided a visual and psychological balance to the increasingly mechanized and instrument-filled operatory. Primarily shaped by instruments, techniques and the controlled environment required to carry out dental procedures, the multi-room office and its laboratory developed out of the ideas and expectations of the dentist, patient and dental equipment manufacturer. Offices, like homes and work places, often reflected the individual preferences and idiosyncrasies of their proprietors. Since the end of the 19th century dental offices have been arranged "to minimize labor, save time for the busy dentist and his patients and diminish their discomforts."[54]

During the period when the office was becoming the focus for the dentist, his role as a medical professional was changing from that of an itinerant tinkerer or handy craftsman with a few skills, who traveled from town to town with his tools, to a technician with scientific training, medical sophistication and sensitivity to the patient. The new approach to dentistry required a variety of apparatus installed in a permanent location, consisting of at least one room divided by screens and partition walls, and preferably, extending to a suite of rooms.

The dental exhibit of the 1876 Centennial Exhibition in Philadelphia displayed a sample of the equipment the American dentist could purchase to set up one of the earliest offices outfitted with mass produced furniture and equipment. The S.S. White Company of Philadelphia put up the largest and most complete display of dental equipment, furniture and supplies, including the latest S.S. White chair and a foot engine, powered by water or by electricity for those dentists who installed batteries to power their instruments. Another manufacturer with a full assortment of dental office equipment on exhibit at the centennial was Codman and Shurtleff of Boston, which also manufactured surgical instruments and continues to provide instruments to medical and dental professionals. In 1876 Codman and Shurtleff displayed highly polished forceps, excavators and pluggers, newly designed floss silk holders, and gold foil carriers, mouth mirrors, ether, chloroform and nitrous oxide inhalers, chairs, brackets, spittoons and a compact operating case. Over a dozen other American manufacturers displayed a variety of patented appliances and specialized tools, so that any dentist who visited the exhibition or read a description of its contents could have selected all the items needed to set up a well-equipped and up-to-date dental office. Only two women, Mrs. Dr. F.C. Treadwell of Philadelphia and Dr. Anne D. Ramberger who exhibited examples of their gold fillings and gold plate-work were among the many dentists represented at the first major American technology celebration.[55]

Late in the 19th century, cleanliness, and then, in the 20th century, sterility, became the earmarks of a first class dental office. Achieving a clean office prepared the way for extending the process to include sterilization of instruments, hands and all auxiliary apparatus and medicaments applied to the patient. In setting up a clean office the dentist removed or covered up those things which offended his patients. He learned the sights, smells, tastes and attitudes his patients rejected and "the tranquilizing effect of the beautiful and the refined." Some dentists became oblivious to conditions in the office which they had learned to live with, in the course of their intense concentration on the mouth and teeth. Foul odors emanating from the spittoon, waste system, bloodstained instruments and clothes were contaminants in even some of the best dental offices. An observer's description of how one patient was treated after an extraction in 1887 tells us what patients endured. He wrote:

> In a large city we saw a first class dentist go through a very bloody operation, when there was no spittoon attached to the chair. The dentist said, 'The spittoon is a very dirty thing, and therefore I never have one about.' This lady patient was given a little old, dirty-looking tin-cup to spit in. When he was through, her lap was bespattered all over with blood, and the cup was a disgusting sight. The dentist's hands were covered as though he had been butchering. He had been thoughtful enough to wipe them now and then on a cloth that became more and more bloody; but when through he did not seem to see any necessity of immediately cleaning himself, or of seeing that his patient was cared for. He must first go through a learned expatiation on what he had done, and convince his patient and us that he had shown remarkable skill, and ended her long suffering *without much inconvenience*. And there she still sat besmeared from head to foot, holding the disgusting cup![56]

Emptying the spittoon regularly was a habit many dentists learned after repeated instruction in dental journals, texts and popular magazines. D.W. Barber of Brooklyn urged in 1893 that

> The spittoon should be emptied and washed as soon as the patient leaves the chair. If an odor exists it may be removed by filling the vessel with pulverized charcoal and allowing it to stand over night; a small quantity of copperas or washing soda put in the vessel each day is a good disinfectant. A porcelain spittoon is better than metal, being much easier cleaned.[57]

To avoid the bloodstained equipment and soiled clothes experienced patients scheduled their appointments in the morning when clean water and washed instruments were more likely to be available.

Female patients commented on other changes they expected in the dental office to make their visits more comfortable. Some of these suggestions were published in 1886 in a note entitled "A lady's suggestions to dentists." Women noted the uncomfortable quietness of dental offices and a lack of books and papers in the waiting room, as well as novelties upon which to cast their eyes in the operating room. While in the dental chair the lady patient wanted "something pretty to look at, to keep from thinking how slow the dentist is, also how that clamp hurts."[58]

After the need to sterilize was accepted, dental and surgical instruments were made completely of metal, so that they could be boiled in water and subjected to sterilizing chemicals which disfigured wood, bone, shell and ivory. Furniture in the operating room was designed to provide fewer surfaces for germs to infiltrate and made of materials suitable for repeated cleaning. Metal chairs and wooden and metal cabinets with shelves, as well as, inserts for instruments, which could be washed with chemical solutions, became commonplace. Strong chemicals such as phenol used on patients, while kept in tightly sealed bottles when not in use, remained open while the dentist finished his work on the patient, subsequently the dental office became permeated with characteristic offensive medicinal odors.[59]

Foremost among all conditions desired in the dental office was the availability of sufficient light without glare in all seasons. Dentists continued to place the dental chair and cabinet in a position to receive the best natural light even after artificial lamps were available. Offices were placed in bay windows, built out over areaways or covered with a ceiling of glass to let in sunlight. Until electricity became available in the late 19th century, coal, gas and kerosene lamps were employed with varying results to light the dental office and added their own unpleasant odors.

Specially designed lamps provided light directed into the mouth, but it took a series of designs to provide a convenient lamp for both the patient and the dentist. Thomas L. Gilmer (1849-1931) of Chicago, a meticulous dentist who practiced for over 50 years, in 1893, placed a small, pea-sized lamp of half a candlepower in the patient's mouth. To keep it from overheating and annoying the patient he turned it off periodically. With its use he discovered cavities he had not suspected and could determine whether a pulp was dead or alive. With a five candlepower lamp he could diagnose pathological conditions in the antrum sinus over the upper molars.[60] This technique when carried out with an improved lamp in the early 20th century provided the basis for dental diagnosis and treatment of diseases affecting the whole body.

CHAPTER EIGHT

Who Practiced Dentistry in the Office

At this juncture the reader is well-served by being informed of the educational background which dentists brought to their practices. Professionally trained American dentists began to appear after the first preceptorial dental school was organized in Bainbridge, Ohio in 1827 and the first dental college in the world was established in Baltimore, Maryland in 1840. The four pioneering physicians who opened the Ohio school and taught courses were the physicians and dentists Chapin Harris, Horace Hayden, Thomas E. Bond and H. Willis Baxley. The first class enrolled five students who attended for two years, repeating the same courses in the second year. The dental degree was granted after passing the courses which convened for four months each year. The remainder of the year was spent in a dental office developing skills. Small classes graduated for many years. American dentists, most of whom were not graduates of any dental school, but had been trained by dentists who acted as preceptors to them were fairly numerous by 1845 when there were from one to 20 dentists in every town with a population of from 2,000 to 5,000 inhabitants.[61] Between 1850 and 1890 dental school graduates doubled in every decade and in the next decade the number tripled so that in the 1880s, there were 5,781 graduate dentists and in the 1890s 14,878 graduate dentists in the U.S.[62] William Gies reported that at the turn of the century of the 28,142 dentists who began practice in 1840 or later, 11,311 were not graduates of a dental school.[63] Five thousand dentists graduated from 50 schools in this year. By 1900 the number of dentists in the U.S. rose to 29,665. These dentists, of whom 60 percent were dental school graduates, served a population of 70 million people for a ratio of 39 dentists per 100,000 inhabitants, which, compared to other nations, was among the highest per capita.

For comparison, in the same period, 5,000 dentists in Britain treated a total population of 40 million. Beginning in 1878, through an Act of Parliament, British dentists were required to attend a dental school before practicing. However all those in practice, regardless of their training at the time of the Act, were permitted to continue their practices. These untutored dentists could not apply the term dentist or dental practitioner to themselves, but they did use the terms dental specialist, dental consultant and dental expert which impressed the layman enough to bring these "specialists" many patients.[64] Therefore, even at the end of the century a number of unqualified dentists treated patients in the British Isles as they did in the U.S., primarily by extracting teeth, rather than conserving them through the various methods in vogue.

Untutored dentists convincingly advertised their skills and ability to treat dental diseases. Furthermore, lacking a sufficient number of trained dentists the services of the uneducated were in demand. Their methods and the offices of the less skillful were mistaken for those of the professional dentist, thus contributing to the mixed heritage of dentistry and certainly confusing the patient, who only rarely sought the services of a dentist. The problems created by the ineffective and unscrupulous "dentist" play a major role in popular versions of dental history, which has provided substance for the stereotypical dentist represented in cartoons, jokes and movies, which will be the topic of a later section in this essay. The dentist's exploits form his image with the result that the common caricature of a dentist is a buffoon who inflicts pain and is generally feared. These, by and large, are not the dentists who practiced in the offices discussed here. But then, patient perception has also contributed to the dentist's reputation, so that only when dentists are discussed within their total communities are their practices better understood.

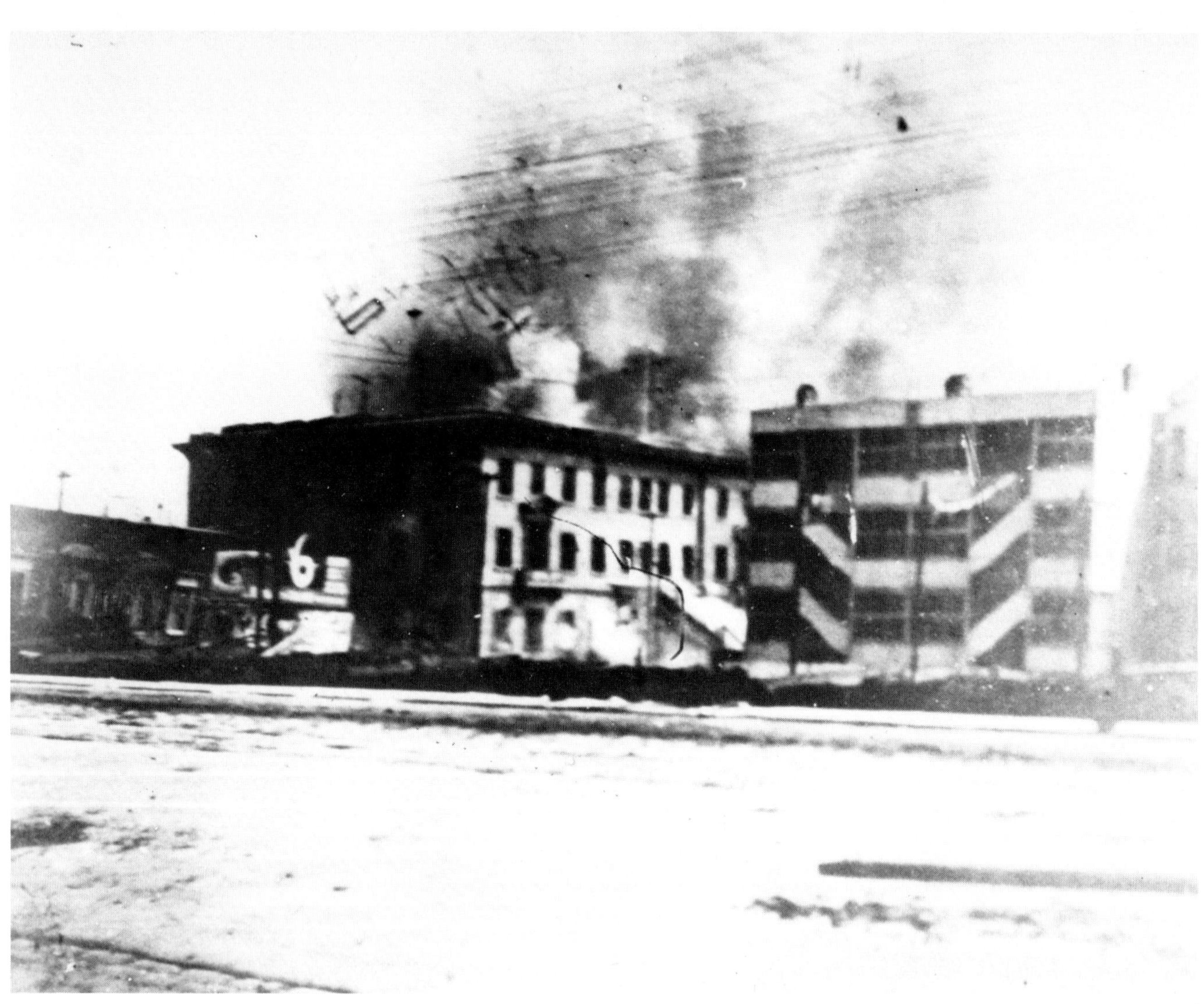

The college of Physicians and Surgeons on 14th Street, forerunner of the School of Dentistry, University of the Pacific, is shown shortly after the earthquake in 1906 when devastating fires swept through the city of San Francisco. The building was subsequently reconstructed of wood and later the school moved to a new building at the Presbyterian Medical Center. From the A.W. Ward Museum, School of Dentistry, University of the Pacific.

CHAPTER NINE

Dental Education in America

The first method of teaching students the practice of dentistry was the preceptorial system which consisted of a practicing dentist who, for a fee varying between several hundred dollars and $1,000, for periods extending from a few months to a year or more, signed up a student who showed promise of becoming a dentist.[65] There were few books and the length of study depended on the knowledge of the preceptor and the appetite of the student for information and knowledge of his future profession. Introduced into America from Europe in the 18th century, the system continued well into the 19th century, even after dental schools were founded. The preceptorial system was criticized by those who believed that theory, in addition to practice, was important in educating the dentist. Similar discussions cropped up in the education of physicians. A major incentive for retaining the preceptorship system was the income which the dentist-tutor earned in an age when patients were irregular and unpredictable.

The training which the apprentice received could be very thorough as Dr. Joshua Tucker, a preceptor, explained in 1840:

> When they entered our [Boston] office to lay a good foundation for a future thorough knowledge of dentistry, they were first introduced into the laboratory, handed the blow-pipe, hammer, and file, and were taught to copy, fashion, make and temper their own instruments. This was to improve their mechanical skill, and educate the hand equally with the head. They were also taught to carve and manufacture mineral teeth, and the rules and art of modeling, so as to give a natural expression to the face. Lastly, they were taught to use the instruments they had made to manipulate and pack gold foil against the walls of the dental cavity so as to completely stop exudation from within, and ingress from without, and then to restore carious teeth to health. We insisted upon their studying at the same time the science of medicine generally.[66]

Dentists lacking a formal education in a dental college sometimes defended their careers. Occasionally preceptor educated dentists, such as H.A. Hibbard of Connecticut, justified their professional contributions and asked for acceptance by their younger colleagues who profited from a formal theoretical preparation. Regarded as an "old wheel horse" by the Connecticut Valley Dental Society, in 1890, Hibbard described his practice at a time when "it was a severe task for most of us to do halfway justice to the patient, and I am quite sure many of mine didn't even get that."[67] One memory remained of the time Hibbard put a gold filling into his younger brother's tooth when he did not have a rubber-dam, engine, annealed gold and other items, invented since then. He had to do his own laboratory work including grinding teeth and "blowing out his lungs" before attaching them to a metal plate. Hibbard claimed his trials as a dentist without the advantages of formal schooling and recent inventions and techniques, required more patience than Job. Consequently, he believed that he had learned a good deal and spoke for "a large majority of dentists in the U.S." when he requested that "the same privileges be given to those who have been in the traces since 1860, that are granted to many who possess a diploma, and feel obliged to call on us for advice."[68]

The first American dental school evolved out of the preceptor system and therefore is a preceptor dental school. John Harris, a physician in Bainbridge, Ohio, a town along the major route to Cincinnati and the west advertised in the local newspaper for students on November 1, 1827 under the heading "Medical Instruction." He offered to prepare students to enter a medical college. The students he attracted were interested in dentistry. Having acquired new supplies of medical and dental instruments in the spring of 1828 he taught a group of nine men. Until 1830 he taught in the living room/office of his school, using candlelight to supplement natural light. He used a rocking chair for patients and alcohol as an anesthetic. Among his resources were an Indian skull and text books imported from England. All of his students became outstanding dentists and his brother, Chapin Harris, became a co-founder of the first dental college in the world. Another student, James Taylor founded the world's second dental college in Ohio, a few years later.[69]

American dentists, many of whom were physicians,

The Baltimore College of Dental Surgery

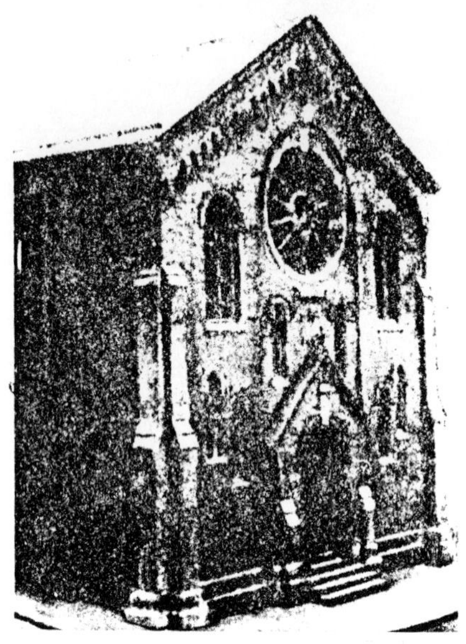

Picture of the Baptist Church in which the first lectures were given at the Baltimore College of Dental Surgery.

Baltimore College of Dental Surgery.

THE INTRODUCTORY LECTURES in this Institution will be delivered in the Baptist Church in Calvert, between Lexington and Saratoga streets—commencing TUESDAY, November 3d, at 7¼ o'clock in the evening, to which, the Board of Visitors, the Reverend Clergy, the Medical Faculty and public generally are invited to attend. The following is the order in which they will be delivered.

TUESDAY,	Professor	H. H. HAYDEN.
WEDNESDAY,	"	THOS. E. BOND, Jr.
THURSDAY,	"	CHAPIN A. HARRIS.
SATURDAY,	"	H. WILLIS BAXLEY.

n3-tf CHAPMAN A. HARRIS, Dean.

Announcement of introductory lectures, Baltimore College of Dental Surgery, November, 1840

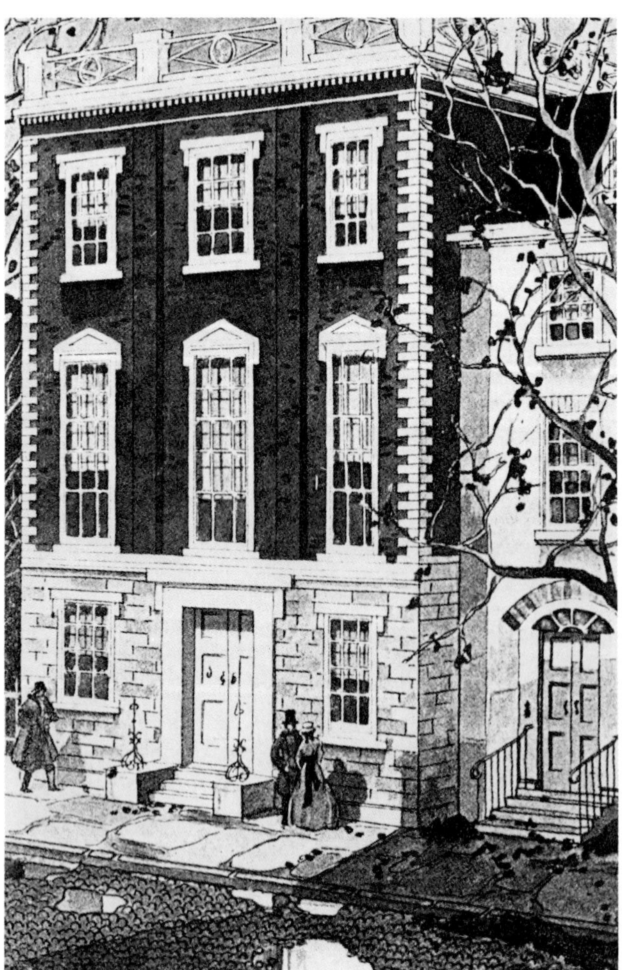

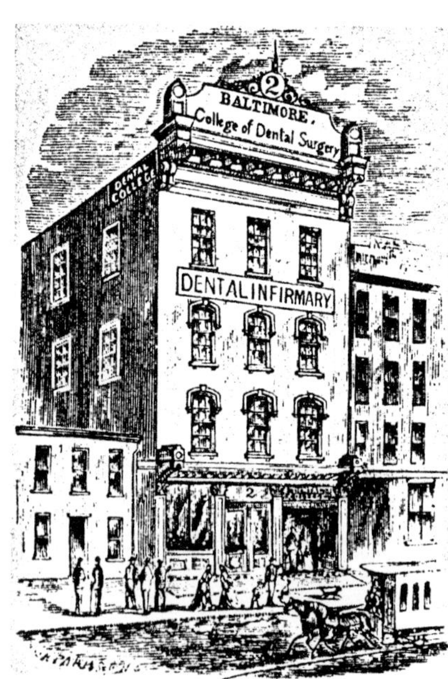

Etching of the Baltimore College of Dental Surgery building, 1872-1875

Drawing of Baltimore College of Dental Surgery. The first class of five students was given introductory lectures in a local church by Drs. Horace Hayden and John Harris' brother, Chapin Harris, who organized this school, as well as by Drs. Thomas E. Bond and Jay Willis Baxley. According to Dr. Baxley, when the new building was available lectures were delivered in a small room and practical anatomy was taught in a secluded stable.

opposed the establishment of dental colleges, and not without good reason, for they knew that practical experience was crucial to the effective treatment of dental diseases and the reconstruction of teeth. Under a preceptor, the novice had an opportunity to participate in patient care from the beginning and to observe an experienced dentist at work everyday. However, in 1840 the blueprint was drawn for future American dental education through special schools. With the founding of the first dental school, the Baltimore College of Dental Surgery, the separation of the dental school from a medical school became a reality. Forced by the refusal of the University of Maryland medical school to accept a dental school as part of its program, the Baltimore College of Dental Surgery course of study did not correspond with a medical curriculum. The rift was enlarged when the American Medical Association, founded in 1848, refused to admit delegates from dental colleges to its meetings. Although dental leaders were displeased with the separation of dentistry from medicine, the die was cast in the pattern of American dental education for several decades and only partially redressed when the first university affiliated dental school was founded in 1867 at Harvard University.[70]

In 1845 in Cincinnati, Ohio, James Taylor, a colleague of Chapin Harris, founded the second dental college, the Ohio College of Dental Surgery. The charter of the college stated that "no branches of medical science shall be taught except those necessary to dental surgery." The courses taught included dental anatomy, physiology, pathology, therapeutics and practical dentistry. The Ohio College gave credit towards graduation to those who had studied with a preceptor before attending the college. The preceptorial system was undermined gradually by resolutions such as one taken by the Massachusetts Dental Society in 1860, which stipulated that dentists could only take on an apprentice if they agreed to teach him for at least two years, and only if the student agreed to complete his education by graduating from a dental college.

The Ohio College of Dental Surgery, unlike the Baltimore College, operated out of a building specifically erected for the dental school. The building contained a general lecture room with elevated seats that accommodated 100 students. Other rooms were equipped to teach anatomy, chemistry, mechanical and operative dentistry. In the period before central heating, a stove in the center of the room provided the heat for the students who worked at chairs lined up facing large windows for maximum light.

Students in another dental school, the Michigan School of Dentistry, complained about the extremes of heat, which depended on their distance from the stove. Russell W. Bunting, dean from 1937 to 1950, described the room as it appeared after 1875 when the school opened and the subsequent ingenious solution to the problem. He explained:

> The class rooms and clinic were heated by central wood stoves which in the extreme winter weather consistently baked those in their immediate neighborhood and allowed those in the outlying portions of the room to suffer with the cold. It was here that we see the inventive ability of that fine old character who is closely associated with the Dental College by every student and alumnus, that of Henry Purfield, the janitor, dispenser, accountant and spiritual advisor, since the beginning of the Dental College even to the present day. Mr. Purfield invented one of the first hot air furnaces by making a circular metal shield to extend about each stove, which was raised a few inches off the floor and extended up to the level of the top of the stove. This gave protection to those nearby and created a draft of circulating air which passed under the bottom of the shield, over the heated stove, and out of the top to circulate to the farthest corners of the room. This very materially aided in the protection of those nearby and in the warming of the more remote portions of the room.[71]

Purfield was the janitor when the school opened and remained on the staff for 69 years.

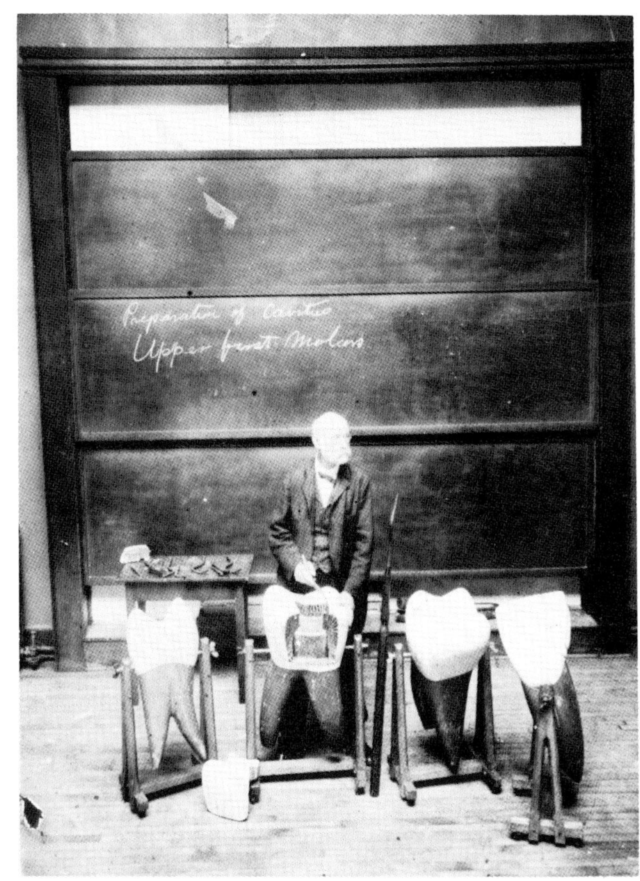

G.V. Black demonstrating his tooth models to a class at the Northwestern University Dental School. Note section of tooth on the floor in front of the model he is pointing to. From Northwestern University Dental School.

Harvard Dental School, (founded in 1867, oldest university affiliated dental school in the U.S.), first department of Mechanical Dentistry, second floor, Cambridge Street, Boston. President Charles Eliot of Harvard University claimed in 1878 that "No form of professional education is so little endowed in this country as dental education."

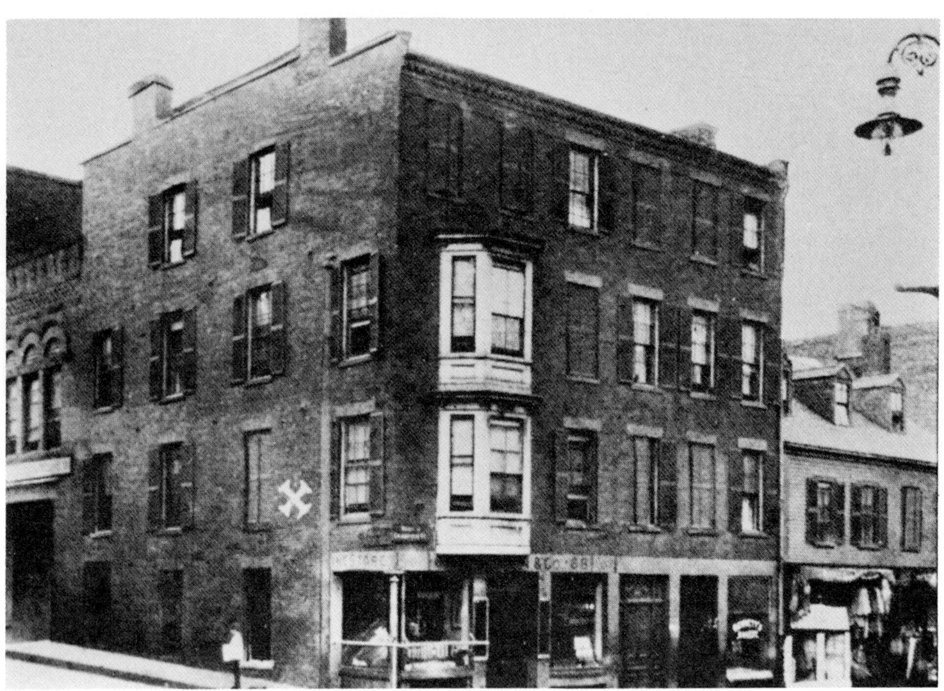

HARVARD UNIVERSITY.

DENTAL SCHOOL.

Admit A. S. Hill

To the Course of Lectures

For the year 1874.

Thos B Hitchcock Dean.

Boston, Feb 14 1874

Harvard Dental School.

DAILY ORDER OF EXERCISES, SPRING TERM, 1874.

Hour.	Monday.	Tuesday.	Wednesday	Thursday.	Friday.	Saturday.
9	Dent. Lab.	Dent. Lab.	Dent. Lab.	Dent. Lab.	Chem. R.	
10	Chem. L.		Phys. R.			Phys. R.
11	Phys. L.	Surg. L	M. G. H. Operations.		Phys. L.	M. G. H. Operations.
12	Surg. L.			Surg. R.		
1	Anat. L. till May.	Anat. L or R till May.		Anat. L. till May.	Anat. R. till May.	
2	Infirmary.	Infirmary.	Infirmary.	Infirmary.	Infirmary.	

Practical Anatomy in the Dissecting-Room daily till May. Chemistry taught daily in Chemical Laboratory. The Demonstrator is present in the Dental Laboratory every forenoon, and in the Infirmary every afternoon.

By 1854, in a larger building, the Ohio College of Dental Surgery became a center for the training of dentists in the Midwest. After dental colleges began to be linked to state supported universities, the private dental college no longer had sufficient resources to compete for students. The *coup de grace* came with the report of William Gies on the state of American Dental Colleges in 1926, a counterpart to the Flexner Report on Medical Schools. The Ohio College closed in 1926. In the first six years of its existence more than half the graduates of this college had practiced from four to 20 years before they entered dental school. State licensing laws became a factor in sending dentists back to school, as well as the fact that systematic instruction developed a reputation for improving the skills of the dentist.

The first three university affiliated dental schools were Harvard University, which opened in 1867, the University of Michigan, (1875) and the University of Pennsylvania, (1878). In the 80s and 90s some students received both medical and dental degrees, however, when the medical and dental curricula enlarged it became difficult to study for both degrees.[72] The separation of the dental school from the medical school had a major impact on the American dentist's knowledge. Dentists became unusually proficient in mechanical processes and manipulation of instruments and techniques and demonstrated superior skills to those of dentists in any other country. Contributions to the dental literature by American dentists between 1850-1875 emphasized mechanical techniques and advances. Manual dexterity was a characteristic of the most prominent dentists.[73] Between 1875 and 1890 the building of tooth crowns and installation of bridges of artificial teeth developed markedly.

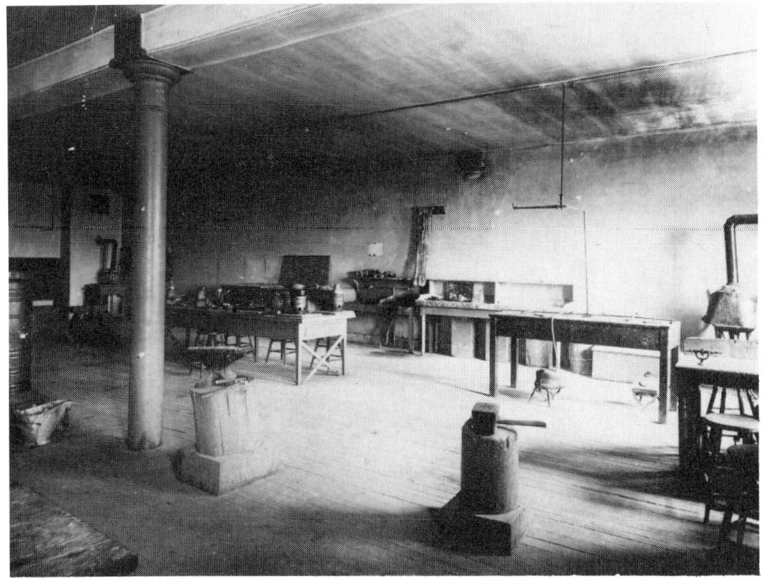

The mechanical laboratory of the University of Pennsylvania School of Dentistry, as it appeared in 1878, the year the school opened. The school was located in the basement of Medical Hall from 1878-1896. From University of Pennsylvania School of Dental Medicine.

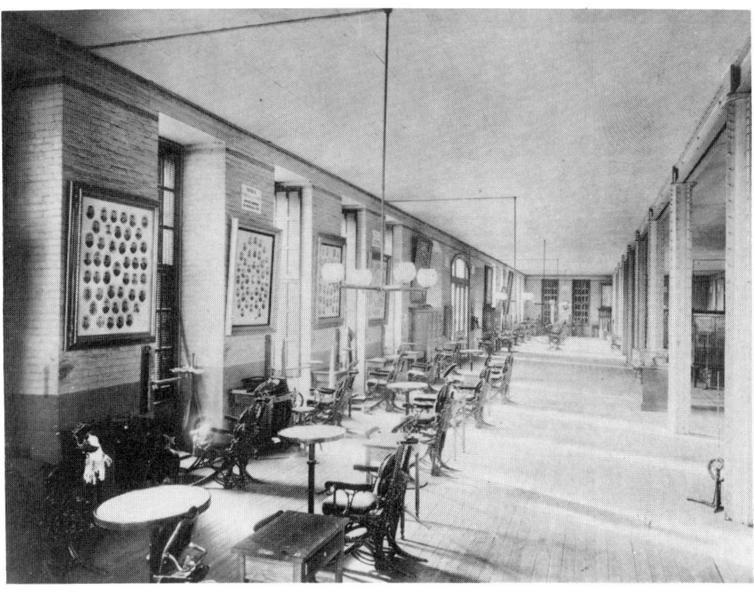

Department of Dentistry Operating Room in Hare Laboratory, University of Pennsylvania School of Dentistry, 1880. In this public setting of Morrison chairs arranged in a row beneath large windows, the students worked on clinic patients. Each student used a foot-pedal drill and a spittoon was attached to the chair for the patient's use in this period before electricity and plumbing were available. From University of Pennsylvania School of Dental Medicine.

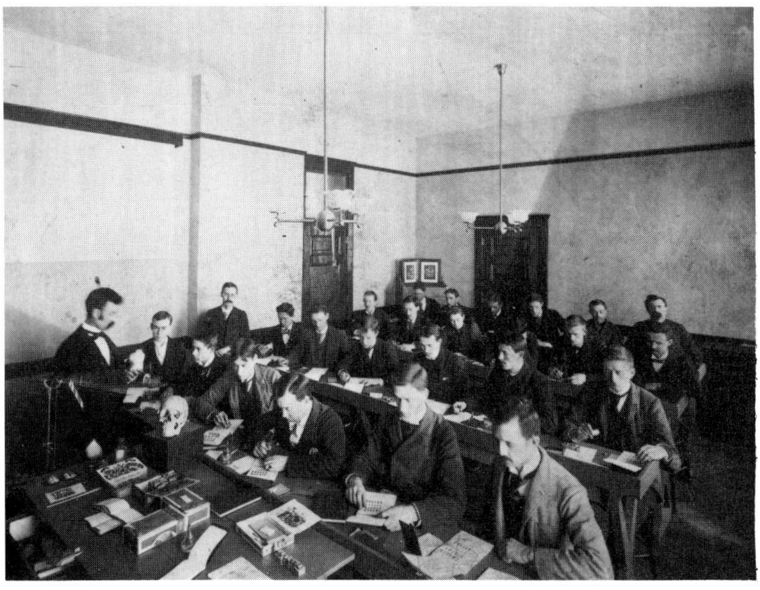

A class in dentistry at an unknown dental school, circa 1892. Students refer to a chart of the teeth at their desks, while the teacher instructs them in the anatomy of the teeth. Cigar boxes often were used to transport artificial teeth and hand tools when dentists traveled to the homes of their patients or from town to town. From Minnesota Historical Society, No. 32266.

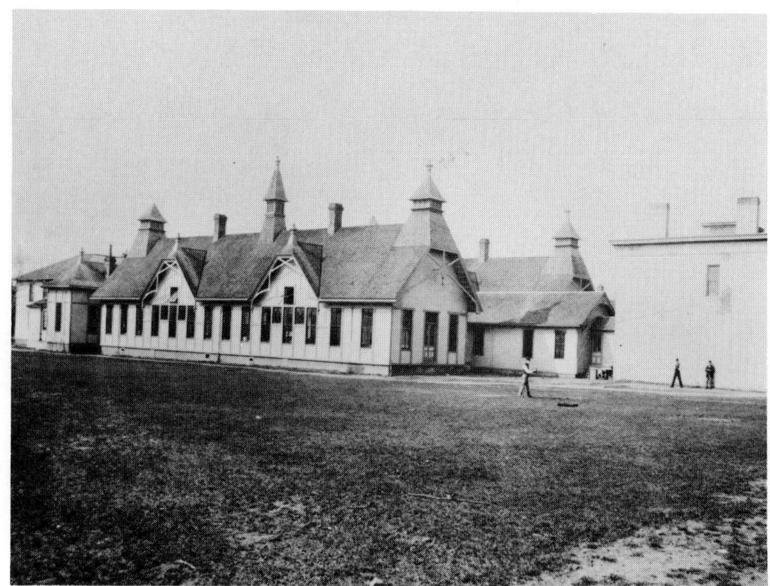

Third building, University of Michigan (1891-1908). Not atypical of the earliest buildings employed as dental schools is this one, originally a professor's home. Two frame wings were added to the stucco house. The building was equipped to accommodate 150 underclass students and 54 chairs were available in the operating room for senior work. From University of Michigan School of Dentistry.

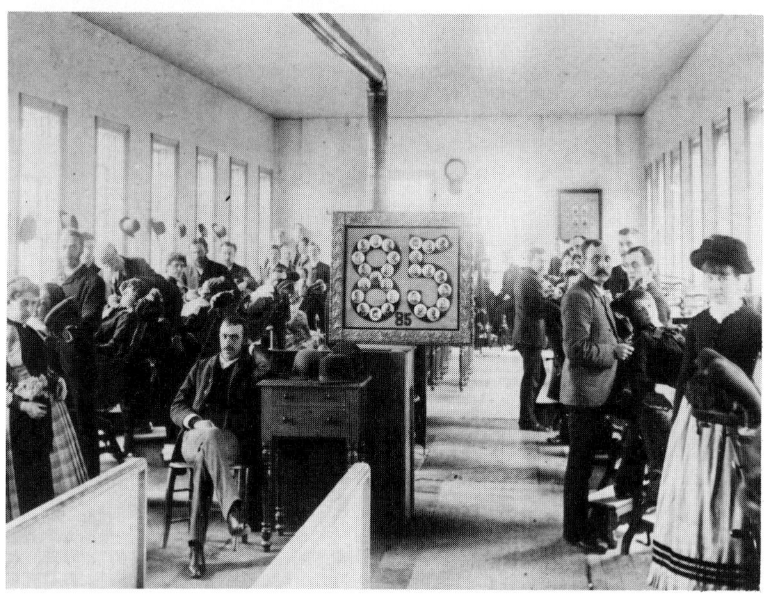

The Operating Room of the University of Michigan School of Dentistry on its 10th anniversary. This is the earliest picture of the dental school clinic. The stove behind the sign "85" is described on page 74. From University of Michigan School of Dentistry.

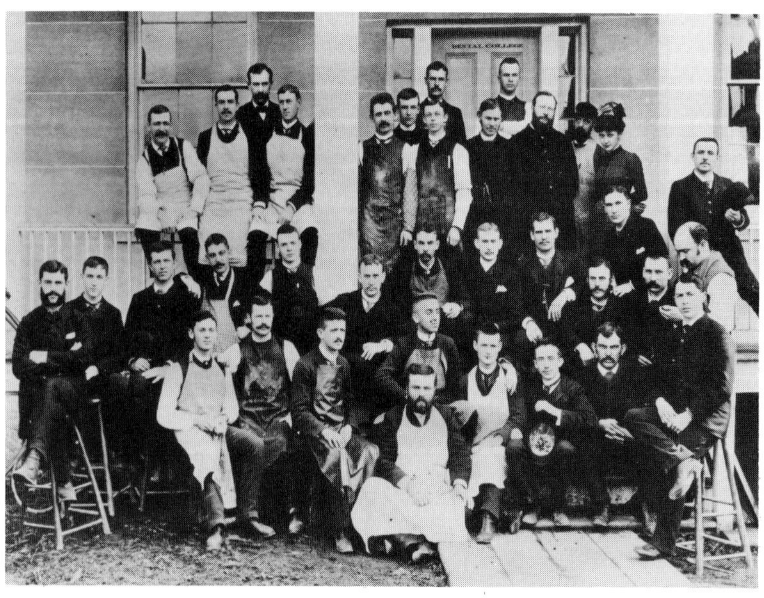

Prosthetic Laboratory class (late 1880s) in the rear of the second building of the University of Michigan School of Dentistry, which opened in 1875 (the second university affiliated dental school in the country). From University of Michigan School of Dentistry.

In 1867 a two-year dental curriculum was developed consisting of different courses in each year, rather than repetition of the same courses in both years. Dissection and laboratory instruction in chemistry followed the introduction of laboratory methods in anatomy, physiology and surgery.

Basic techniques were taught in dental colleges through repetition, as well as by the example of preceptors. One painstaking procedure was filling teeth with gold. Roy G. Hayward, graduate of the class of 1911 of the University of Michigan, explained during an interview in 1972 at the time he was 84 years old that "Toward the end of our junior year, they took us into the clinic and let us do prophylaxis. In the senior year, of course, we were pounding gold, gold, gold, gold. . . . in the afternoons from one o'clock on, it was gold foil, gold foil. I pounded enough gold foil to sink a ship."[74]

The Kansas City Dental College, founded in 1881, provides an example of the evolution of a private dental school into a university affiliated school. At the time it was organized there were 27 dentists in Kansas City which had a population of 75,000. Six dentists founded and owned the school. They invested in the school to earn profits on the funds collected from the school clinic. The school merged with the Western Dental College in Kansas City, an unusual dental school, in that it had been run by a single owner. The new school became the Kansas City-Western Dental College. In 1922 Kansas City-Western Dental College ceased paying dividends to its owners, and the next year, the college became a non-profit corporation. In 1941 it became a part of the University of Kansas City and was renamed in 1963, the University of Missouri-Kansas City School of Dentistry.

University of Michigan's first graduating class in school of dentistry, 1876. This was the second university affiliated dental school in the country. From University of Michigan School of Dentistry.

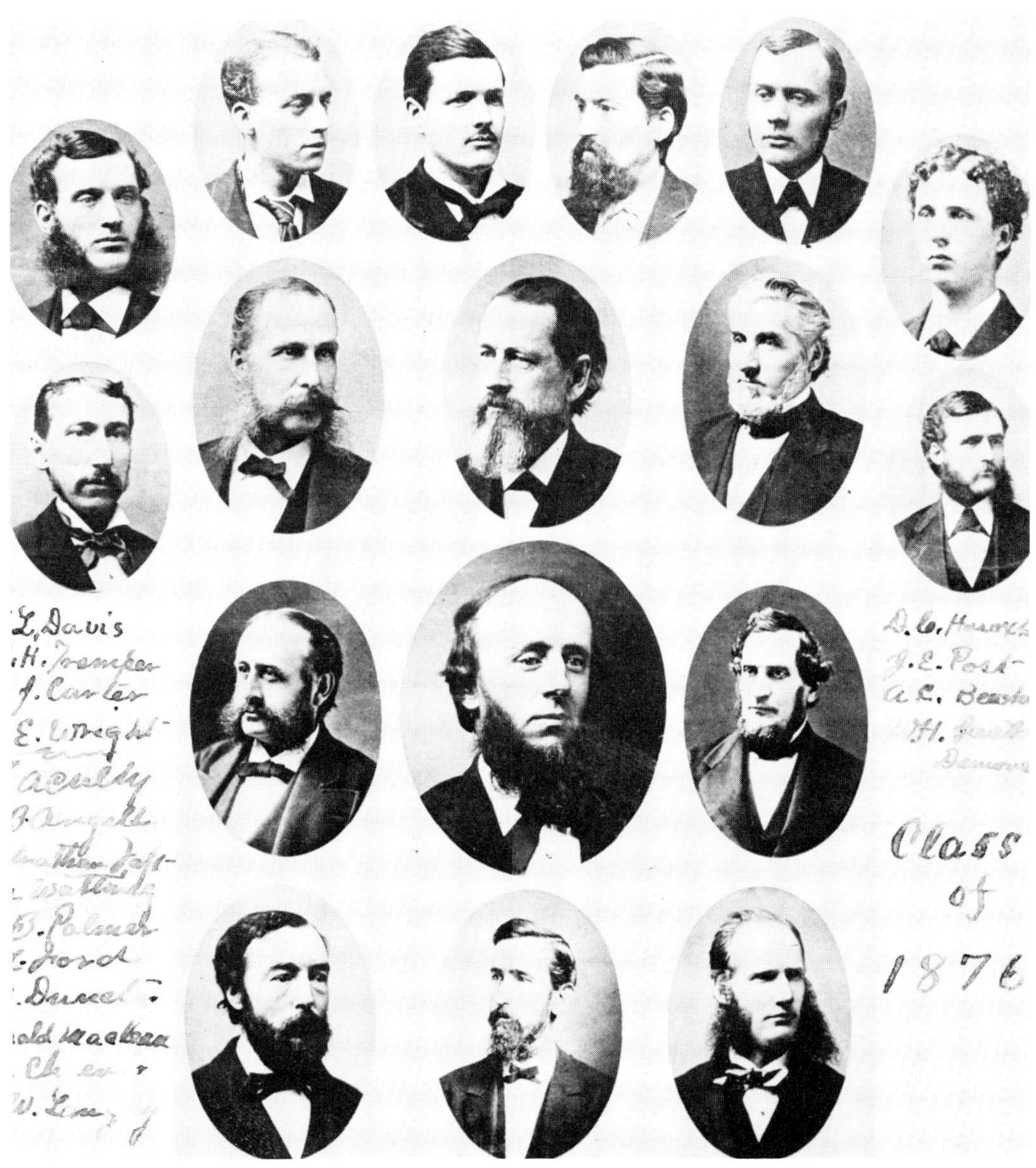

Dental clinic in third building, University of Michigan. Each chair has an electric light suspended from a wire in the ceiling and attached to each bracket table. However, foot-powered dental drills were used and spittoons were provided for each patient. From University of Michigan School of Dentistry.

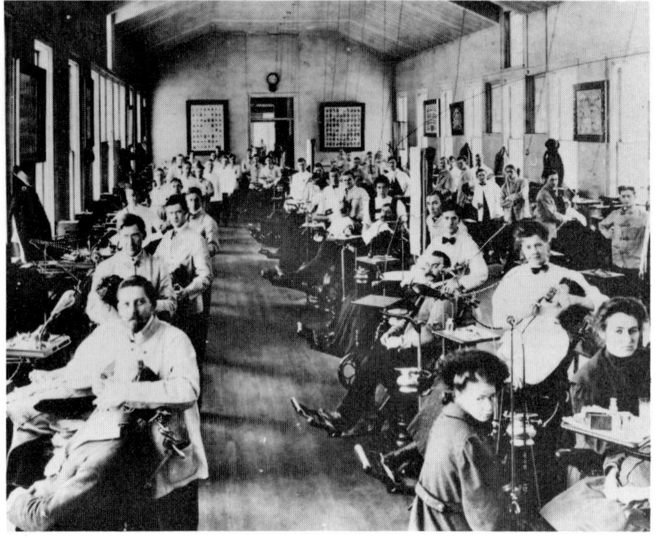

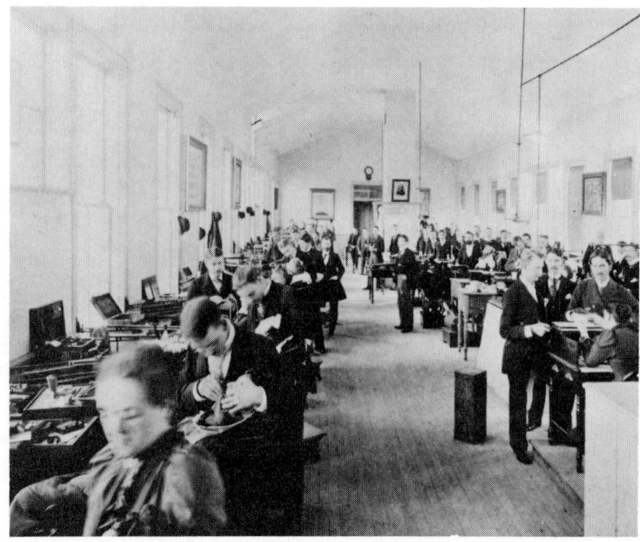

Dental clinic in third building, University of Michigan School of Dentistry, 1892-93. Although there were gas lights in the center of the room, poor lighting for performing dental work was a constant student complaint. Professors voiced another complaint which concerned student practice in 1892: "We again call the attention of seniors to the disinfection of their instruments. Steam jets can be found in the operating room, and we recommend that they be used for this purpose." (pg. 22, *Alumni Bulletin*, 1971) From University of Michigan School of Dentistry.

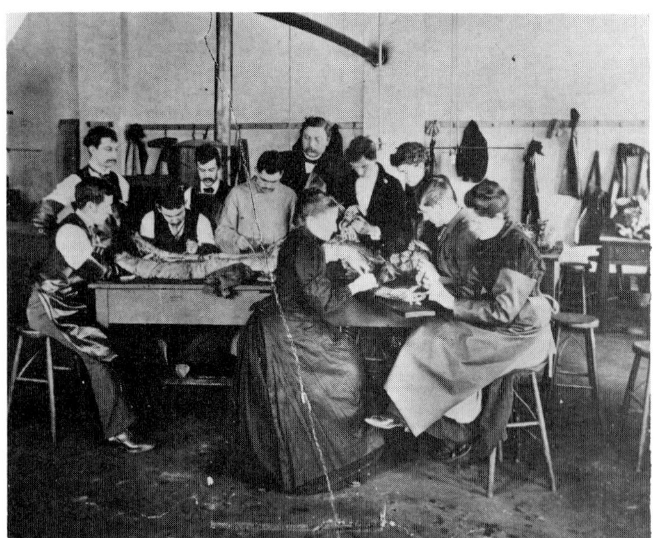

Dental students dissecting. Anatomy was one of the required courses in dental school. A shortage of cadavers hastened the merger of dental schools with medical schools, or at least, the sharing of the basic science courses by medical and dental students within a university. The Pennsylvania College merged with the University of Pennsylvania School of Dental Medicine in the 1920s. From Pennsylvania College of Dental Medicine.

Lecture amphitheater in third building, University of Michigan, 1895-96. The only female student is in the front row. In the class of 1895, F.F. Scott, the first black student graduated. A contemporary claimed: "There is a good place for Mr. Scott in the profession." (pg. 22, *Alumni Bulletin*, 1971) From University of Michigan School of Dentistry.

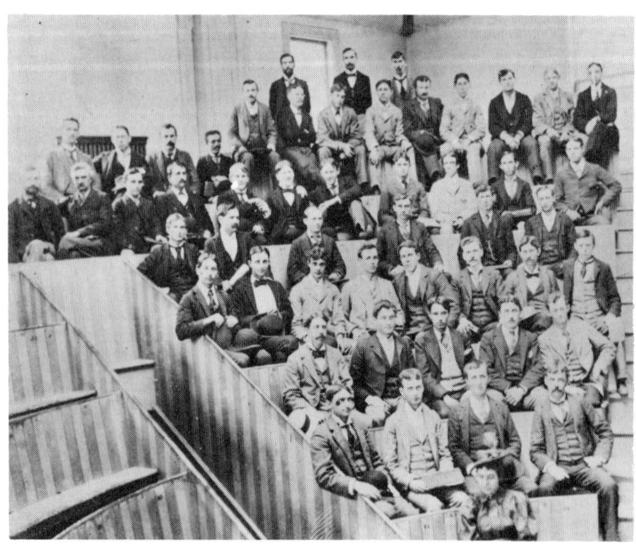

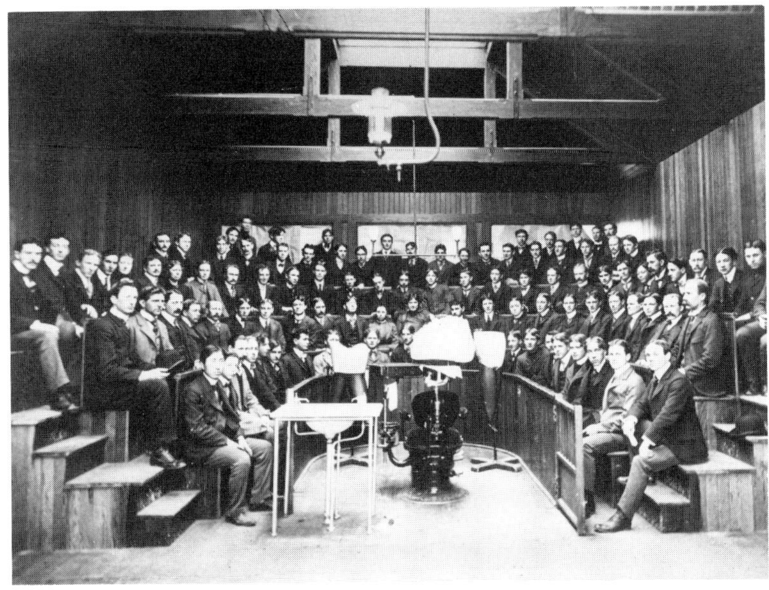

Class in session at North Pacific Dental College, Portland, Oregon in 1900. There are two women in the center of the second row out of well over 100 students. The school was established in 1898 to train young men and women and claimed to have the best facilities for the purpose. By 1913 the school drew students from 33 states. From Oregon Historical Society, Portland, Oregon.

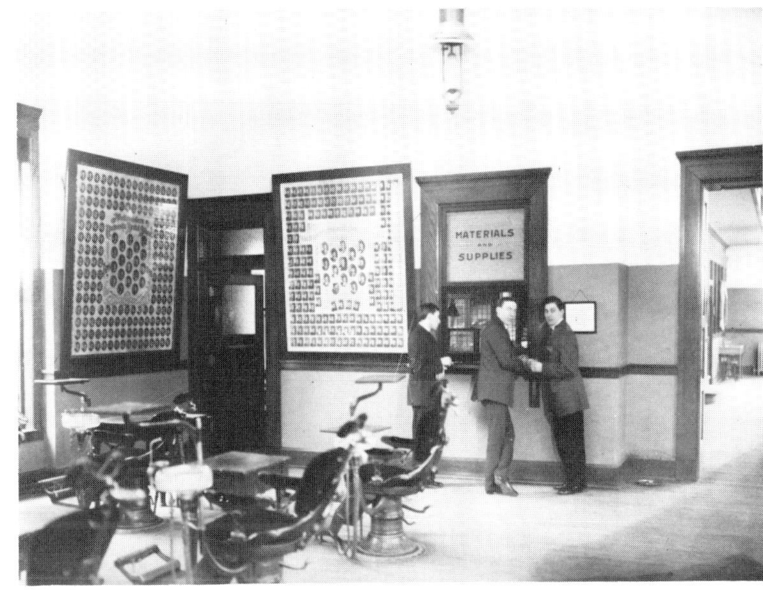

Supply closet at end of the clinic of the Northwestern University Dental School, circa 1896-1902. From Northwestern University Dental School.

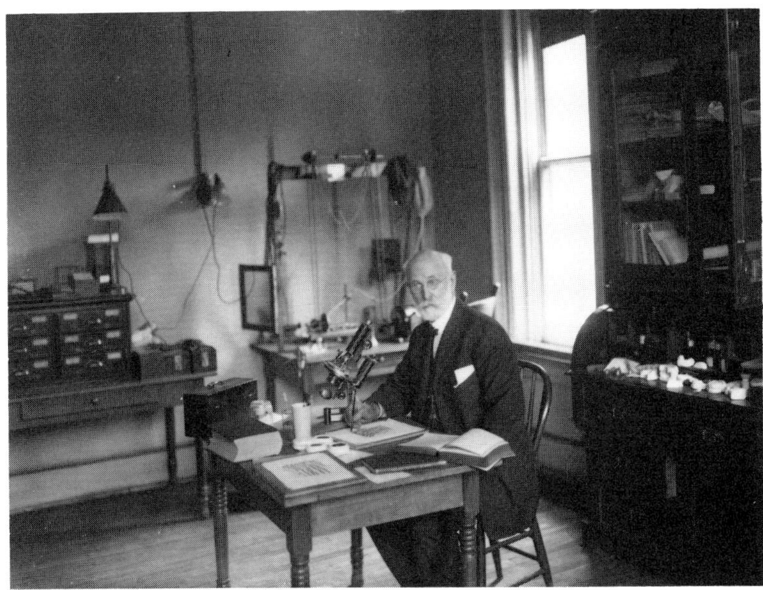

Dr. Greene Vardiman Black in his laboratory at Northwestern University Dental School. Black became dean and was a leader in improving dental school instruction. From Northwestern University Dental School.

During its early years students were expected to provide supplies including a spirit lamp, air syringe, dental syringe, enamel chisel, foil carrier, pluggers, excavators and cavity burs for a dental engine which cost between $20 and $30 dollars.[75]

The dentist educated in a dental school received practical training in a clinic or infirmary. The clinic was arranged in one large room with chairs placed side-by-side in long rows beneath large windows and skylights. The photographs reveal the "crowded" demeanor of the clinic and with little imagination the noise and odor of such a room is apparent. The income derived from clinic patients was important in keeping the school budget balanced, although the purpose of the clinic was to educate the dental student.[76]

In the best managed schools the instructor supervised students who kept records of each stage of the work they performed on a patient. Not until the record card had been marked by the instructor after he had inspected the student's patient, could the student obtain materials, such as amalgam, to proceed with the patient. Throughout the process the student was graded. This method of record keeping also provided a means of preventing the student from using his own material and collecting a fee from the patient. To avoid the problem of a student forgetting his patient's name or vice versa, an index register was maintained for all students and clinic patients.

Students encountered the least problems in collecting payments from patients when the clinic announced set fees for each procedure and gave the instructors the responsibility of deciding who would receive treatment free or at a reduced cost.[77]

One of the advantages of the dental school being separated from the medical school was the emphasis on tooth reconstruction and prosthodontic techniques that resulted in American dentistry becoming without peer in these procedures. Discussion of the merger of dental and medical schools led to fears that American dentists would lose their special mechanical skills, if they were to spend less time in school learning and practicing. To investigate all dental schools and provide direction for future plans, William J. Gies began to study dental education in 1922 under the sponsorship of the Carnegie Foundation which had supported a similar study of medical schools a decade earlier.[78] The Gies report resulted in the demise of private dental schools which could no longer compete with university affiliated schools and pay the expenses of the clinic out of student tuitions and patient fees. Whereas in 1900, 50 percent of the 60 dental schools were proprietary, after the Gies report the number of dental schools was reduced to 38 by 1934.

Dental schools introduced new courses as the demands on the dental practitioner changed. In 1905 the Northwestern University Dental School began a course on dental economics. Students no longer had firsthand experience under a preceptor in a dental office, and therefore, it was important for them to receive instruction in the business side of dental practice. The course included practice building techniques, setting and collecting fees, and keeping accounts.[79]

Tufts College of Dental Medicine was among the first to introduce a course on Social Dentistry in 1961. The purpose of the course was to make the dentist aware of his environment, the dentist-patient relationship and the relation of the dentist to other health professions and institutions, as well as the dentist's responsibilities to society.[80] Later we will see how many dentists, who had not received formal instruction in the social aspects of their profession, discovered the issues raised in the Tufts course, through their own office experiences, and then, how they solved the problems they encountered.

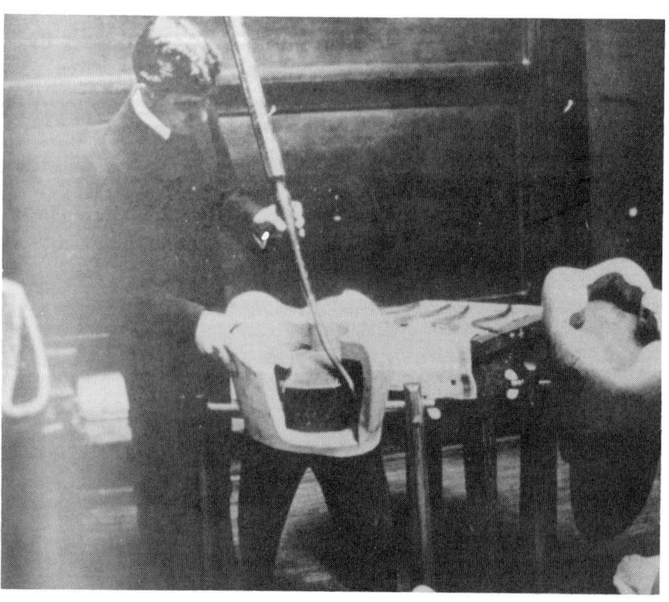

Northwestern University Dental School student in the 1890s demonstrates the correct way to prepare a tooth cavity for a filling using oversized model and instruments designed by G.V. Black. From Northwestern University Dental School.

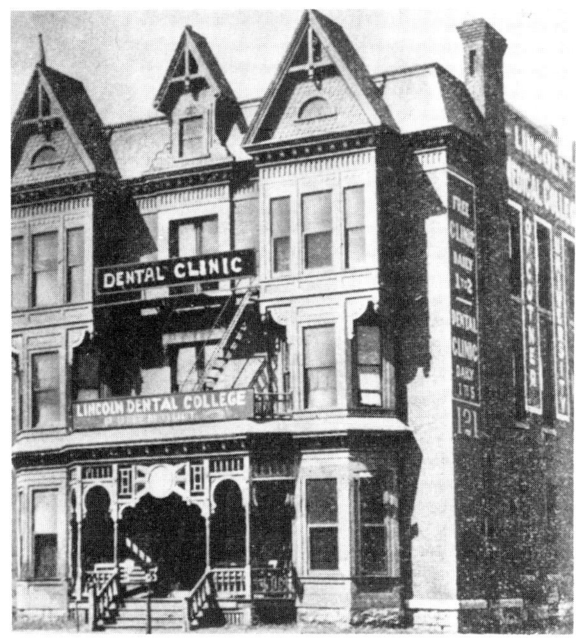

First building of Lincoln Dental College, (1899-1902), forerunner of the University of Nebraska College of Dentistry. From University of Nebraska College of Dentistry.

Students in the Dental Department of the College of Physicians and Surgeons at the turn of the century. From the Abraham W. Ward Museum, University of the Pacific School of Dentistry, San Francisco. The Ward Museum is dedicated to Dr. Ward, 1902 graduate of the College of Physicians and Surgeons and professor of Oral Hygiene from 1918 to 1925. Ward was a pioneer periodontist.

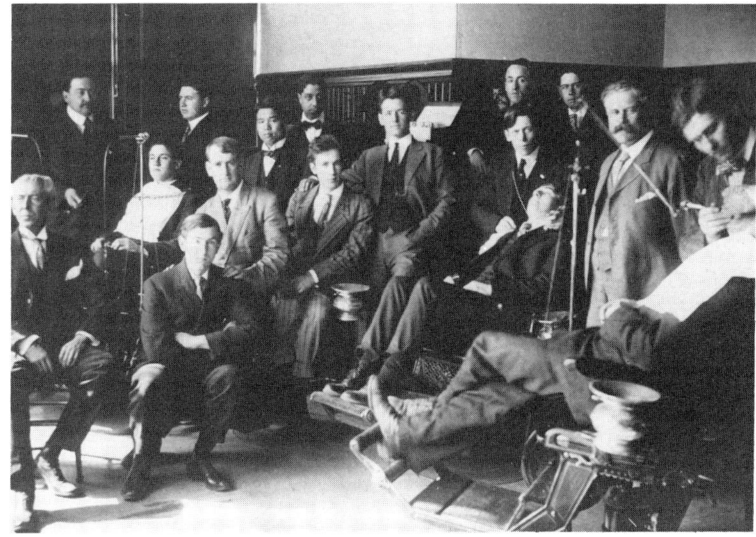

Dissection room of class of 1904 of the College of Physicians and Surgeons, San Francisco. Founded in 1896, the College, in 1962, joined the University of the Pacific, as its School of Dentistry in San Francisco. From A.W. Ward Museum, University of the Pacific School of Dentistry.

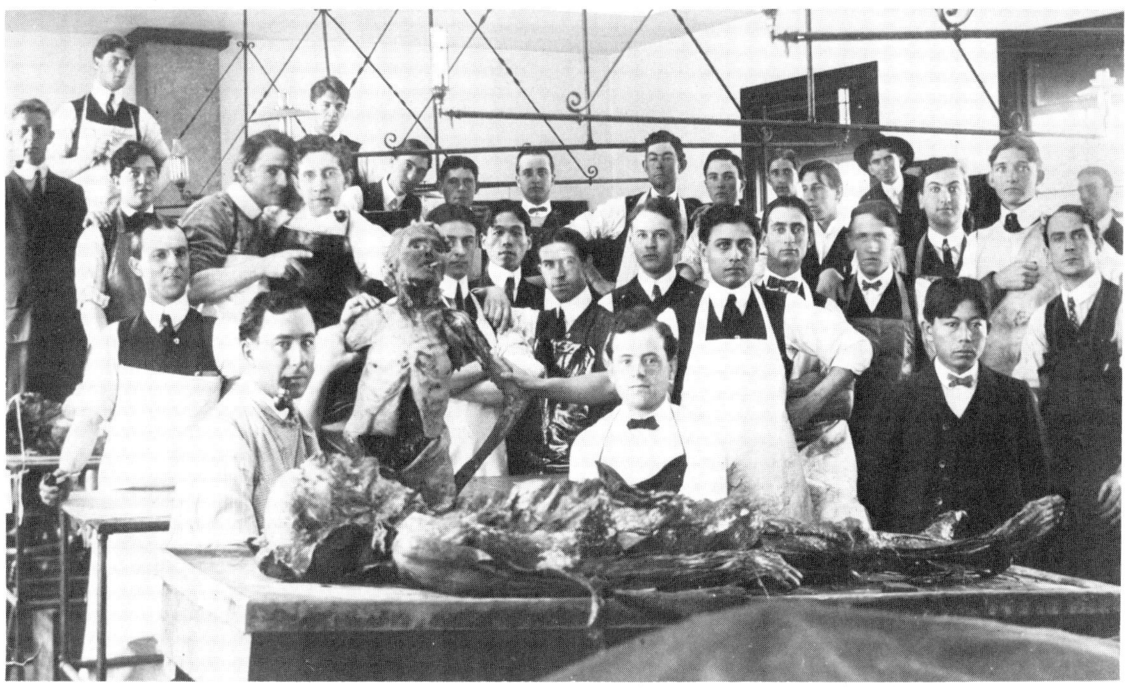

Learning preclinical technique, 1910. Dental students are working on their dentiforms (dentex is the trade name used in some schools for an artificial jaw). They perfected their skills by preparing artificial teeth on model jaws mounted on poles raised to the height that they would be expected to work on their patients seated in a dental chair. From Tufts University School of Dental Medicine.

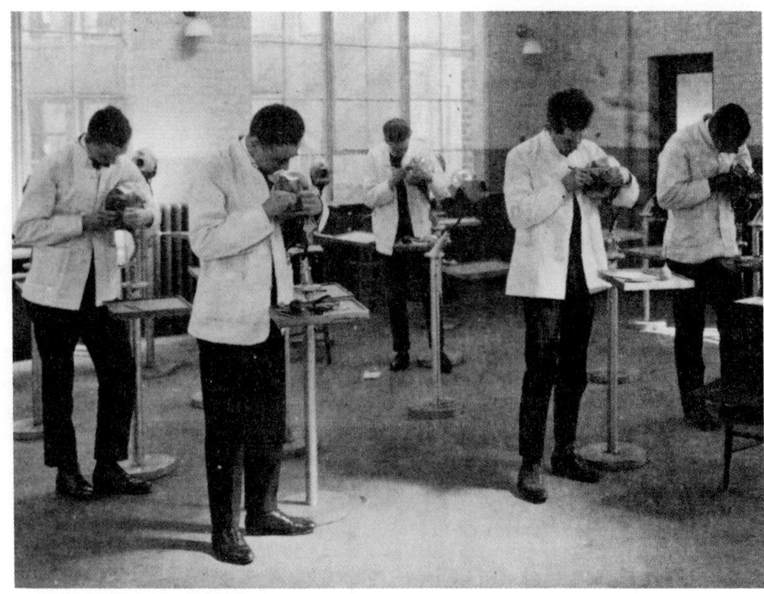

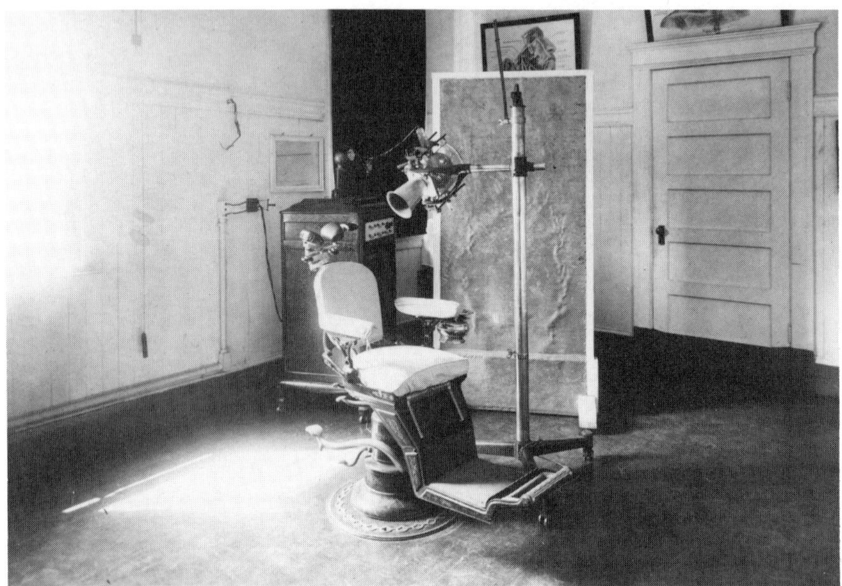

X-Ray Department of the College of Physicians and Surgeons, San Francisco, 1921. The King Wappler Coolidge X-Ray Tube is fitted with the Campbell X-Ray Coil. From A.W. Ward Museum, University of the Pacific School of Dentistry.

Dental Infirmary of the College of Physicians and Surgeons, San Francisco, 1910. From A.W. Ward Museum, University of the Pacific School of Dentistry.

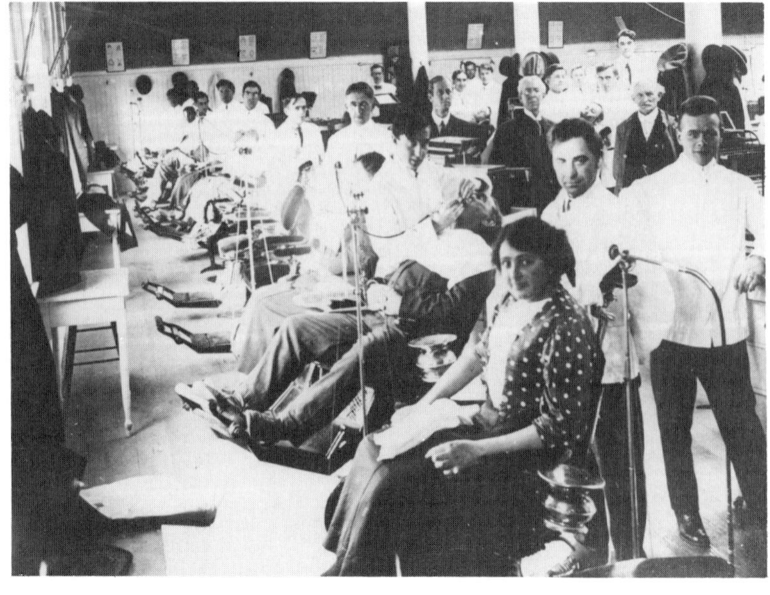

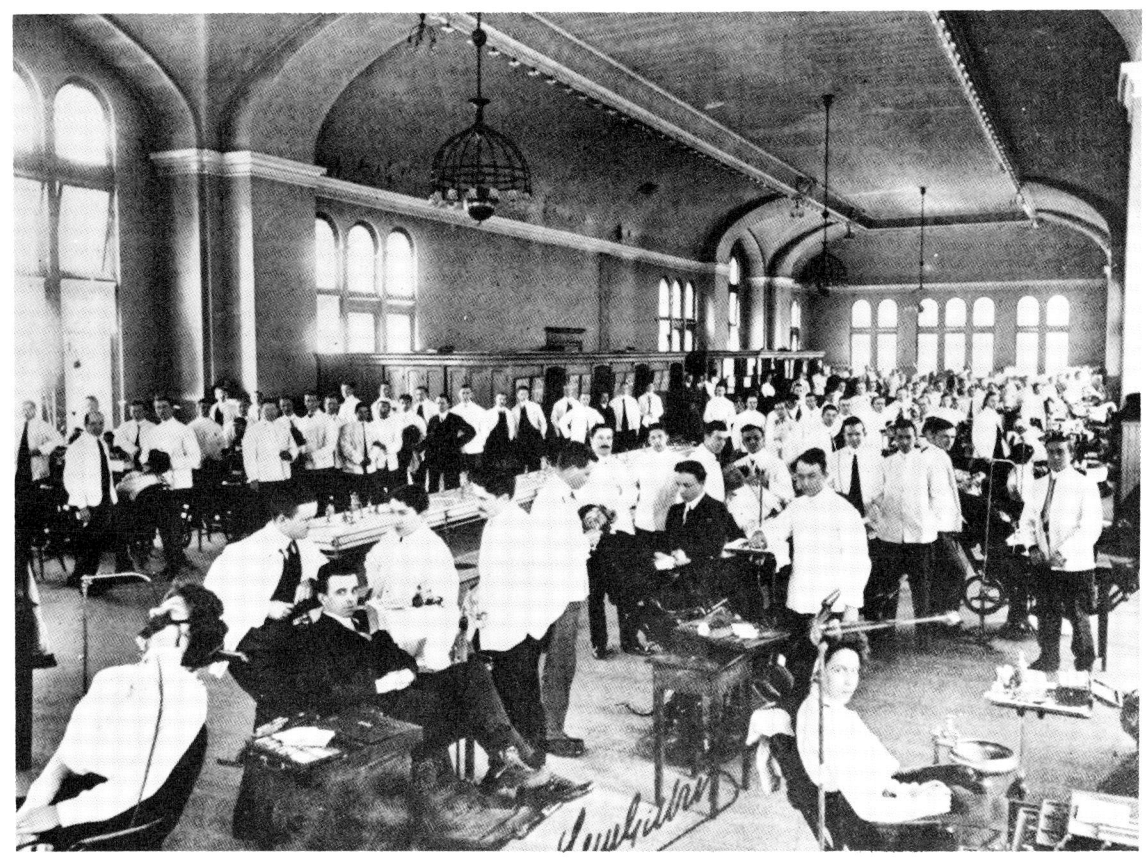

Clinic in Dental Hall, University of Pennsylvania in 1911. From University of Pennsylvania School of Dental Medicine.

Students of the University of Pennsylvania School of Dentistry working in the Evans Laboratory of Bacteriology in 1915. From University of Pennsylvania School of Dental Medicine.

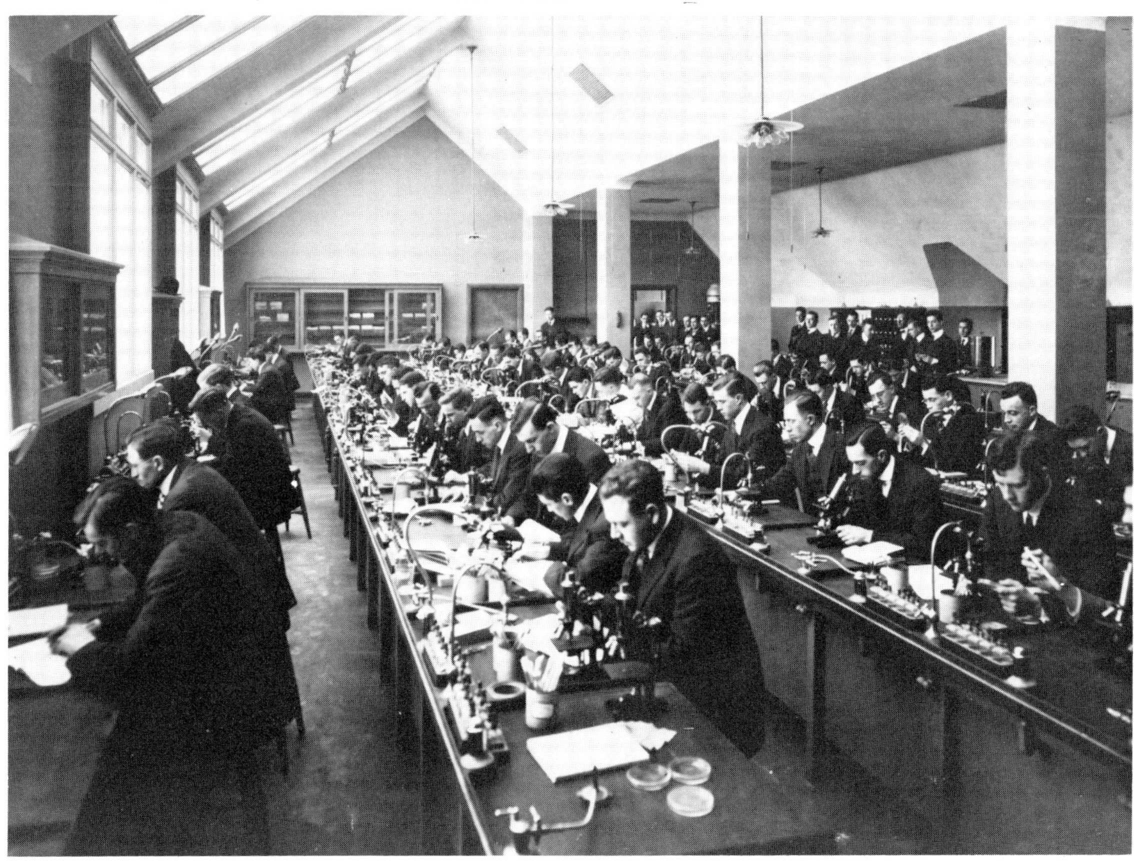

First Oral Hygiene Clinic in the Evans Building, University of Pennsylvania School of Dental Medicine. Established in 1923, the school for dental hygienists taught women students techniques of cleaning teeth to prevent loss. Dental hygienists were hired by the school board when the wisdom of prevention programs prevailed over the rationale for economy in the school budget. Costs were minimized by using portable dental chairs set up in an empty room. Lacking running water, spittoons were installed on each chair. Sterilizers were shared: Note the small unit in front of the chair on the right. The dentist examines a boy's mouth on the right. From University of Pennsylvania School of Dental Medicine.

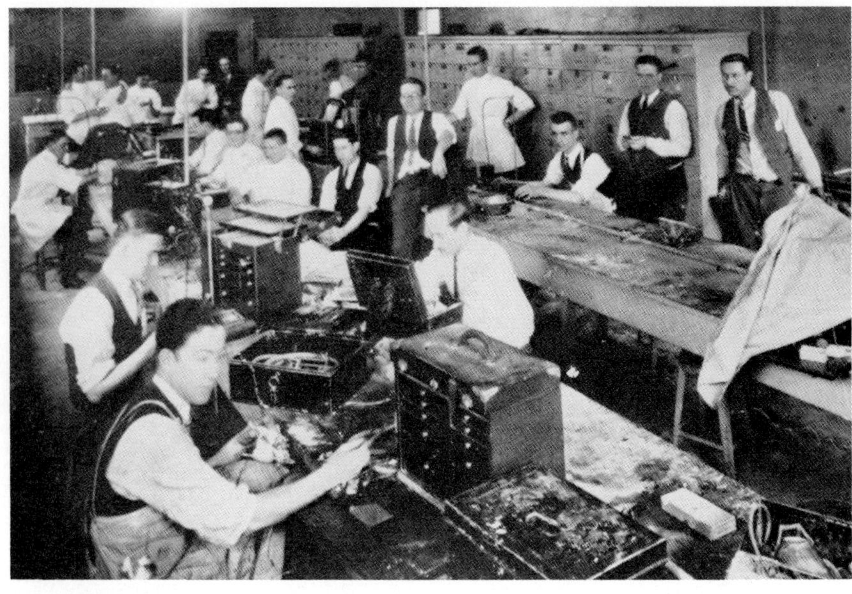

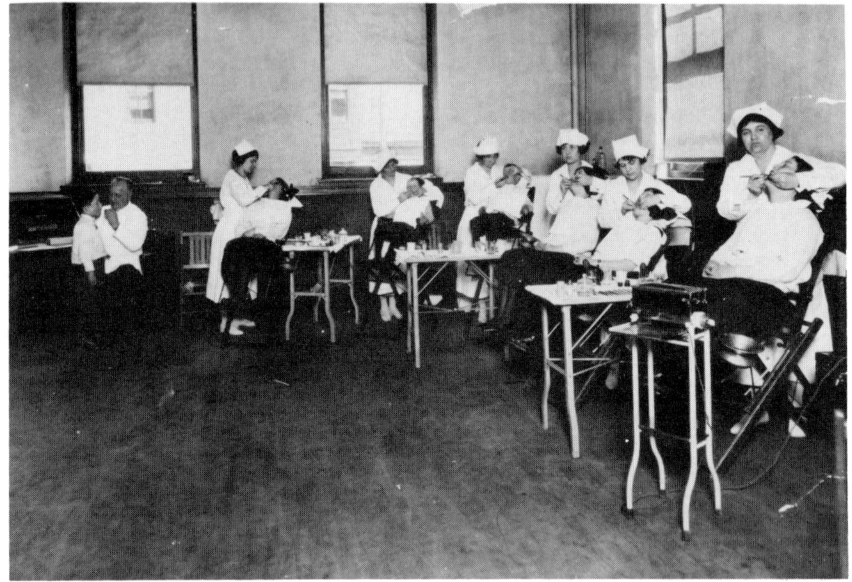

Each student with a chest of supplies and instruments is learning to make artificial dentures in the laboratory in 1925. From Indiana University School of Dentistry.

Student dental hygienists at the Eastman Dental Dispensary work on employees of the Eastman Kodak Company, Rochester, New York in 1926. From Eastman Kodak Co.

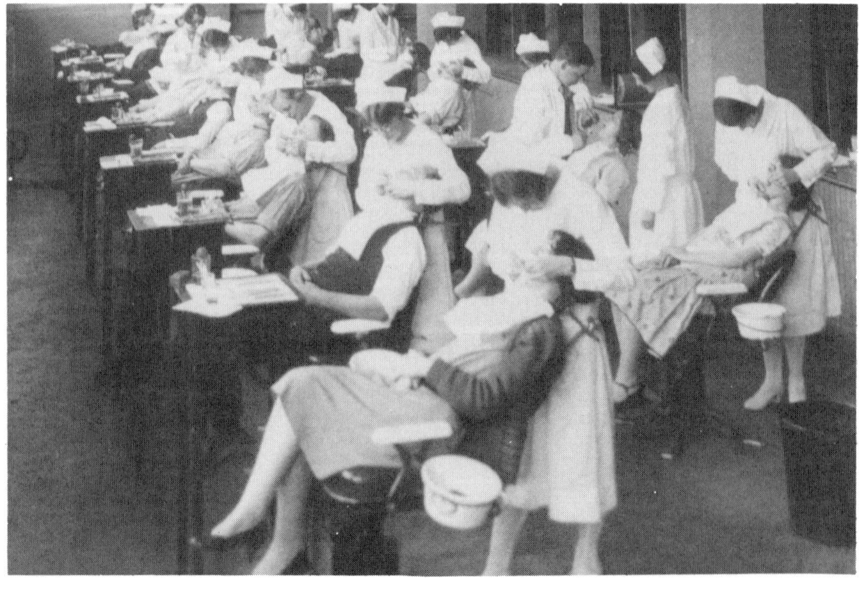

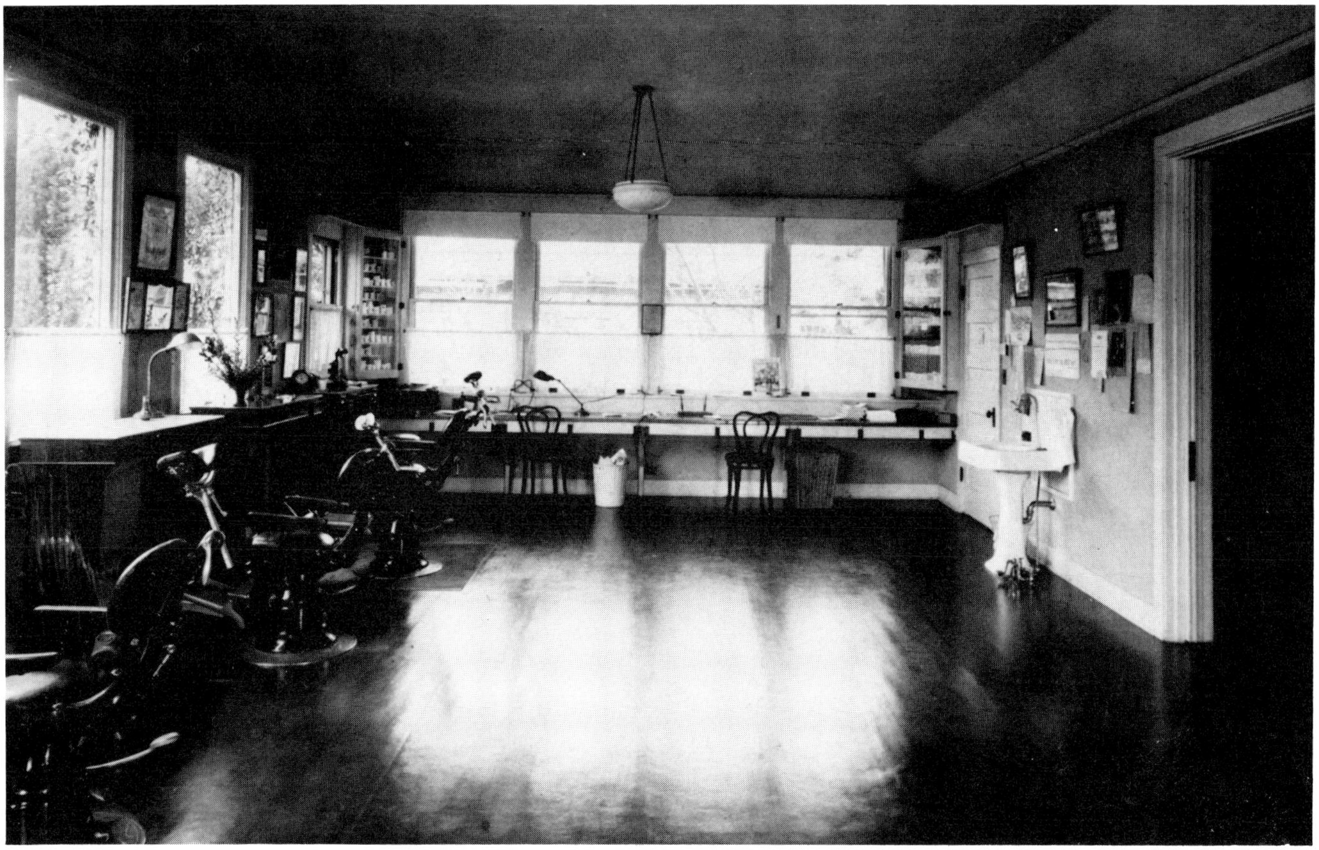

Edward H. Angle (1854-1930) Orthodontia Clinic in Los Angeles, California, circa 1920s. Angle developed unique principles of orthodontia (straightening the teeth) after graduating from the Pennsylvania College of Dental Surgery in 1878. He patented a dental appliance in 1889. His students followed him from St. Louis, New York and Connecticut until 1914, when he settled in California. This school, presented to him by his students, the first of its kind, was established to teach the Angle method of teeth re-alignment. From Smithsonian Institution, Neg. No. 83-4871.

Orthodontia flourished in Hollywood where film-stars needed to keep their teeth in excellent condition or, on occasion, have them altered to play special roles. These photographs of Shirley Temple show her teeth before and after receiving caps. Ms. Temple describes how she sneezed and lost her two front caps in the grass. Without them filming could not continue, so she had her dentist replace them. Black, Shirley Temple, *Child Star: An Autobiography,* McGraw Hill, New York, 1989, p. 103-04.

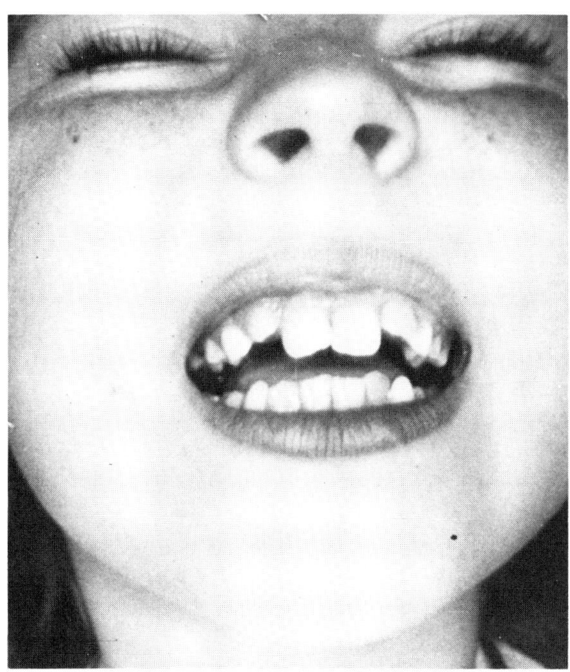

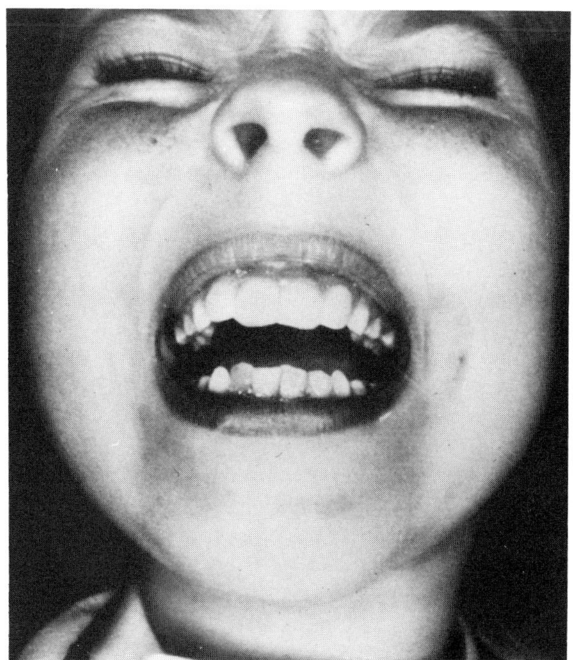

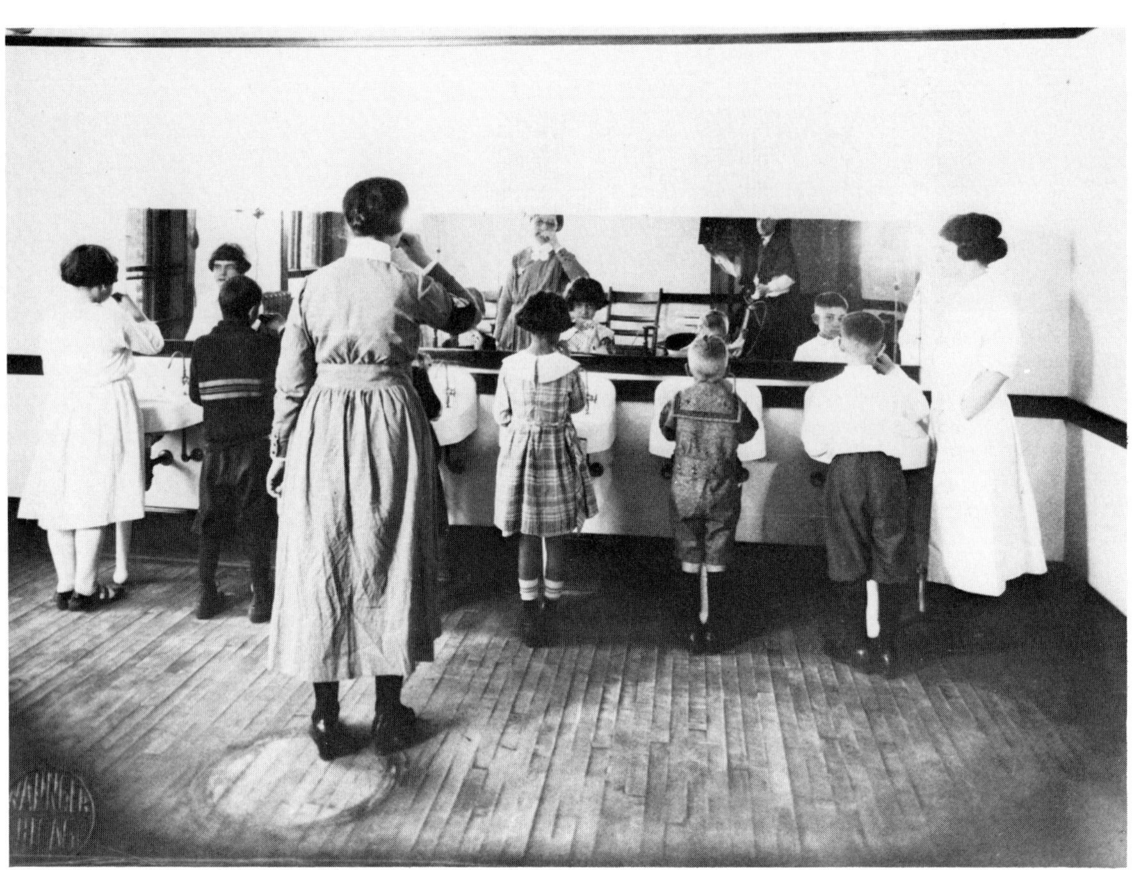

Teaching children how to brush their teeth in the Northwestern University Dental School Clinic, 1923.
FROM NORTHWESTERN UNIVERSITY DENTAL SCHOOL.

Children's Clinic at the Northwestern University Dental School. From Northwestern University Dental School.

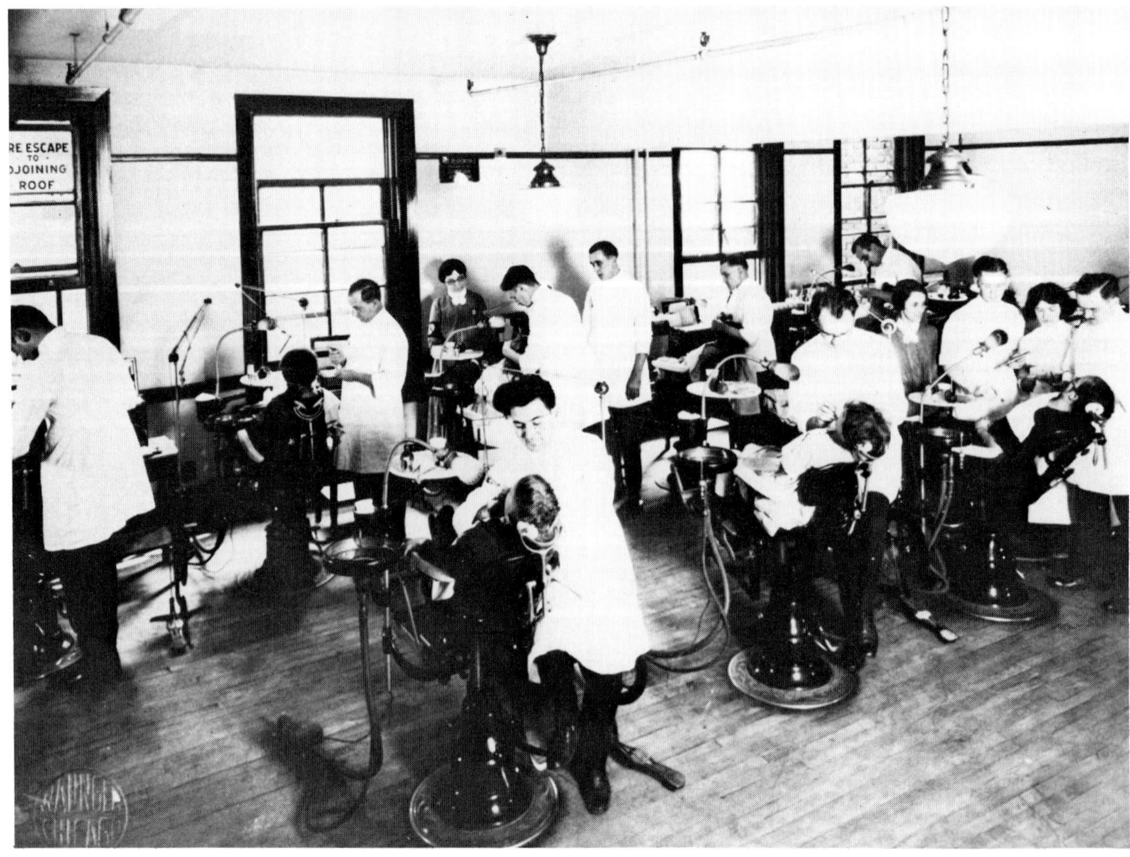

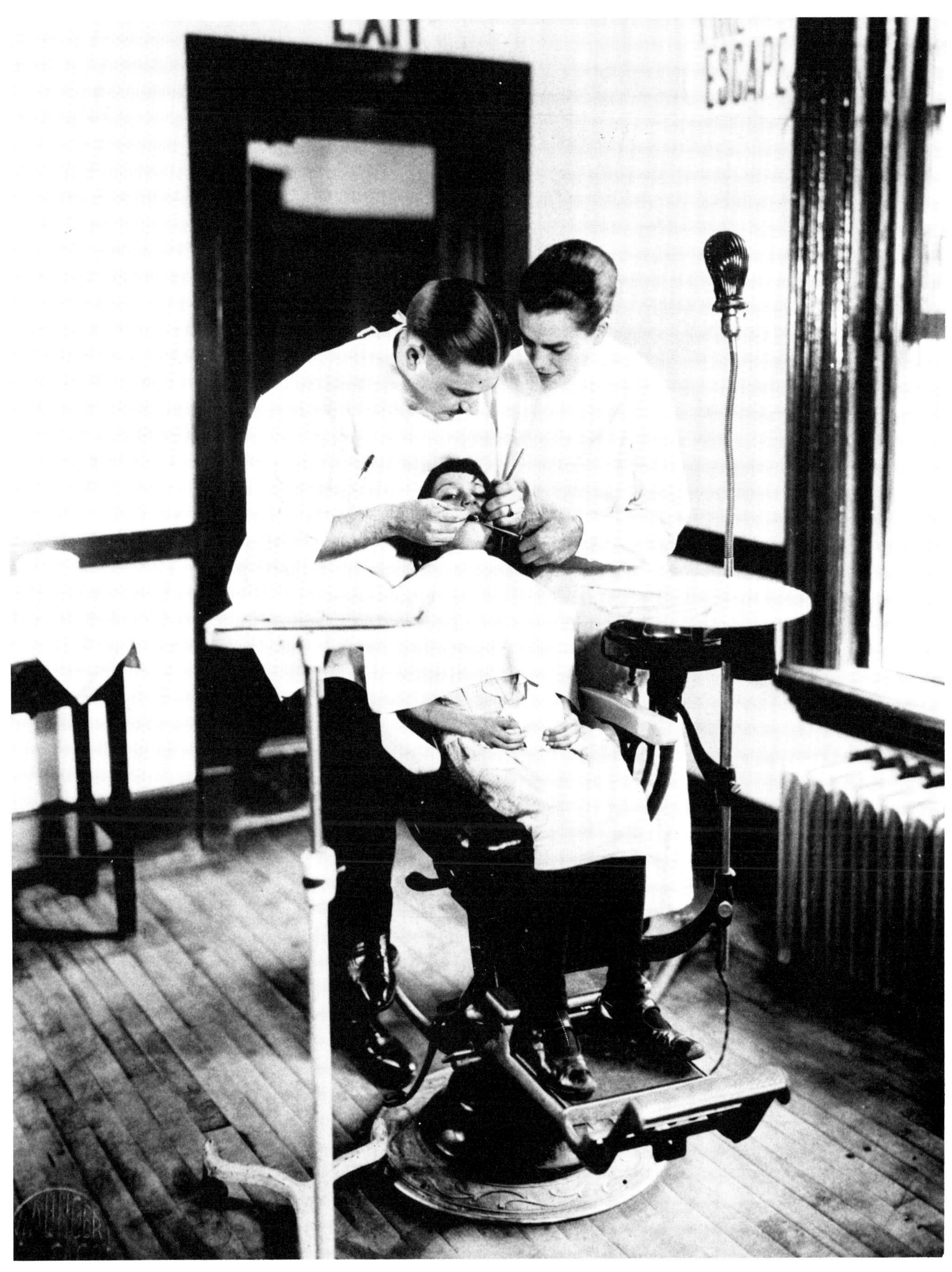

Board of Public Health Dental Clinic at 1008 Nicollet Avenue, Minneapolis, Minnesota, Nov. 1923. The dentist engages the attention of the child patient before he proceeds. From the Minnesota Historical Society.

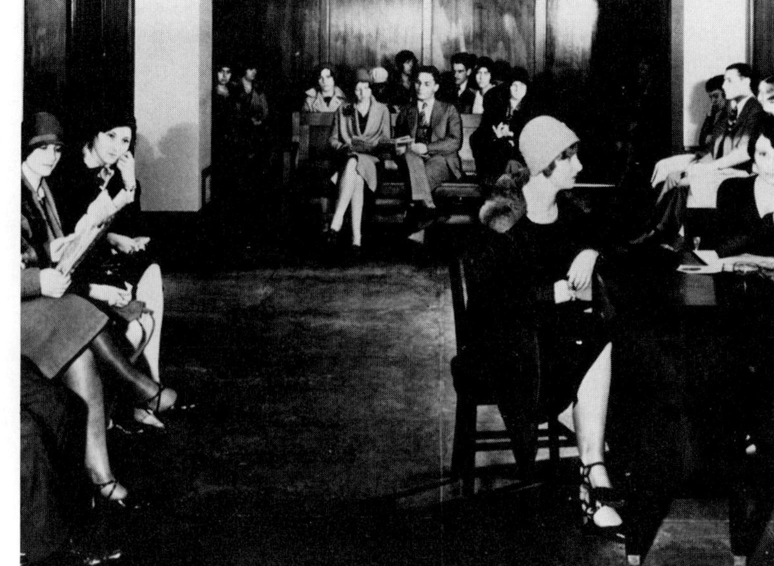

The waiting room of the Columbia University Dental School in 1928. From Columbia University Dental School.

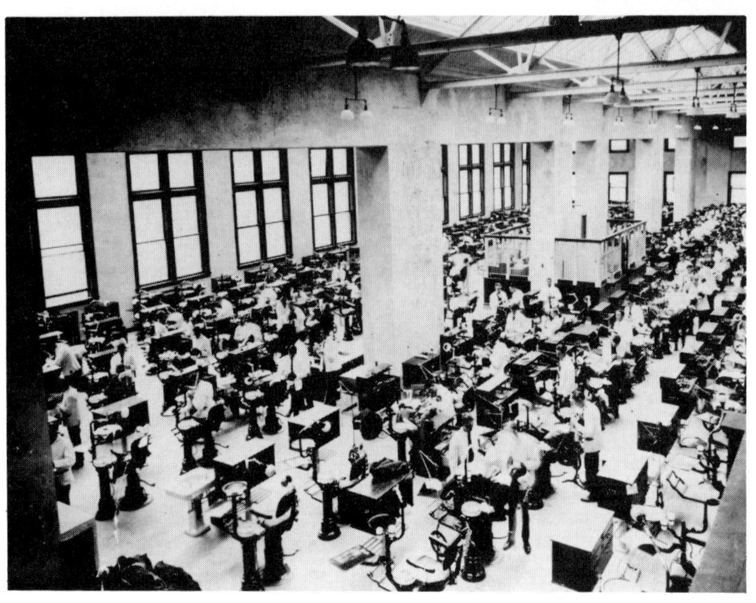

The Dental Clinic in the fourth building, University of Michigan School of Dentistry circa 1920s. The size of the school doubled in 1923. From University of Michigan School of Dentistry.

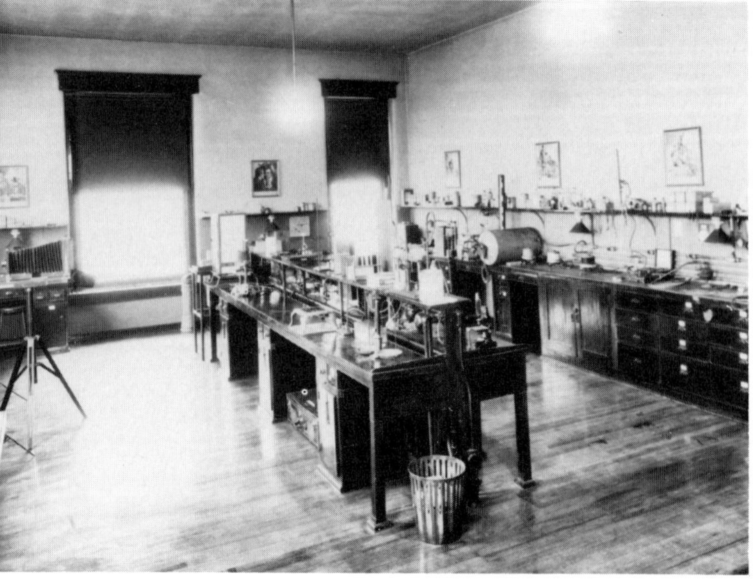

Dr. Raymond Myers' dental casting research laboratory on the third floor of the Broadway Building circa 1930. The Louisville College of Dentistry was founded in 1886 as a private school. In 1918 it became the School of Dentistry of the University of Louisville. From University of Louisville School of Dentistry.

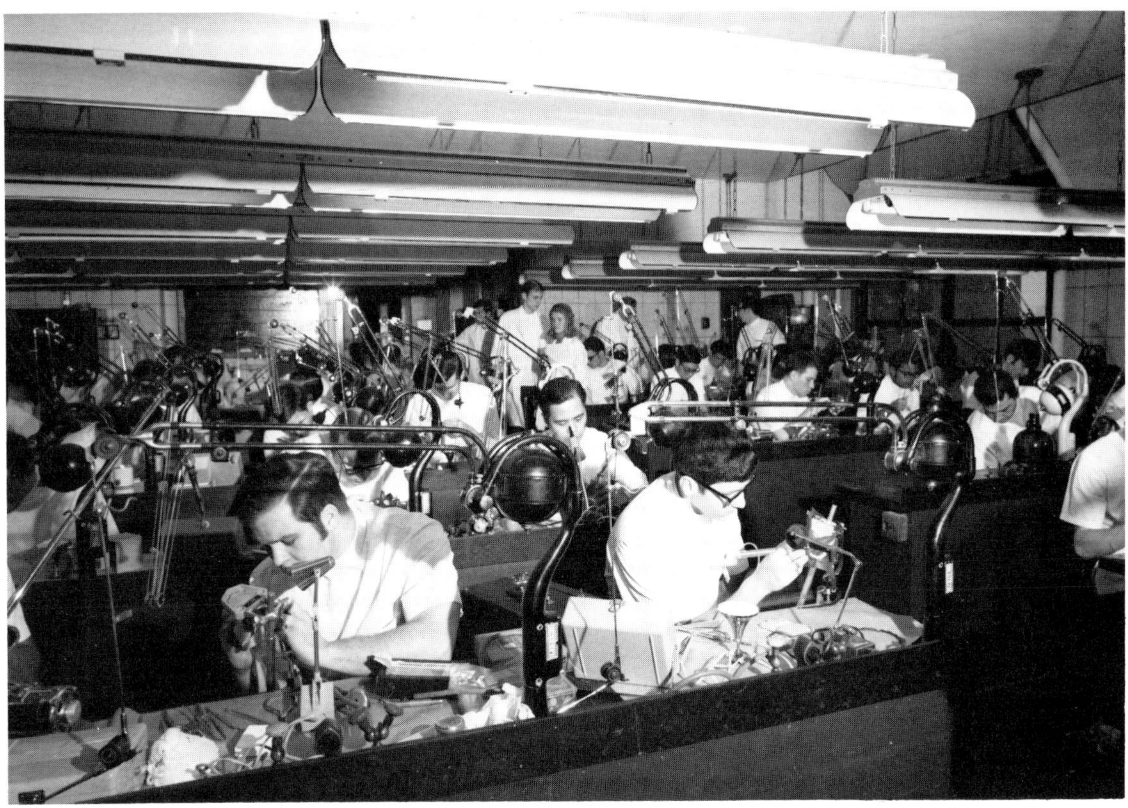

Dental students of the College of Dentistry of the University of Illinois at the Medical Center working on their dentiforms in a technique laboratory in the late 1960s. A dentiform is a mock-up of the dentition and alveolar structures which is also known under a trade name as a dentex. From College of Dentistry of the University of Illinois.

Pedodontic or Children's Dental Clinic of the University of Indiana in 1962. Pedodontics became a specialty after the turn of the century. See text in section on the female dentist, Evangeline Jordon, for the beginnings of this specialty dental practice. From Indiana University School of Dentistry.

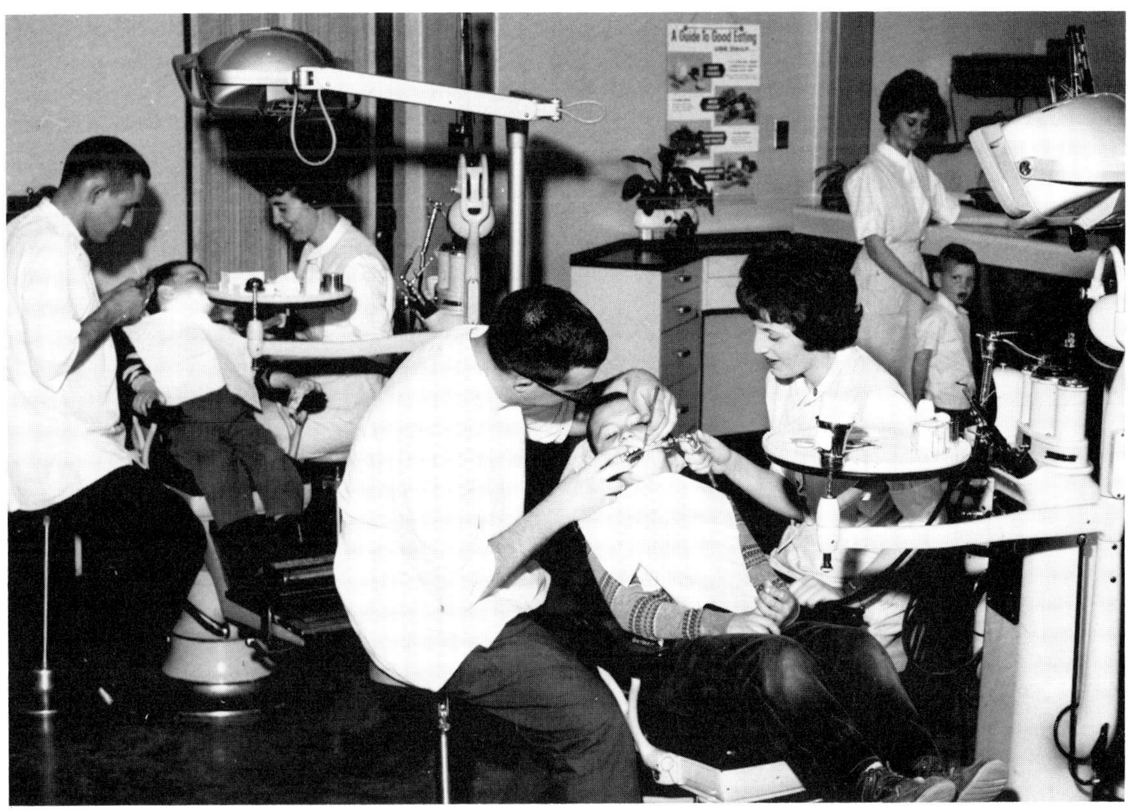

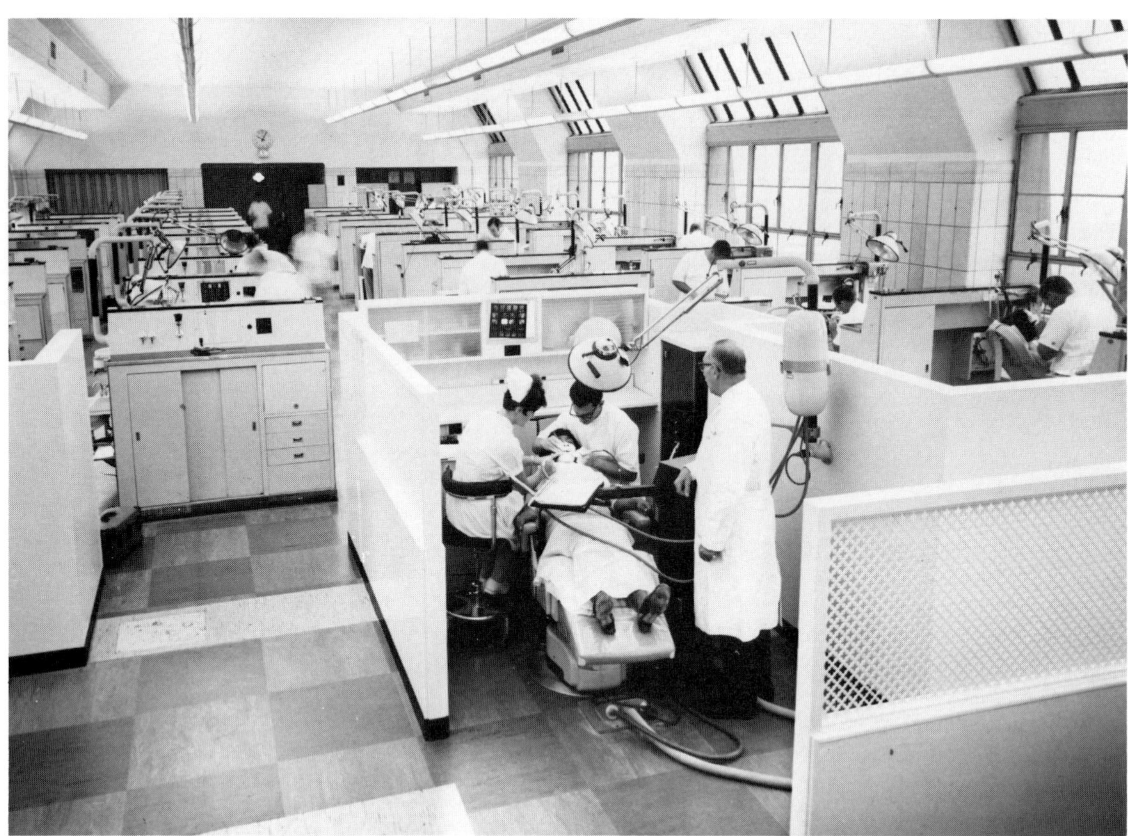

The operative dental clinic in the older building of the University of Illinois in 1969. The cubicle concept was tried out as the enclosure in the foreground indicates, while the remainder of the students work in the usual way standing up beside their patients. The instructor observes a student and his assistant working on a patient. This cubicle concept of dental care was adopted as new dental schools were built. From College of Dentistry of the University of Illinois.

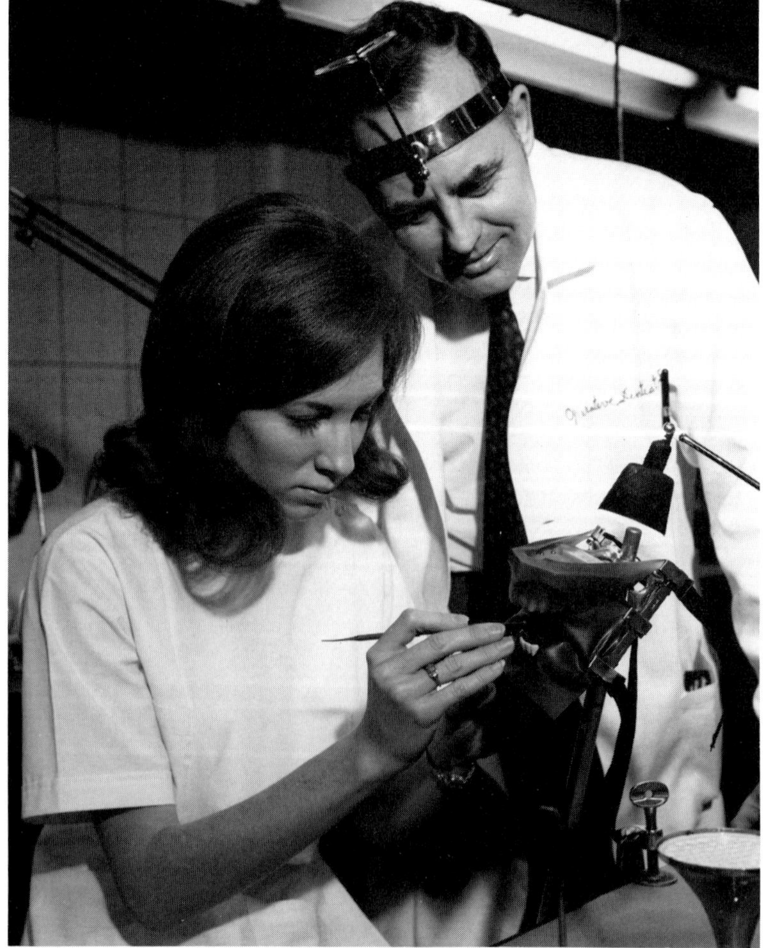

Dental student working on her dentiform in the late 1960s. The dentist is wearing a magnification loup. From College of Dentistry of the University of Illinois.

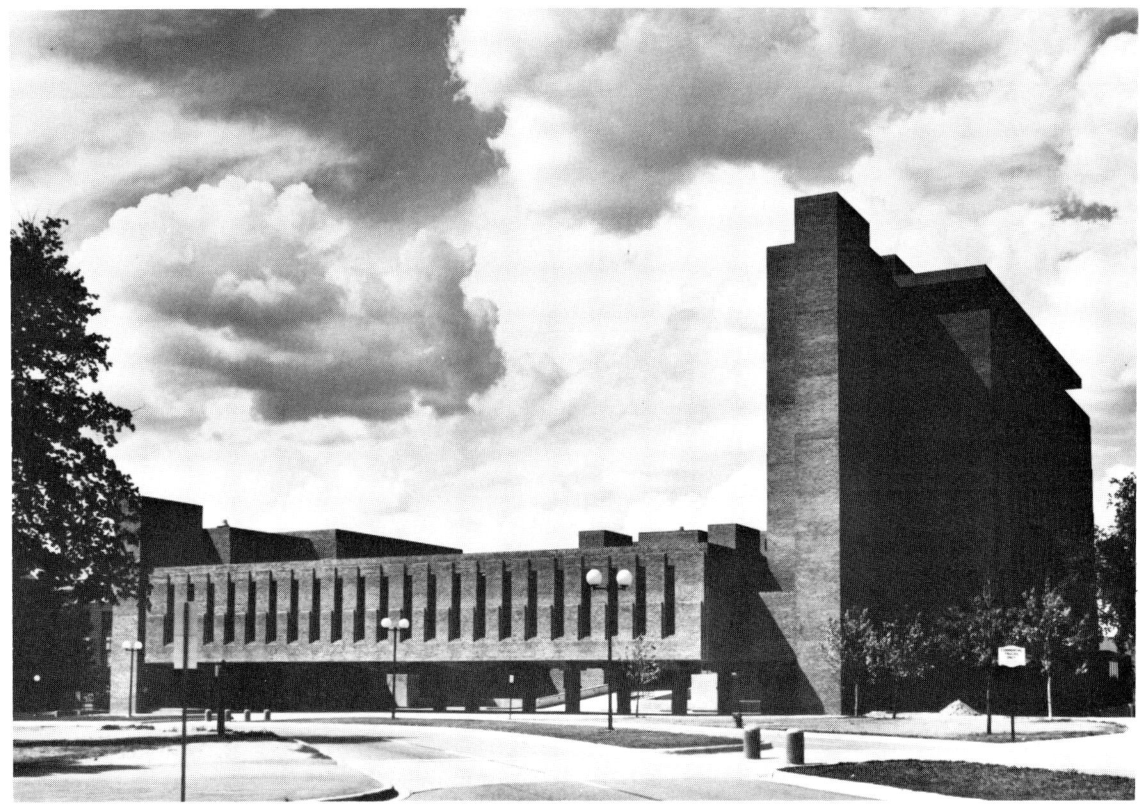

School of Dentistry, University of Michigan, in its sixth building, erected in 1969. The fifth building, the W.K. Kellogg Institute was the first building in the world to be devoted exclusively to graduate and postgraduate teaching in dentistry. From University of Michigan School of Dentistry.

Student operatories in 1971. The junior and senior clinics are divided into four quadrants containing 36 operatories each. Each operatory is partitioned to give patients and students privacy during treatment. All units may be adapted for the use of right- or left-handed students. From University of Michigan School of Dentistry.

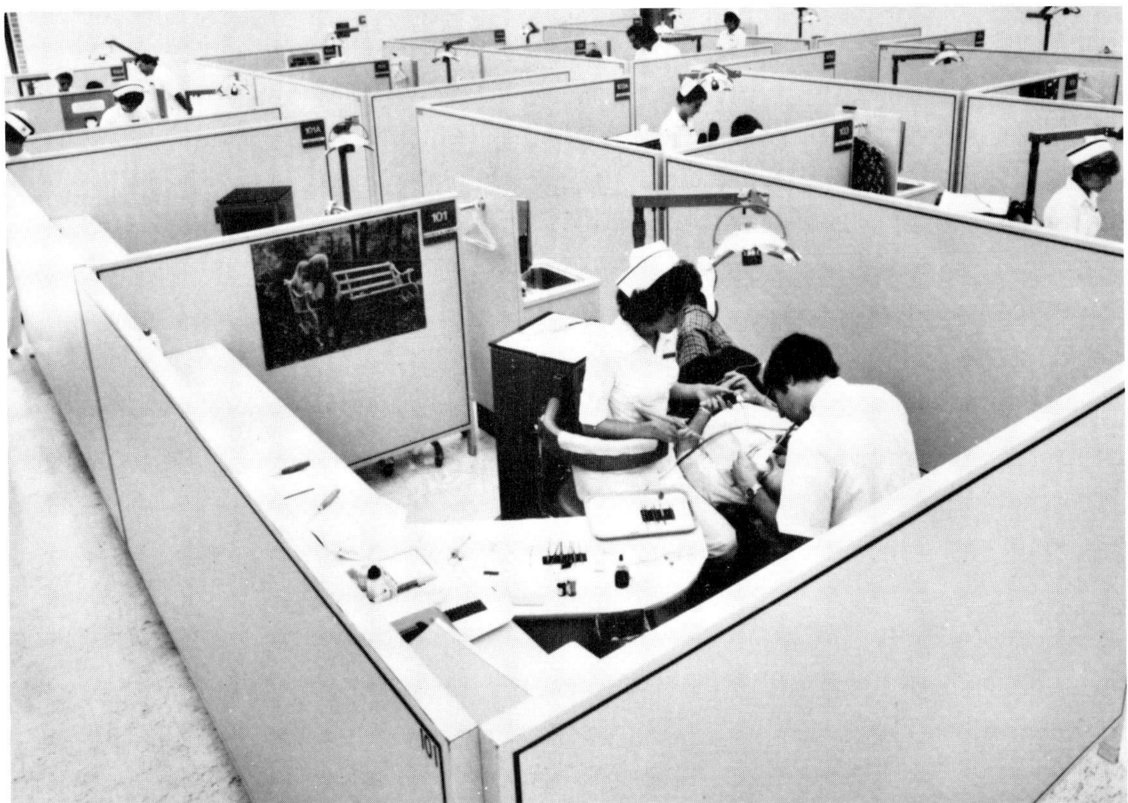

Student with patient and assistant in 1986 at Howard University College of Dentistry. This school was founded in 1881 as the first dental school to educate blacks, women and other minorities. From Howard University College of Dentistry.

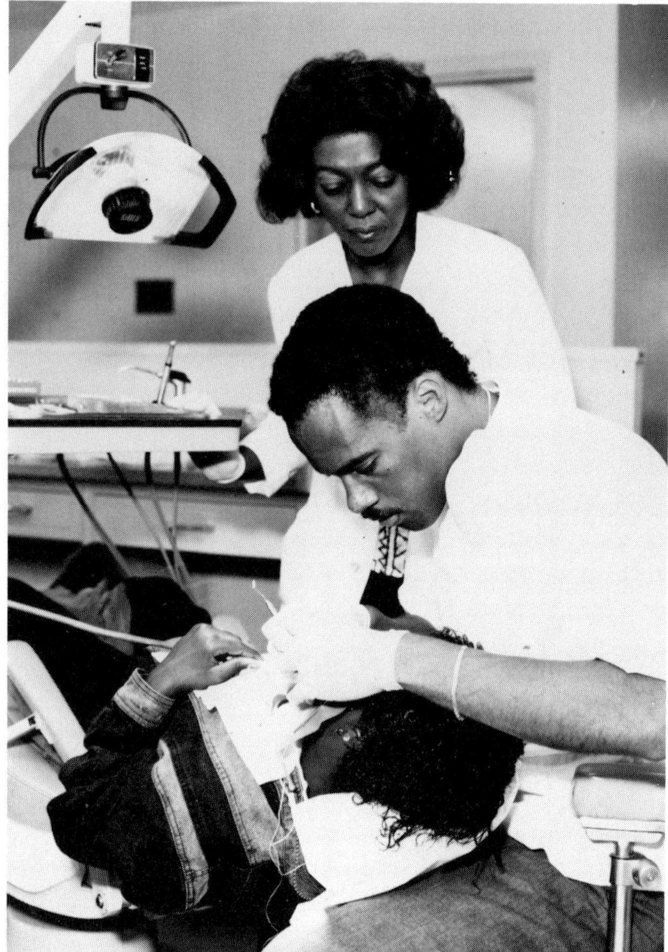

Freshman and sophomore preclinical laboratories contain 154 work places in 1971. Television monitors are connected to the main studio, but may also be used for viewing live television demonstrations made in the laboratory. From University of Michigan School of Dentistry.

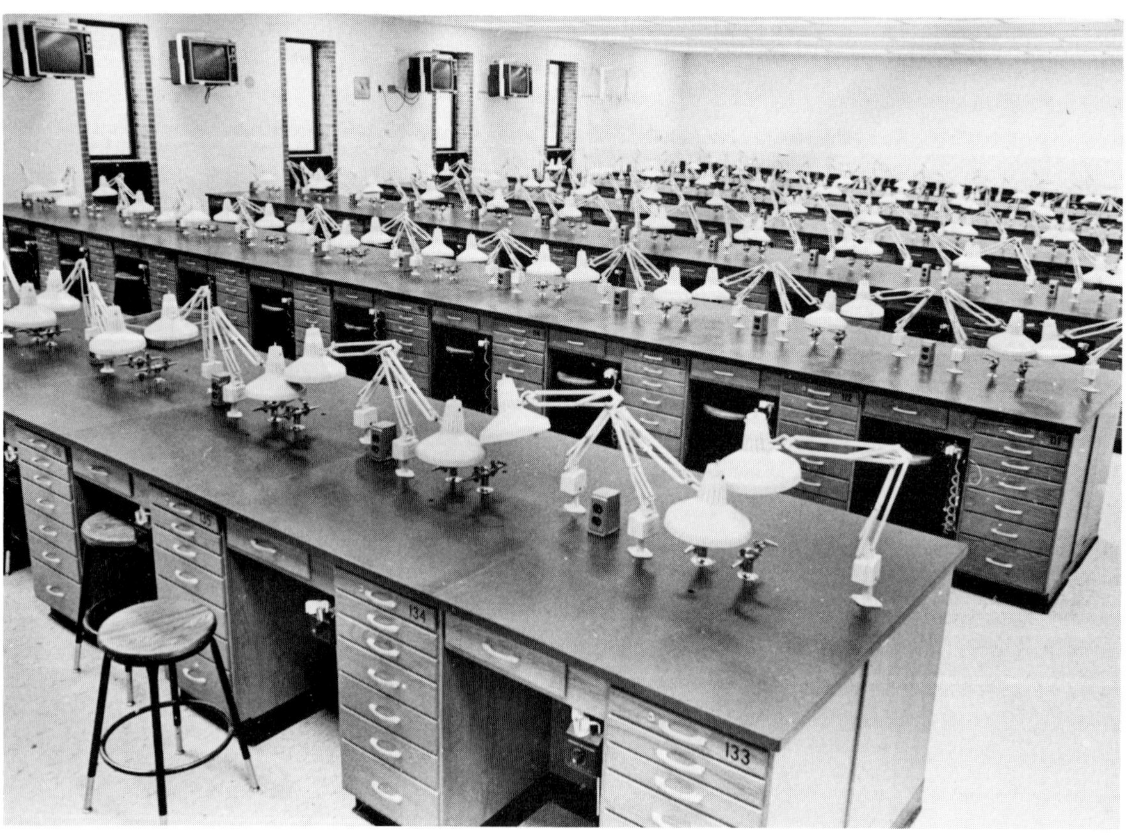

CHAPTER TEN

Women Become Dentists

An important benefit of the system which permitted those without a dental school education to practice dentistry was to allow talented women and men to become dentists who lacked the resources to attend a dental school. In a period when women were denied access to professional schools, they could demonstrate their skills by practicing under the supervision of, or serving an apprenticeship to, a dentist. Among women dentists who did not attend dental school were a few outstanding practitioners. By taking advantage of the opportunity to enter the dental profession before they were permitted to attend dental school female dentists proved their capability and "earned" the right to become graduate dentists.

The first female dentist, Emeline Roberts Jones began to practice in 1854, after being instructed by her dentist husband. She convinced him that she had the talent to practice dentistry by learning to fill the extracted teeth she obtained from his office, without revealing what she was doing until she had filled hundreds of teeth successfully. Without ever attending dental school she carried on her husband's practice for half a century after his death. Her excellence in dentistry was rewarded by her election to membership in the Connecticut State Dental Society. The National Dental Association made her an honorary member in 1914.[81]

Lucy Hobbs Taylor (1833-1910) learned dentistry as an apprentice before she became the first woman to receive a dental degree in the U.S. She began her dental career in 1859 after a three month apprenticeship with Samuel Wardle, a young graduate of the Ohio College of Dentistry. While assisting Wardle she supported herself by sewing. Her skill in carving teeth was rewarded with a first prize in the Mechanics Fair held the same year in Cincinnati. Twice she was refused entrance to the Ohio College of Dental Surgery but was advised by Wardle to practice dentistry without a degree, as so many others were doing at the time. She opened her first office in a small, red-brick building on West Fourth Street in Cincinnati on March 14, 1861. A month later, the Civil War began and her practice deteriorated. Hoping to treat more patients by moving further from the war zone, she moved to a second office in Bellevue, Iowa. Her next location was in McGregor, Iowa. She bought a new dental chair and set up her third office, in which she practiced until November 1865, when she was admitted to the Ohio College of Dental Surgery. Due to her experience she soon fulfilled the requirements for a degree and graduated on February 21, 1866. Dental schools with a longer history were slower to allow women to graduate as dentists. The first woman to graduate from the first dental school, the Baltimore College of Dental Surgery was a Prussian, Emilie Foecking, who received her degree in 1873.

Hobbs Taylor's fourth office was opened at 93 Washington Street in Chicago. The following year she married James Myrtle Taylor. To live in a better climate they moved to Lawrence, Kansas, where she settled in her fifth and last office and taught her husband dentistry. Together they practiced until his death in 1886, having achieved the most lucrative dental practice in Kansas by 1874. She continued to practice until her death on October 3, 1910.[82]

At the time Lucy Hobbs Taylor graduated there were about two dozen women practicing dentistry in America. By 1880 there were 611, and then, a decade later, the number decreased to 337.[83] There were 10 times as many female medical students as dental students at the end of the century.[84]

Ida Gray, graduate of the class of 1890 of the University of Michigan School of Dentistry, was the first black woman to receive a D.D.S. degree and the first black woman to practice in Chicago. At the time of Gray's graduation the dental school had matriculated 22 women. Gray (pictured on page 48) was born in 1867 or 1870 in Cincinnati and was encouraged by Jonathan Taft, founding dean of the Michigan school and supporter of women dentists. Her interest in dentistry began as an apprentice in Taft's office. She lived to be 87.[85]

Women dentists also were encouraged to become dentists for reasons other than their dental skills. In 1859, in response to Dr. D.W. Jobson's efforts to bring women into dentistry an editorial in the *Cincinnati Dental Reporter* stated:

> We heartily second [Dr. Jobson's efforts]. Even now we almost imagine ourselves seated in what is usually termed the "chair of Torture" — dreaded now no more — by our side a beautiful lady, with sweet breath and glowing cheek, her delicate arm encircling our head, our cheek resting against a bosom still more soft, looking up into her eyes, so tender in their gaze — they take away all dread, and in their sympathy even divide the pain itself. With such a dentist, we would want our teeth examined every twenty-four hours.[86]

Women dentists who practiced in the 19th century usually treated women and children.[87] Female dentists were thought to have a special "touch" with children. This skill, helped to stereotype women as dentists for their own sex. The first dental practice devoted entirely to children, which was established in California by a female dentist in the early 20th century is discussed on page 125-26.

Women joined the staff in the dental office even before they became dentists. There are instances of women assisting dentists, not uncommonly, their husbands or fathers, in the first half of the 19th century. In 1843 Dr. N.W. Kingsley discovered that

> When she becomes familiar with the details of practice, she will perform all operations required upon deciduous teeth, including fillings with any of the plastics, she will take entire charge of the regulating cases, and that branch of practice, so dreaded by all because of the apparent waste of time, in the rearrangement of splints, becomes in her hands a valuable source of income. In short, it is impossible to enumerate in detail the acquirements she will come to possess.[88]

Splints made out of wood, gutta-percha and vulcanized rubber were used to treat fractures of the maxillary bone.[89]

The next instance of a dentist employing a woman assistant occurred for another reason — to overcome the fears of the unescorted female patient. C Edmund Kells, whose office is discussed below, made a striking change in his office by employing a woman in 1885 to replace a black man, who had served as his assistant. A female assistant in the office calmed women patients, who now felt more comfortable going alone to the dentist. Kells advertised his accommodation to his patients on a sign placed outside the office which read "Lady Attendant"[90] Fifteen years later Kells employed a female secretary in his office.

The specific chores of the assistant demanded the skills of a dexterous and orderly person. Assistants were drawn into those aspects of the practice of dentistry which were tedious to the dentist. Cleaning teeth was monotonous and even annoyed the dentist. Relief from these procedures rested on the woman assistant. Myer L. Rhein, whose office and practice also is described on page 101, employed a "dental nurse" in 1903 to carry out prophylactic treatments, a practice which he innovated. Rhein's first attempt to get assistance in cleaning the patient's teeth was to employ a recent dental graduate as his assistant practitioner. The young dentist soon left to establish his own practice. Rhein explained the dentist's position:

> . . . It certainly is the consensus of professional opinion that the busy practitioner cannot give up his valuable time for this tedious monotonous, and irksome labor, however important it may be for the salvation of the human teeth. A small number of us have tried to solve this important problem by employing an assistant practitioner to attend to this department. In twelve years it has failed to satisfactorily solve the problem.[91]

In 1913 the term "dental hygienist" was applied to the woman assistant, a term derived from the term "dental hygiene" which was used initially by Dr. A. Arthur of Baltimore in 1871, to mean the effort on the part of the public to maintain a clean mouth.[92] After we discuss the intervening evolution of the dental office, primarily without dental assistants, we will return and discuss the expanding role of the female dental assistant.

CHAPTER ELEVEN

Equipping the Dental Office

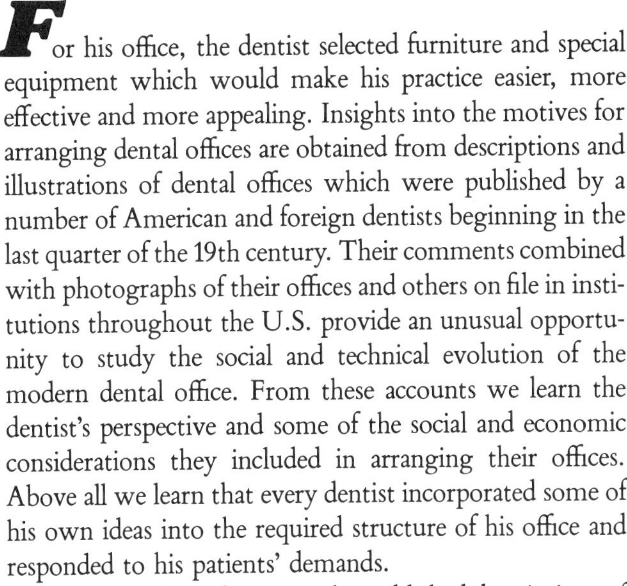

For his office, the dentist selected furniture and special equipment which would make his practice easier, more effective and more appealing. Insights into the motives for arranging dental offices are obtained from descriptions and illustrations of dental offices which were published by a number of American and foreign dentists beginning in the last quarter of the 19th century. Their comments combined with photographs of their offices and others on file in institutions throughout the U.S. provide an unusual opportunity to study the social and technical evolution of the modern dental office. From these accounts we learn the dentist's perspective and some of the social and economic considerations they included in arranging their offices. Above all we learn that every dentist incorporated some of his own ideas into the required structure of his office and responded to his patients' demands.

Among those dentists, who published descriptions of their offices, in the American dental journals, *Items of Interest* sponsored by the Wilmington Dental Manufacturing Company, and *Northwestern Dental Journal, Dental Survey* and *Journal of the American Dental Association* were a cross section of the successful and average practitioners who expressed their enthusiasm for certain aspects of their offices, as well as their discontent with their shortcomings. From their descriptions and the rationale provided for specific physical arrangements, we can begin to understand how the dentist viewed his role as a professional and as a person seeking the confidence and patronage of the public for his services. We also learn how the dentist articulated the economic, social and cultural issues which entered into his decisions and compelled him to make choices among furnishings, equipment and locale. Among the dentists with the most admired offices were those who led the profession in making the public more conscious of their own role in dental hygiene, as well as, expanding the office and those employed in it to provide a variety of services to reach the goal of healthier teeth and gums for more people.

Rodrigues Ottolengui of New York City, the new editor of *Items of Interest* in 1896 introduced a regular feature in the journal which he called "Office and Laboratory." He invited all dentists with planned offices to send in descriptions and photographs of their offices. After accounts of several offices had been published and others had been received which he found less informative than he had expected, he published in 1897, a description of his own office to demonstrate the type of information he was seeking.[93] It was his belief that a dentist wishing to attract "the better classes" should place his office in a residence on a private street. However, he acknowledged that within all cities except New York, it was also permissible to establish an office in an apartment or commercial building. At this time dentists were beginning to install offices in multi-purpose commercial buildings within the city, rather than in their private residences, although some dentists continue to maintain offices in their homes.

The main feature in Ottolengui's office was his dental cabinet. Designed and arranged to embellish the office, as well as, serve its purpose of storing the myriad of dental instruments and supplies, Ottolengui claimed that his cabinet was superior to the most complete cabinet for sale by a dental manufacturer at $125, which he criticized as "a hideous piece of walnut furniture." Ottolengui bought a sideboard from a furniture dealer and converted the pedestals on each end into a medicine closet. He removed the ornaments from the pedestals and applied them to the closet doors. "The three large drawers of the sideboard were replaced with eight drawers of increasing depth, the shallower ones at the top for small instruments, and the others for appliances."[94] The contents of each drawer were determined by its location and the ease of access to it.

Models of teeth and regulating cases were stored in the upper closets for immediate access. The lower drawer, of least use, became a depository for unread articles, "unarticulated models of irregularities, sent by dentists seeking advice which they deem of too little value to send stamp for reply, and other things of a similar nature, all of which are cleaned out once a year."[95] The drawers containing instruments were constructed without a bottom so that the in-

Latest Dentistry

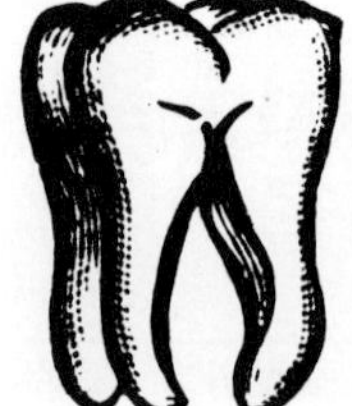

SET TEETH, $5.[50]

BEST SET, $8.[00]

No Better Made at Any Price

Gold Fillings and Bridge Work a Specialty

TEETH EXTRACTED

Positively without Pain

DR. C. L. HILL has secured the exclusive right to use "*TONALGIA*" for his Albany office. It is the most satisfactory local anæsthetic ever used.

Teeth Extracted, 25c.; Local application or Vitalized Air, for the painless extraction of teeth, 50c.; Teeth filed with Amalgam, 25c.; Alloy 50c.; Silver 75c.; Gold $1 00 and up.

If you wish GOLD CAPS on your teeth or teeth without plates called BRIDGE WORK, call and get our prices and references from the best people in this country.

DR. C. L. HILL'S DENTAL CO.

34 North Pearl Street,

Opp. John G. Myers ALBANY, N. Y.

LADY IN ATTENDANCE

A typical late 19th century dentist's advertisement. Note the last line "lady in attendance," a practice provided by dentists to attract female patients and make it convenient for them to go to the dental office, unaccompanied. From the Warshaw Collection, National Museum of American History Archives, Smithsonian Institution, Neg. No. 74-6514.

struments were placed on a sheet of blotting paper which could be replaced when soiled, and the drawers cleaned without allowing dust to remain in the corners. The top of the lower half of the cabinet was covered with a piece of olive green leather which the owner found most serviceable and able to withstand constant use. Ottolengui used the cabinet while sitting or standing and to do some operations normally carried out in the laboratory. He worked without an assistant.

Charles Edmund Kells (1856-1928), a pioneer in the use of X-ray equipment to determine the extent of decay in teeth in 1896 and one of the first dentists to employ a female dental assistant in 1885, provided a description of his office in 1897, which garnered 50 requests for his floor plan in the month after it was published. Kells stated the underlying criterion all dentists should use in arranging their offices when he wrote: "There is no reason why a dentist should not be in the midst of as pleasant surroundings in his office as he is at home; and, as the nature of his work and his callers permit it, he should take the same pride in one as in the other."[96] Other dentists such as F.P. Cronkhite of St. Joseph, Missouri agreed with Kells and broadened the position the dentist should take in furnishing his office. For Cronkhite the "office may be furnished in such a manner as not to attract the attention of any particular class of patients. This is the best proof of good taste."[97] Based on his practice Kells assumed that most patients were women, a statistic that remains accurate today, and he believed that a dentist would obtain more female patients if he set up an attractively arranged and well-lighted reception room.

Kells joined most other dentists of the period in stressing good light and ventilation in the rooms of a dental suite. In an office structure where space was rented, it became economically essential to organize within the smallest space, a series of rooms to be used to receive patients, to operate, to consult, to relax in, and as a laboratory and storeroom.

Kells' father, who was a noted dentist in New Orleans, exposed him to some of the rigors of dentistry. Kells' experiences as a child gave him early insights into the changing methods in dentistry and some of their consequences. One episode impressed him with the dangers of dental practice and the unusual expectations of the patient. Kells related in his autobiography published in 1926 the incident of a man who went one evening to have a tooth extracted from a leading dentist, not his father.

> The patient was seated in the chair, and besides the ordinary gas jet in the room, a candle was held by someone in order to light up the mouth.
>
> The ether spray was started, and the first thing the dentist knew, he saw everything enveloped in a flame. He was 'scared to death,' as the saying is, and the candle holder 'liked to have dropped dead with fright,' and started to back away from the chair.
>
> As soon as the candle was removed a little distance, the blaze went out—it was the vapor of the ether that had caught fire.
>
> Then composure was regained, and the operation was concluded (more carefully, as far as the candle was concerned) satisfactorily.
>
> Meanwhile, the patient had never 'batted an eye.' When all was over, the dentist began complimenting the patient upon his nerve upon not being frightened by the fire. 'Fire? What fire?' 'Why, when the flame shot up.' 'Oh, I thought that was part of the process.' Can you beat that for a *real, true story upon local anesthesia*?[98]

A lesson Kells learned so dramatically, others learned in the dental school classroom. Edward Cook Mills, graduate of the University of Michigan Dental School in 1889 wrote in the margin of his notebook on the subject of ether anesthesia "do not use at night, for light use (gas) may cause explosion."[99]

Kells began to assist his father in 1874 before he graduated from the New York College of Dentistry in 1878. While in New York he became friends with Thomas Edison's assistant in Menlo Park, New Jersey, which sparked his life-long interest in electricity that he later incorporated into his practice of dentistry. Kells' first dental office was located on the fifth floor of a building in New Orleans. He had leased the space before construction of the building, and therefore, had an opportunity to have rooms designed according to his special needs. His first operating room in 1878 was simply furnished with "a chair, operated by hand cranks, old-fashioned cuspidor, a Morrison foot engine, cabinet and a washstand . . ."[100] Electric lighting, fans, call bells, hot-water heating and plumbing were arranged to allow the "maximum amount of work to be accomplished with the expenditure of a minimum amount of time and worry," and thus, "the work of the day [was] a pleasure."[101]

When the Edison Electric Light Company first supplied electrical power to large firms in New Orleans, Kells arranged to have electricity supplied to his office. He wired the office by himself and connected it to the power source on the street. He became the first dentist in this city to use street current to power a motor to run dental instruments

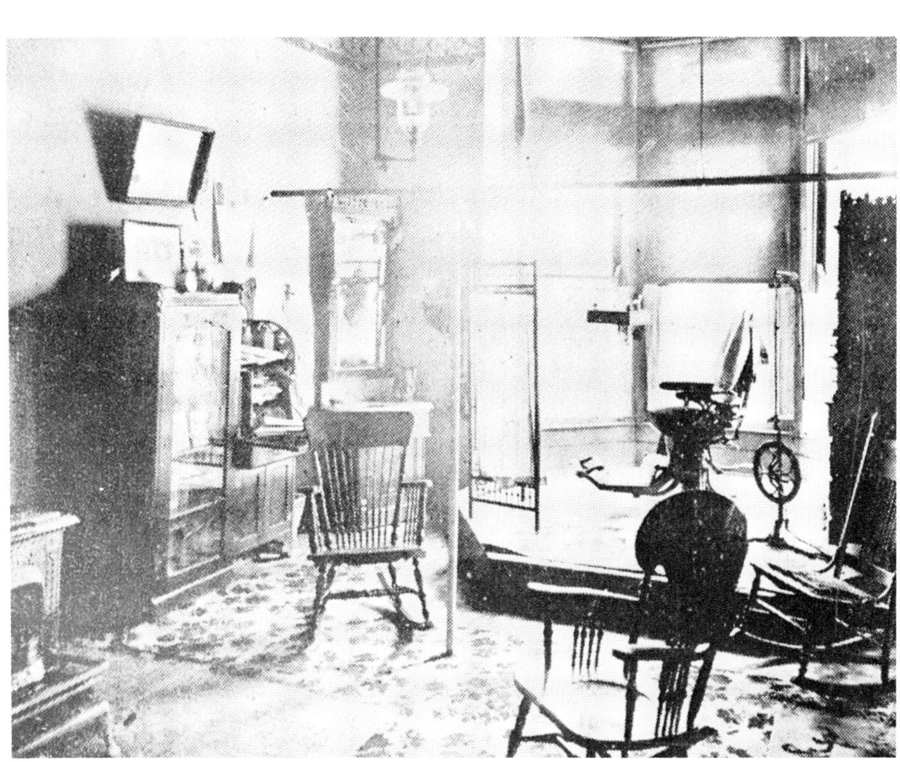

Dental parlor of Dr. Smith of Rushville, Indiana. This dental office is typical of an early to mid-19th century office located in the dentist's home, in which the dental chair is placed on a platform in front of the bay window (sunlight being the best source of light until electric lamps became available at the end of the century). The shades provided the only method of regulating the light entering the room. The foot-pedal drill stands to the right of the chair and the bracket table which holds the dentist's instruments is attached to the wall between the windows to the left. Screens separate the operatory from the waiting room in the foreground. A gas lamp is suspended from the ceiling in the waiting room and is located in the upper left center of the picture. Gas lamps were sometimes used to provide light for the dentist while working on a patient's teeth, occasionally with tragic results when ether was used for an anesthetic. From Indiana Historical Society and published in *Commercial History of Rushville and Rush County*, compiled by George L. Johnson, 1899, pg. 91.

The dental office in Kendallville, Indiana in 1874 was a residence with the office on the first floor and the family quarters upstairs. This office was unique because it contained a separate waiting room, there was more than one operatory and it used a commercially manufactured dental chair. A stove heated the office. From Indiana Historical Society and on pg. 8 of Richard Glenner's, *The Dental Office*.

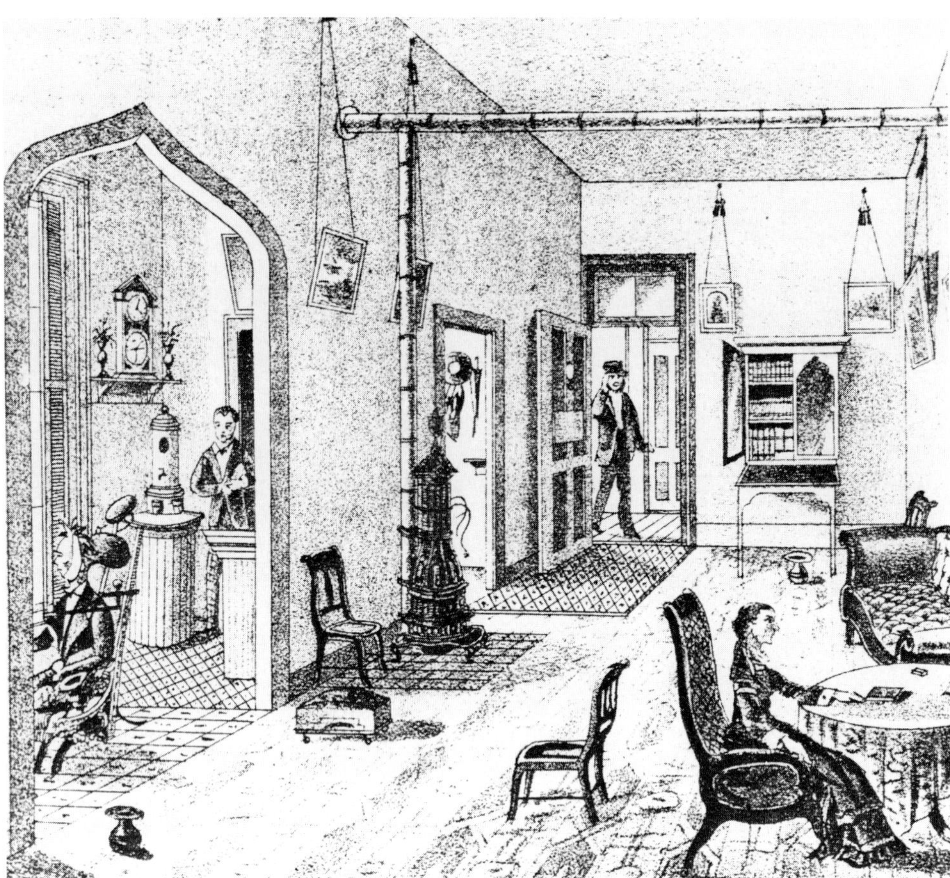

and machinery. Kells designed a rheostat to control the current to his instruments, an electric cabinet to store the instruments, and an electric lamp to use while working on the patient. He arranged the engine belts, pulleys, rheostat and foot control in one dental unit. A prolific inventor, Kells obtained over 30 patents including those for an electric thermostat, fire extinguisher and alarm, electromagnetic clock, automobile starter, sanitary faucet and a drinking fountain.

The most significant equipment Kells applied to dentistry was the X-ray machine to diagnose tooth and gum disease. In 1896 with the help of a physics professor at Tulane University, Brown Ayres, Kells acquired a Crooke's tube and a Tesla coil to use in his office to take skiagraphs (radiographs) of his patient's teeth.[102] Kells installed the first commercially made X-ray unit specifically designed for dental use which was sold in 1913. These original items and some of Kells' office equipment are on exhibition in the National Museum of American History where they were placed, along with G.V. Black's office, 25 years ago.[103]

Among his inventions which were most widely adopted by dentists, physicians and surgeons was a suction apparatus used to remove fluids and irrigate body cavities during surgical operations. This apparatus replaced the method of mopping up blood and fluids with surgical sponges.

Kells designed his dental cabinet. It was 3 feet long, 3 feet high and 20 inches wide, containing 26 drawers, varying in depth from three-fourths of an inch to 4 inches. There were two compartments with doors. Six drawers and both compartments opened from either side, so that the dentist's assistant could also use them. The assistant's items included napkins for wiping the instruments and strops, and polishing powders for keeping the instruments shining. Kells fitted one of the drawers, with a removable bench block for use as a temporary laboratory bench.

Among the thoughtful items Kells provided, to use on the patient, was a pot of warm water which he used to syringe cavities, instead of drawing cold water directly from the tap that inflicted discomfort in addition to the tooth under treatment.

Kells remained in this office for 13 years, and then, practiced for 17 more years on Canal Street in the Maison Blanche building, in a 12th floor suite, built to his specifications in 1907. This office offered two excellent views, one of the Mississippi River from the reception room. The operatory window opened out on Lake Pontchartrain.[104] Major B. Varnado joined Kells in 1918 and practiced until his death in 1971 in the same office.[105] In keeping with his views that the office, and especially, the operating room was the center of the dentist's working space, Kells insisted that the colors in the room not be harmful to the dentist's eyes. Thus he rejected the fashion for light-colored or white walls, which developed during the pre-World War I years,

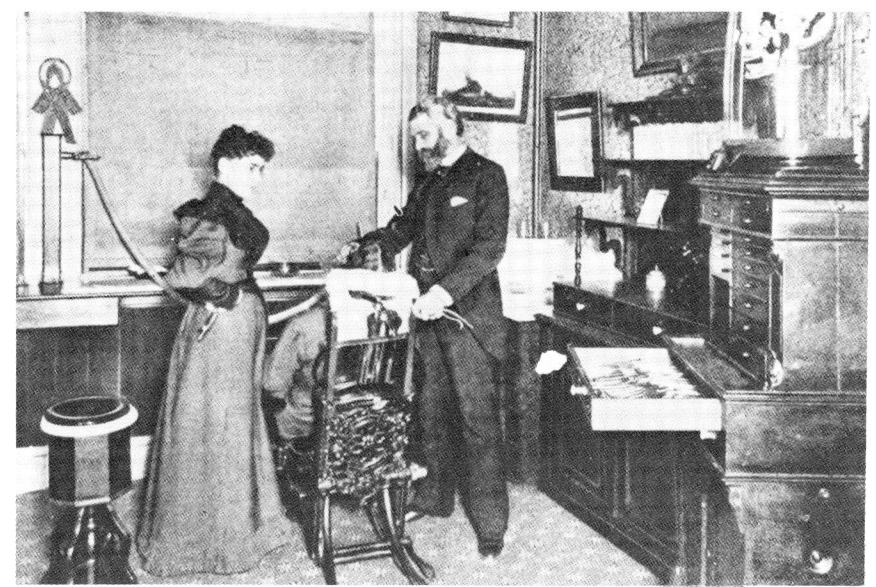

Office circa, 1880-1890. In this office the dentist wears street clothes, a patient is seated in the Morrison chair, and a female assists the dentist. The Morrison chair, produced in 1872, was the first to allow sufficient vertical movement to permit the dentist to work standing up or seated. Note the dental cabinet on the right with one drawer open and a human skull under a bell jar on top of the cabinet. A few female dental assistants were first employed in dental offices in the 1880s. They were trained by the dentist until the first school for dental assistants was opened in 1913 by Dr. Alfred Fones in Bridgeport, Connecticut. The first graduate, Irene Newman received license Number One in Connecticut, the first state to issue a license to dental hygienists. Fones insisted on distinguishing the dental assistant or hygienist from the dentist by keeping the duties separate. From *History of the Connecticut State Dental Association*, 1956, pg. 82.

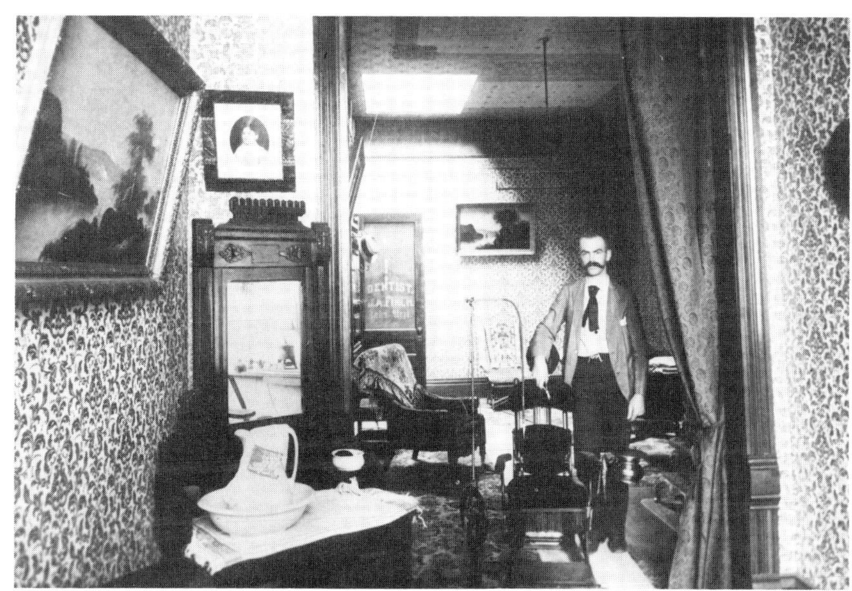

Dr. D.A. Finch in the early 1890s in his office in Grand Island, Nebraska. The German words for dentist "Zahn Arzt" are lettered on his office door, reflecting his ethnic background and that of his patients. He holds a forceps in his right hand and his chair is flanked by a foot-pedal drill on the right and a spittoon on the left. From Stuhr Museum of the Prairie Pioneer, Grand Island, Nebraska.

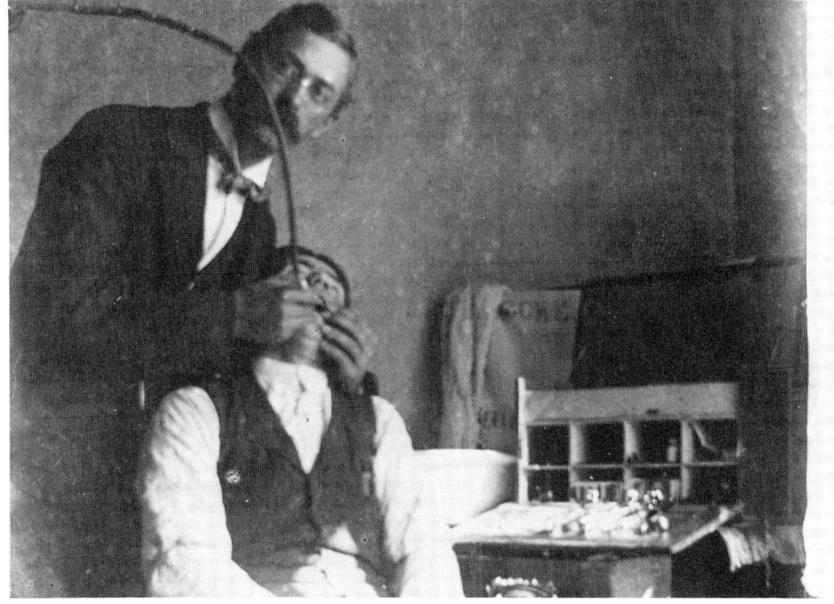

Frank Bloom, dentist and Alfred Jonason, patient in Chicago City, Minnesota, circa 1895. This rare frontal view of the dentist and patient in the course of treatment with the dental drill, also shows a small cabinet with eight compartments for storage and a surface for placing the instruments and items needed to clean out and fill a decayed tooth. The basin to the left of the cabinet indicates the dentist worked without running water and, of course, did not take precautions to minimize bacterial infection by wearing a clean white office jacket, rubber gloves, etc. American dentists, by and large, did not try to keep instruments bacteria-free and the office environment spotlessly clean until the early 20th century. From Minnesota Historical Society, Neg. No. 17846.

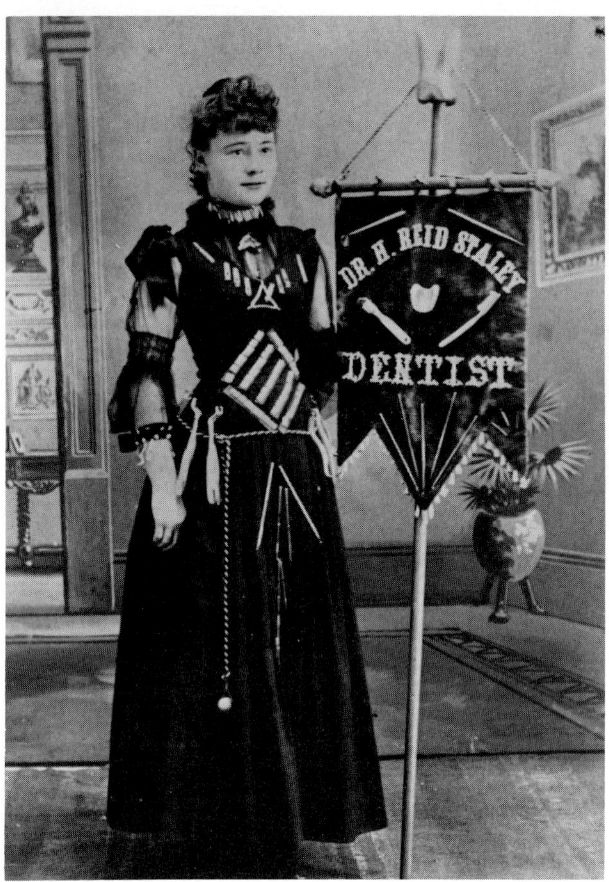

Female dentist or dental assistant advertising for a dentist.

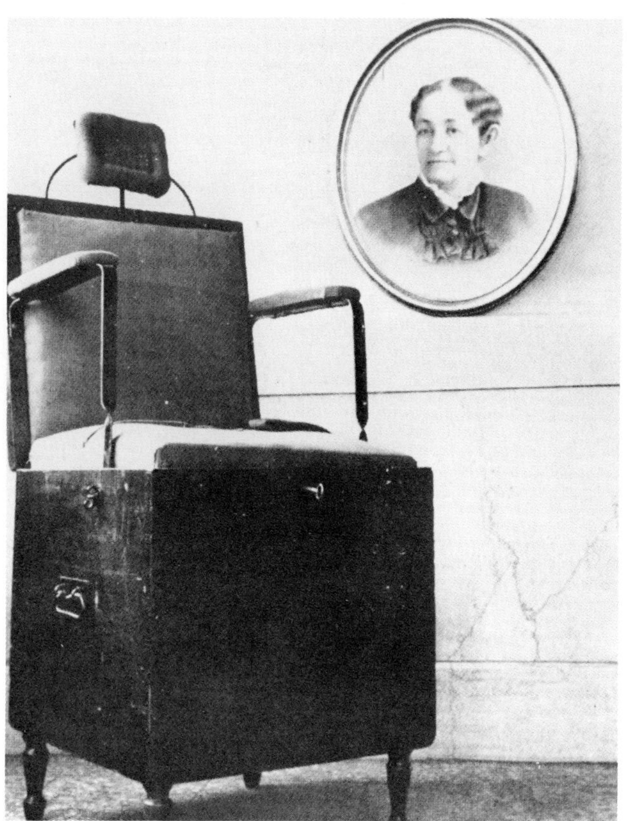

Emeline Roberts Jones, first female dentist in America. She married a dentist in 1854. Although she wanted to learn dentistry he would not support her effort because he believed that women did not have the stamina and dexterity to become dentists. She perfected the techniques of preserving teeth, in secret, by filling hundreds of extracted teeth, and then, was allowed to join her husband's practice. Ten years later, upon her husband's death, she took over his practice which she continued for another half century. She was elected to membership in the Connecticut State Dental Association and the National Dental Association in 1914. From *History of the Connecticut State Dental Association*, 1956.

in an effort to create a sterile office environment. The upper portion of the walls of his operating room were painted a mat green beneath a cream-colored ceiling. The lower four feet of wall space in the room was covered with a green tile wainscoting. On the floor he placed a dark rug which reflected little light. The woodwork was made of mahogany. The color of mahogany wood was considered restful to the dentist's eyes and was promoted by a leading dental manufacturer, The Ritter Dental Manufacturing Company. In a manual published in 1924 entitled, *Practice Building Suggestions*, mahogany finished equipment was suggested as a restful color for use by nervous dentists.

> If a dentist is continually working under high tension, mahogany finishes would be most desirable for him, for the reason that mahogany in itself suggests quietness and would help to tone down the dentist. Oftentimes a nervous condition in the dentist can be traced to operating room cross lights playing on the improper wall treatment, and this effect is intensified in the light finishes of equipment used."[106]

Kells accepted the Ritter Dental Manufacturing Company suggestion of providing a retiring room for female patients furnished with a mirror and dressing table.[107] Amenities included sterilized combs in onionskin envelopes, individual books of powder (papier poudre), cotton balls and pins for their hair. In this room they could apply make-up and re-style their hair after a session in the dental chair. However by the mid-20s, Kells noticed that women no longer insisted on having a special room to apply their cosmetics, but would hastily make adjustments in the elevator. For patients who might become faint he provided a small lounge to recline upon.

Neatness and order pervaded Kells' laboratory as well as the office. He commented on the excellent laboratories he had visited and advised dentists to keep them as clean as the rest of their office by employing a housekeeper. Maintenance included polishing the vulcanizer regularly and taking items off the shelves and wiping them down periodically. The Ritter Company recommended putting a wire net over

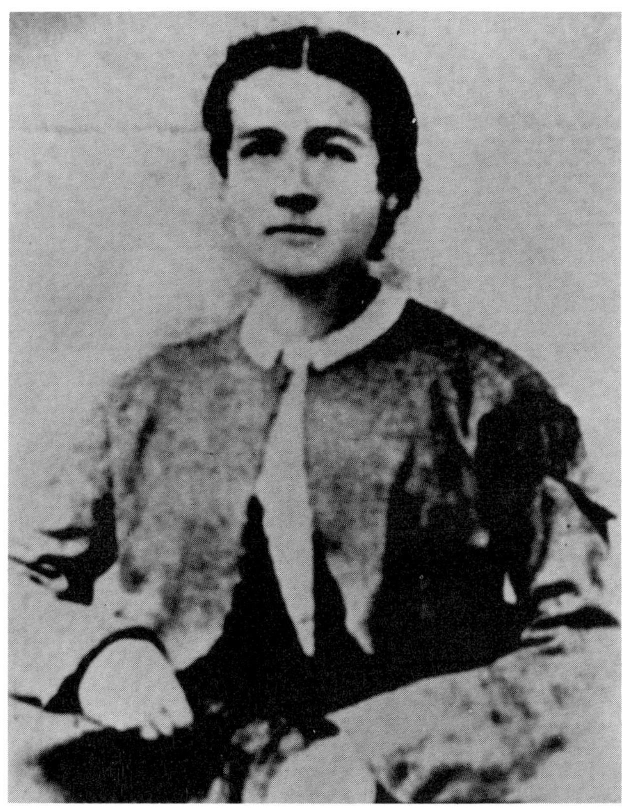

A pioneer female American dentist, who had to win over the male dental establishment by herself, Lucy Beaman Hobbs Taylor (1833-1910), who practiced in the Midwest. After many rejections from schools and preceptors, she was the first woman to receive a degree in dentistry in 1866, which was awarded by the Ohio College of Dental Surgery, and in that year, at the age of 33, she posed for this portrait.

the floor to increase resilience and prevent small items, such as a crown, from rolling after it was dropped.[108]

Kells not only promoted total cleanliness in the dental suite, he also urged that as much dental equipment as possible be kept out of sight of the patient. He believed that "The fewer the instruments and mechanical appliances to greet the new patient, the better."[109] Patients who came into the dental office in fear were most apt to respond to an equipment-loaded space, especially when outfitted with bulbs, wires and similar apparatus as if it were "an executioner's stall." One patient remarked to Kells that his office did not terrify her as did another dentist's chair and instruments.

Kells was a frugal and unpretentious dentist who valued simplicity, and favored using the latest dental instruments and methods. Other dentists built up large practices and served a clientele that responded to a gracious and luxurious office setting. An office of this type is illustrated in the practice of Myer L. Rhein (1860-1928) of New York City. From 1881 until his death in 1928, Rhein operated in an elaborate office, which he constructed and outfitted. After apprenticing to his father, a dentist in Albany, New York, Rhein received his medical degree from Albany Medical College in 1880, and then, a year later, his D.D.S. from the University of Pennsylvania School of Dentistry. Rhein participated in dental societies at local, state and national levels. He continued to learn new techniques by attending clinics in Europe. In 1884 in his paper on "Oral Hygiene,"[101] Rhein described a toothbrush with three rows of serrated bristles which he obtained from a Parisian dentist. He improved it by enlarging the hole in the handle so the brush could be hung up after use, thereby shortening the drying time through ventilation to keep the brush fresh.[111] Along with the "Pro-phy-lac-tic Tooth Brush" for which he received a patent in 1884, Rhein advertised waxed dental floss to promote healthier teeth. He also proposed that the local Board of Education begin an oral hygiene program for school children. He became, in 1893, one of the first dentists to use electrolytic medication for sterilization of the gums or periapical areas and root canals.

In a two-story, remodeled dwelling on East Sixty-first Street, Rhein added an extension at the rear for the operating rooms and laboratory.[112] The sumptuous entrance consisted of two oak-framed storm doors, inset with beveled French plate glass, leading to a vestibule lined with quartered oak and a mosaic tile floor. Behind this entrance was a second pair of oak-framed glass doors. A butler greeted the patient and signaled by a call button, Dr. Rhein or his partner, Dr. C.L. Andrews, in the rear of the building.

Through the hallway covered with Oriental rugs the patient passed to the reception room with its papered walls and comfortable chairs. Amber glass filtered the light so that a soft glow of sunlight appeared to shine through continuously. In a bookcase hidden from view was located a safe.

Next to this room was a lavatory. Down a flight of stairs was the dental laboratory and next to it, Dr. Andrews' office, which was opposite Dr. Rhein's office. Beneath the windows in the offices were closets made of antique oak which matched the woodwork of the room.

In one closet a switchboard was connected to a storage battery in the cellar. It was used to operate the electromagnetic mallet, mouth lamp, headlight and cauteries. Rhein, who was noted for the quality of his gold fillings, preferred to operate his electric mallet with an interrupter, which converted the direct current supplied by the city into an alternating current needed to run the mallet, rather than use the latest S.S. White Company model, without an interrupter. Rhein connected a storage battery and a rheostat to provide the interrupted current for his mallet. Nearby he placed a Custer electric gold annealer.

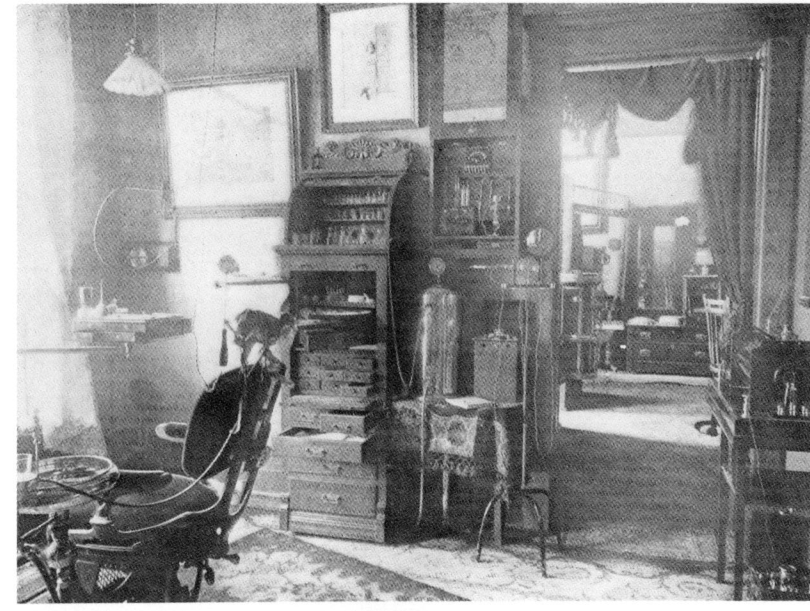

Office of C.J.B. Stephens, Great Falls, Montana, 1897. This well-supplied office contains an electrical panel on the right of the tall dental cabinet. Beneath the panel is a sterilizer and a nitrous oxide dispenser. From *Items of Interest*, Vol. 19, pg. 601.

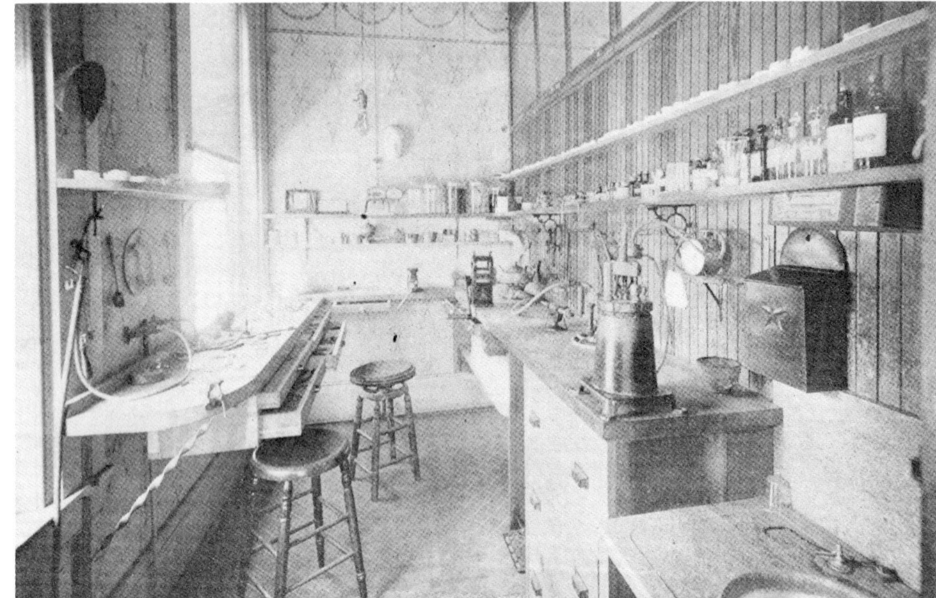

Laboratory of E.S. Fuller, Piqua, Ohio, 1898. This well-supplied laboratory was used for vulcanizing dentures, making repairs and other mechanically related dental projects. From *Items of Interest*, Vol. 20, pg. 387.

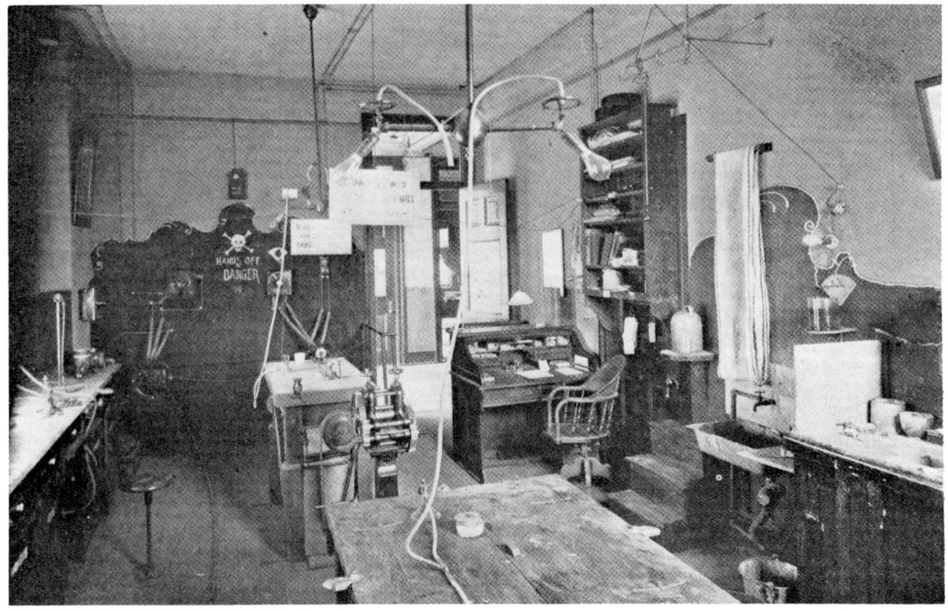

Office of Thomas P. Hinman, Atlanta, Georgia, 1898. A very well-outfitted laboratory with electric lathes, furnaces, lights, etc. Compressed air powers the pipes and furnaces. Each drawer of the laboratory table contains a space to fit each instrument. To prevent slamming, each door was fitted with an automatic closing device. From *Items of Interest*, Vol. 20, pg. 508.

Rhein's office also was stocked with instruments for doing a variety of special dental procedures including douching the diseased antrum sinus (above the upper molar teeth) and medicating the diseased tissues of the mouth. Compressed air tubes leading from the cellar were operated by an automatic water pump. They were used to run a chip blower and attachments to spray chemicals into the mouth. Rhein's reputation for curing cases of bone loss or pyorrhea alveolarus was based on his use of sprayed medicinals. The compressed air spray loosened the debris around the gums and controlled the flow of blood while keeping the diseased periodontal pockets open around the teeth.

Rhein eliminated the foul odor of sewer gas which accompanied the usual installation of a portable spittoon, by passing the pipes carrying the waste water into a sink in the cellar, where the gases passed off into the sewer pipes. This configuration avoided a direct link between the sewer and the office.

Rhein covered the walls of the room with an olive green burlap to provide rest for his eyes. Thus, when he paused during a long procedure of pounding in a gold filling he could avoid the glare of the well-lighted dental chair for a few moments. Rhein designed one of the first cluster-type lights in 1911. Manufactured by the Electro-Dental Manufacturing Company, the lamp consisted of four prismatic shades with enclosed bulbs arranged in a cloverleaf pattern. The lamp directed softly diffused light down and also provided sufficient light for the rest of the office. Cluster lights continued to be used into the 1930s. The arrangement of Rhein's office permitted the inclusion of specialized equipment within the context of a well-designed room.

Rhein and Kells were among the earliest dentists to employ trained nurses and assistants, known as dental hygienists, who would become essential to the modern dentist. In 1898 Rhein trained his "dental nurse" to clean his patient's teeth. Of the many exemplary achievements of Rhein, his advocacy of preventive dentistry and the value of inspecting the dental tissues for diagnostic purposes to detect more general diseases, were among the most important. Widely acclaimed and a leader in various educational projects, Rhein joined many professional organizations and taught at the University of Pennsylvania School of Dentistry.

An equally well-equipped and handsome office was owned by William B. Finney of Baltimore, who employed a black male assistant. His office decor displays the effect of region.[113] Professor of Dental Mechanism and Metallurgy in the Baltimore College of Dental Surgery, Finney's office and home of three stories extended back an entire block and contained 56 rooms. He was a dentist who catered to the upper economic classes. He remained attached to his old instruments and applied them with great skill. His operating room opened into a landscaped courtyard with a fountain, surrounded by plants, ferns, flowers and a pool stocked with gold fish. The laboratory beneath the office also opened into the courtyard and contained a work bench along the length of the window with drawers underneath for storing instruments. A "gold drawer," built like one designed by jewelers, was used to save gold fragments and filings, which for Finney amounted to a considerable amount, since he specialized in making gold crowns and bridges.

Finney's office was powered with water instead of electricity which he considered more dangerous and less reliable. Finney had a choice between water and electrical power, however, others who did not have access to electricity used a water motor to power their dental engines "rather than walk a treadmill all day."[114] Finney designed most of the pluggers, mandrils, scalers and gold filling trimmers that he used. Of particular note was a "set of six beautifully carved pearl-handled gold trimmers, made in sets of two, right and left, . . ." used to "cut down the overlap of gold fillings, instead of sand paper,"[115] which patients found objectionable. A set of 14 hand and electric pluggers designed to Finney's specifications were adopted by graduates of the Baltimore Dental College.

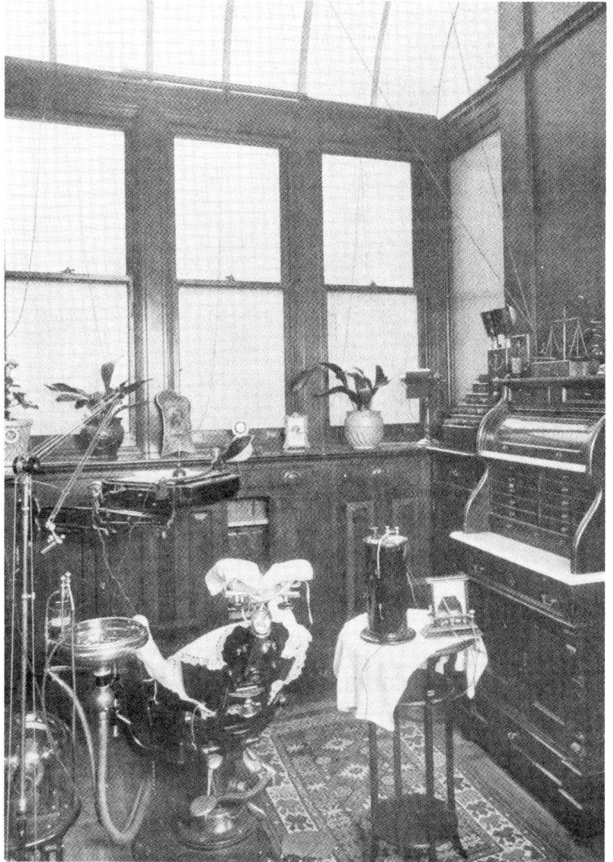

Operatory of M.L. Rhein in New York City, 1897. One of the most sumptuous dental offices in the city at this time was set up in an elaborately decorated town house. From *Items of Interest*, Vol. 19, pg. 517.

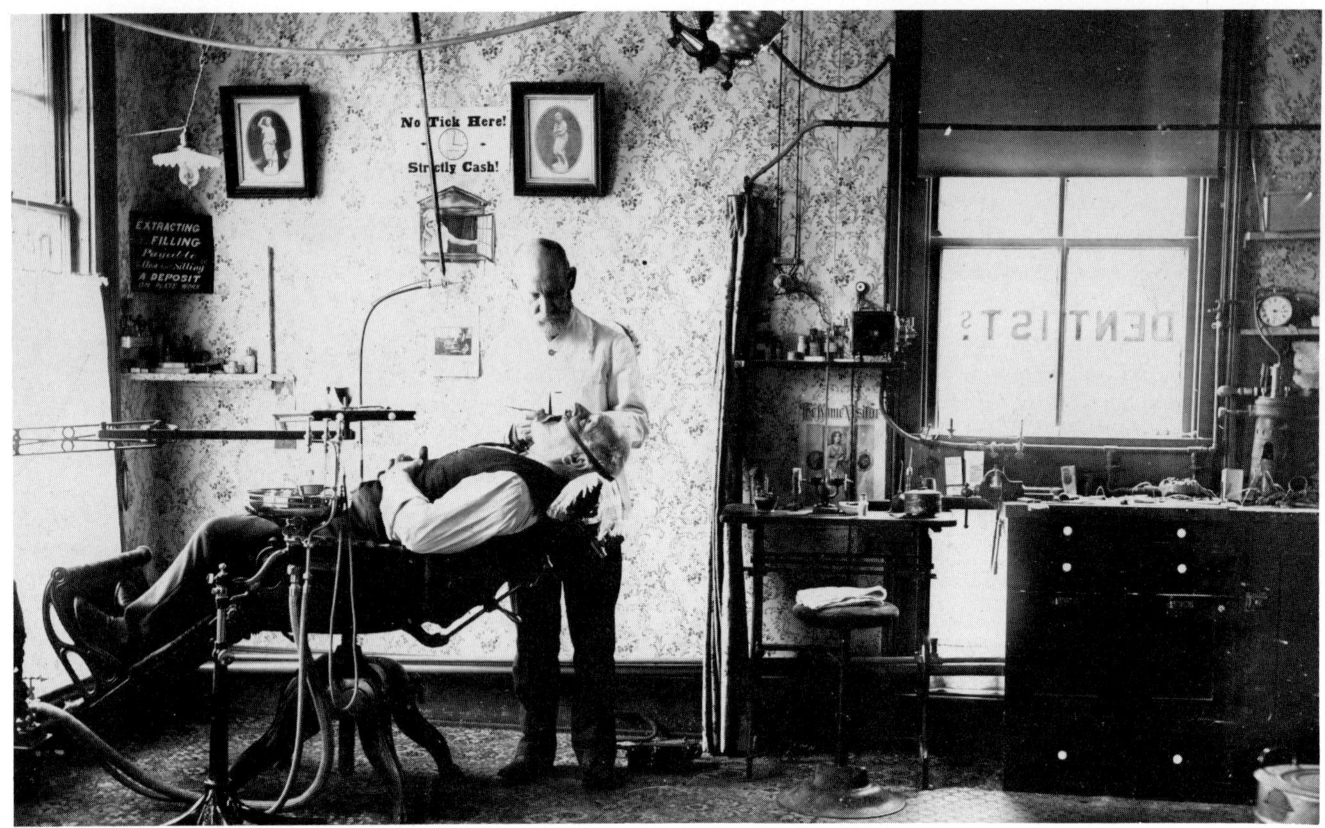

The dentist in this turn of the century photograph works on a patient who wears a band around his head to hold the rubber dam in place in his mouth. Rubber dams were used to seal off the tooth being worked on from the rest of the mouth and its fluids. The laboratory is to the right of the chair and very handy to the dentist. The sign makes it clear "No Tick Here—Strictly Cash." From Gary Lemen, Sacramento, California.

The dentist is in his office at the end of the 19th century. This posed picture shows the dentist's profile reflected in the mirror to his right. Standing beside a female patient in the chair, he rests his hand on the wooden bracket table. Behind the chair is a nitrous oxide apparatus and above it on the wall is a telephone. On the office wall beside the window is a class photograph and diploma. This picture may have been taken by one of the photographers who traveled in this period from city to city, recording offices and shops to earn a living. From Minnesota Historical Society.

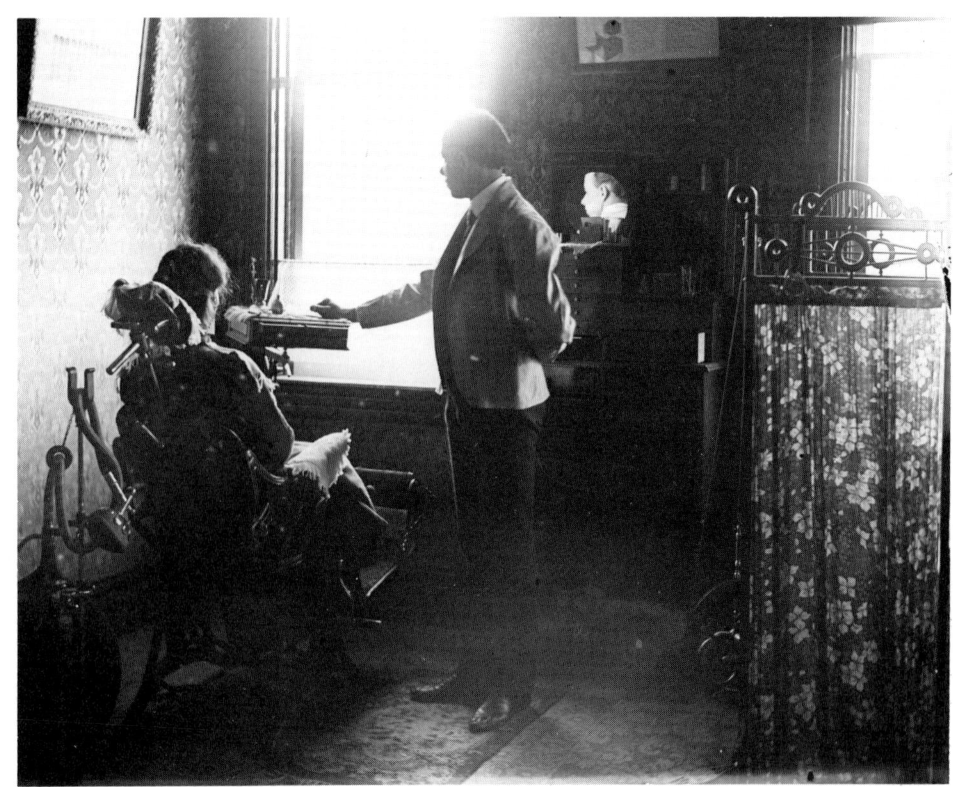

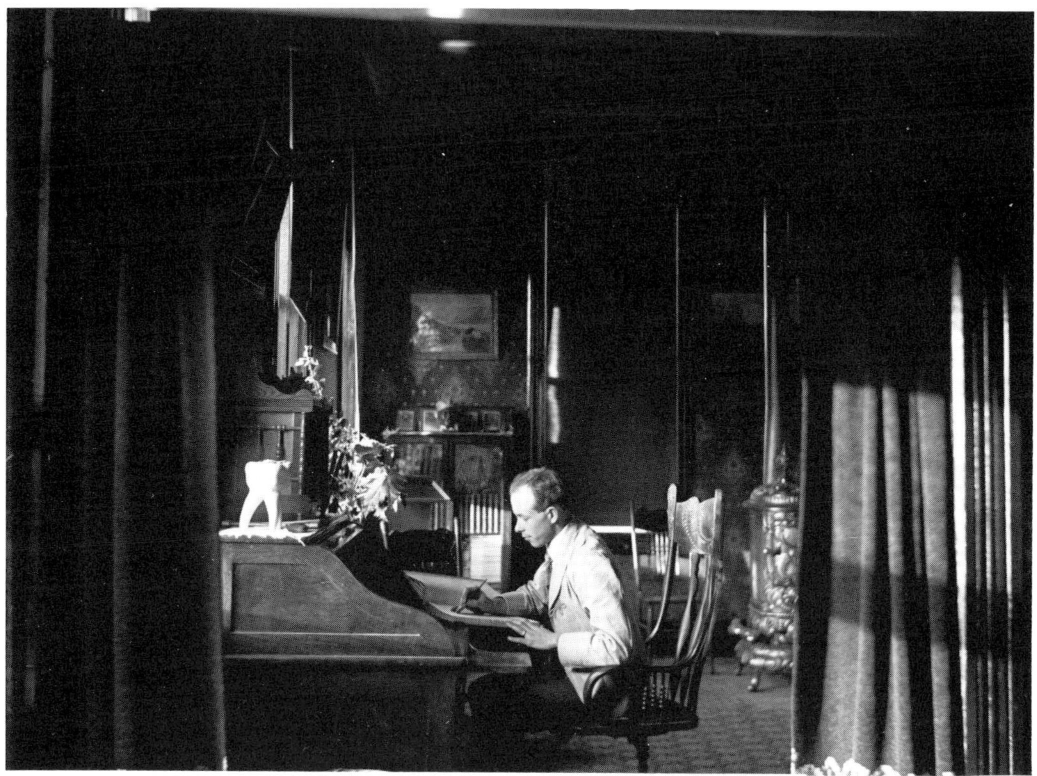

J.A. Morrison in his office in 1900. The model of the tooth standing on the desk reminds us of the film "Greed" which was set in San Francisco at this time. From Minnesota Historical Society.

The office of C.C. Newcastle, circa 1900, in Portland, Oregon, was operated by a dentist and his son. A curtain could be drawn to separate the two chairs. The electrical wiring was recently installed and reflects the make-shift manner in which electricity was supplied to dental offices of the period. From Oregon Historical Society.

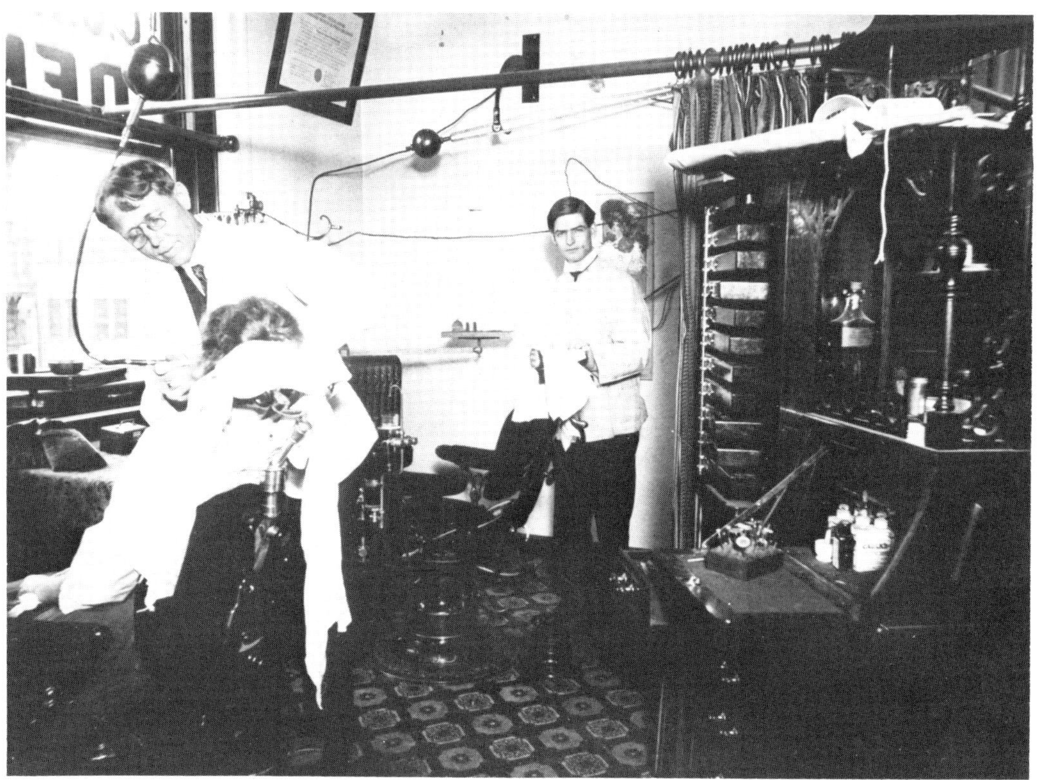

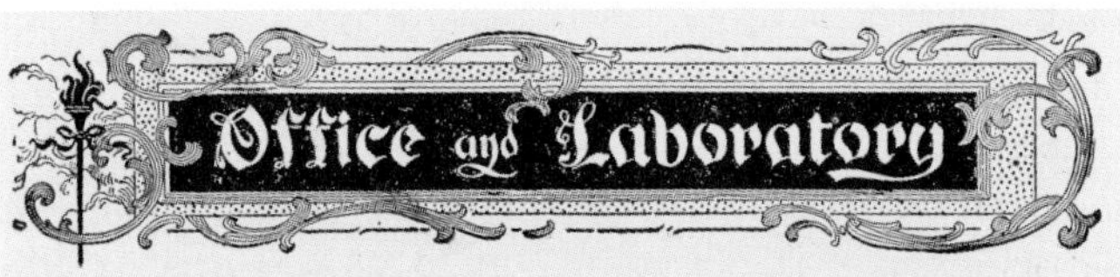

Office and Laboratory

The Equipment of a Country Dental Office.

Office of Dr. T. M. Jamison, Okolona, Miss.

As the readers of Items of Interest have been given several beautiful illustrated and well written articles on office furnishings, we may now discuss the equipment of the country office.

I suspect from a personal feeling, that many of us who are less fortunate in practice and financial ability to supply these convenient surroundings, have looked upon these pictures, and read covetously these articles that have appeared from month to month.

The writer is a believer in all things attendant upon dental practice, and while our income may be small and we cannot afford the outlay of Dr. Rhein or Dr. Kells, we can all provide comfortable and neat office quarters.

My office is located in a small town of twenty-five hundred inhabitants, one-half of this population being negroes, and as I do not work for the "dusky element," the reader can appreciate what a small field of operation I have, when I state further that another dental sign hangs just across the street.

I have two connecting rooms, seventeen by seventeen feet, on the second floor, with north and south exposures. The front and north room I use for operating. This floor is supplied with neat straw matting and rugs, except under the operating chair where I use an oil cloth square,

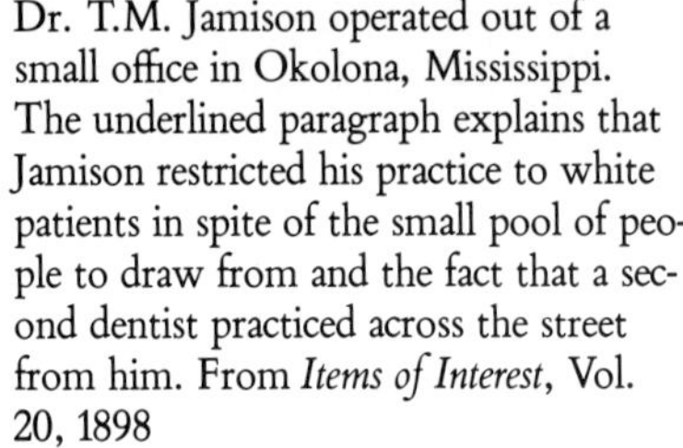

Dr. T.M. Jamison operated out of a small office in Okolona, Mississippi. The underlined paragraph explains that Jamison restricted his practice to white patients in spite of the small pool of people to draw from and the fact that a second dentist practiced across the street from him. From *Items of Interest*, Vol. 20, 1898

For 26 years Finney used a steel-handled mechanical mallet patented by Parmly Brown. Finney's dexterity and power was displayed in his use of this device. He could condense two fillings for every one that could be condensed with an electric mallet. Described in 1897 as a curiosity, the hand mallet bore the traces of Finney's use and "the precision of the blow from force of habit; doing his own malleting, looking at the tooth and striking the blow by guess, the gentle tap, tap of years, has worn a circular depression accurately correct within the circumference of this small hammer, an eighth of an inch deep and not more than a fourth in diameter."[116]

Finney's graciousness was expressed in the methods he used to make the office more comfortable in the hot Baltimore summers. A water motor fan, placed a foot from the fountain spittoon beside the operating chair, blew a gentle breeze across the chair to cool the dentist and patient without noise and without creating an unpleasant draft.

Promoting the emotional stability of the patient became paramount in setting up dental offices such as that of the prominent dentist Thomas P. Hinman (1870-1931) of Atlanta, Georgia.[117] The son of English-born parents, whose family were well-known educators, Hinman graduated from the Dental Department of the Southern Medical College in 1891 and joined the faculty the next year as professor of Oral Surgery. Active in the American Dental Association for 35 years, he was a founder of the American College of Dentists. He set up the Atlanta Midwestern Clinic in 1911 which continues to be an effective dental teaching forum in the South.

Hinman developed one of the largest dental practices in the U.S. A community leader, he served as director of the Atlanta Art Association, First National Bank (Atlanta) and Atlantic Steel Corporation. He also advised and supported the High Museum of Art.[118]

Hinman's attitude toward his patients grew out of his belief that half the pain the patient suffered was during anticipation of the dental procedure, therefore, he wanted "nothing in the reception room to remind the patient what was to be found in the operating room."[119] Even the non-dental related equipment and furnishings were carefully chosen for their ability to provide a quiet and calm environment. All rooms contained overhead electric fans and automatically closing doors to prevent slamming.

The operating room in facilitating examination and treatment minimized the time the patient spent in the dental chair. Tapping the 500 volts of current supplied by Atlanta, Hinman installed a transformer to reduce the current to 110 volts required to operate his dental instruments. His operating cabinet was 3-1/2 feet high, over 2 feet long and 1 foot deep. Each drawer was molded to the shape of the instruments it contained.

To send objects from the operating room to the laboratory and back, Hinman installed a Lamsen carrier or package tunnel. A speaking tube permitted Hinman to talk to his assistants in the laboratory. One procedure which was facilitated by this exchange between dentist and technician was crown manufacture. After the crown was measured it was "placed in the carrier and shot into the laboratory, and then, the assistant instructed by means of the speaking tube as to the width of band desired; when made it is returned and fitted, cusps articulated and then it is sent back for final soldering and polishing."

Special features of the laboratory included a table surface constructed of Portland cement 1 inch thick to prevent burning. The laboratory was equipped with electric lathes, furnaces and blow pipes.

The drug cabinet contained mirrors on the bottoms, sides and backs of each shelf. Small lights were installed so that when the door was opened they lit up for better inspection of its contents.

An office, located in a smaller city, to the north of

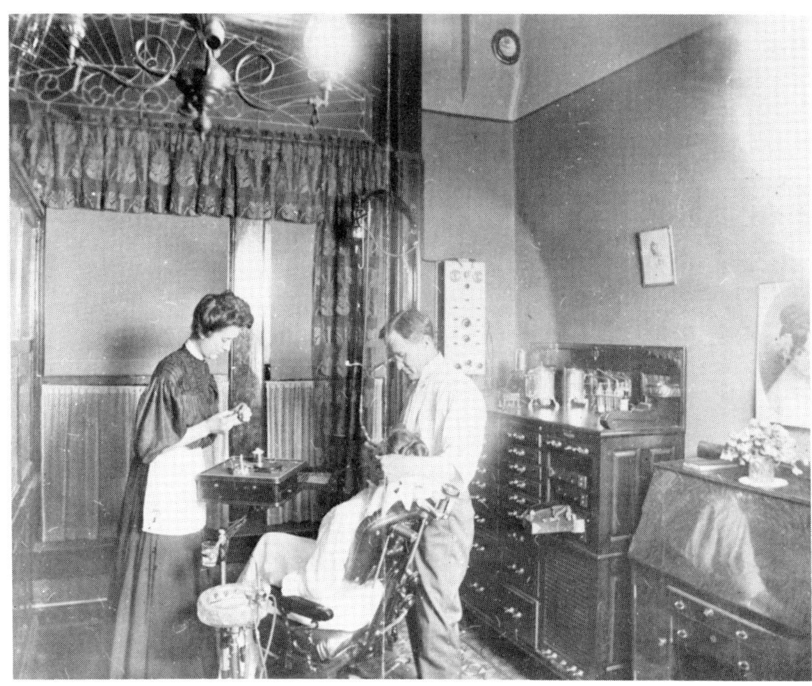

An office in the Midwest at the turn of the century showing an assistant at work with the dentist and a female patient in the chair. An electric panel may be seen over the shoulder of the dentist. From University of Missouri, Kansas City Archives.

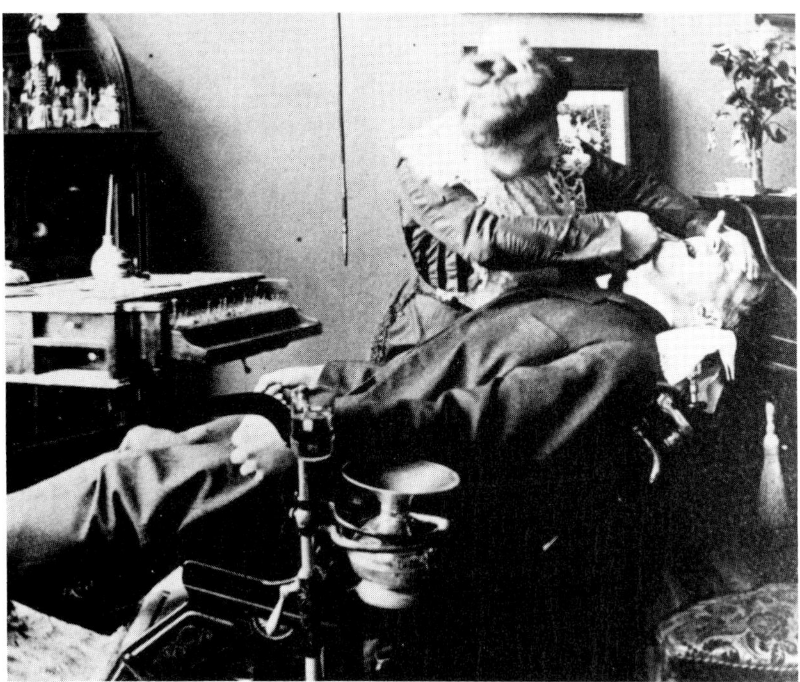

Olga Lentz extracting a tooth in 1910. She practiced until 1926. From Minnesota Historical Society.

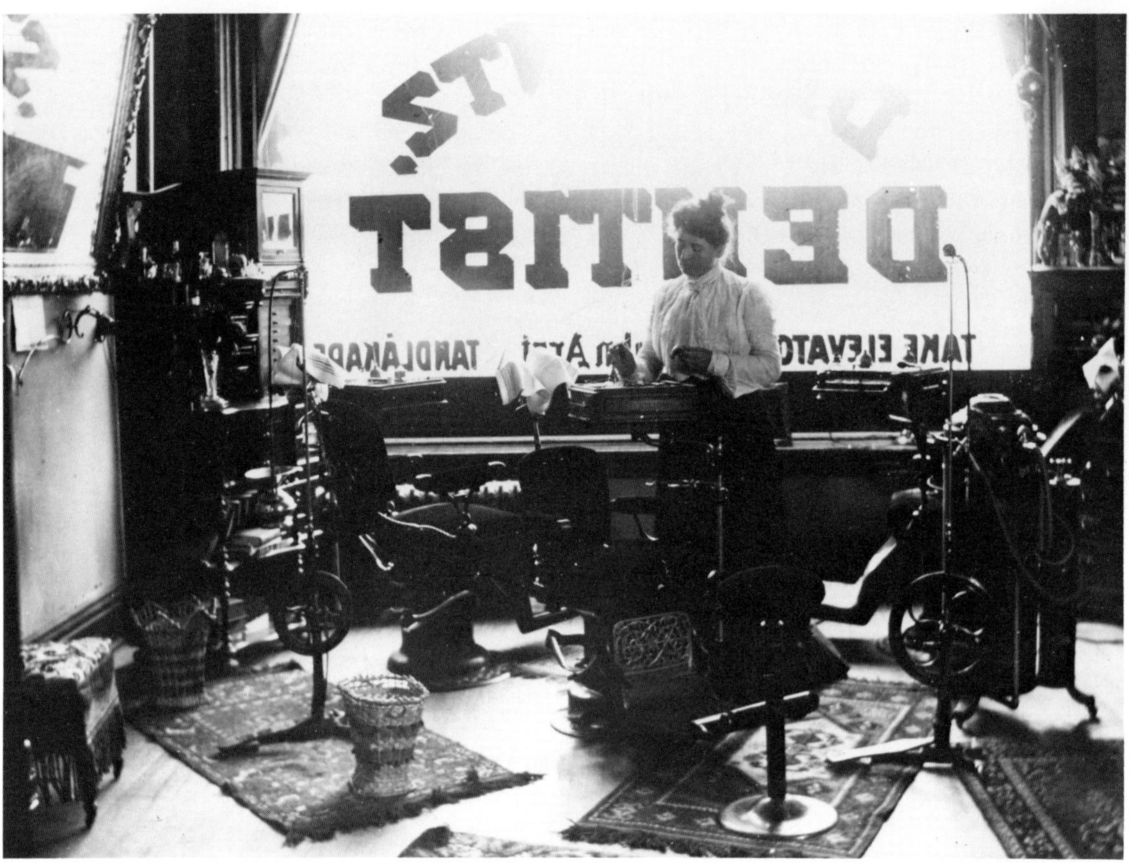

Office of Olga A. Lentz, St. Paul, Minnesota, circa 1905. Dr. Lentz joined her husband, John, in practice, hence the two chairs, tables and foot-pedal drills in the office. The large letters in the sign on the window may indicate that the office was located on the second or third floor. The size of letters used in dental signs became a sore point among dentists who considered large signs a form of advertising not in keeping with a proper professional image. In Connecticut by 1930, the State Dental Association limited the size of lettering to four inches on the ground floor and six inches on the second floor. From Minnesota Historical Society, photograph by Albert Munson.

New York City, was described in 1897 by Charles F. Allan of Newburgh, New York.[120] Allan wanted the assistance of a liberal supply of "machinery and mechanical paraphernalia" but he cautioned that most of these items should be kept out of the view of the patient. He singled out large rheostats with bright metal knobs mounted on a wall and a generous supply of electric bulbs as especially forbidding to the patient. In combination with a dental chair he thought these objects "suggested electrocution." Allan's sensitivities may have been aroused by his location near Sing Sing prison in Ossining, New York, one of the earliest prisons in which electrocution was used for capital punishment.

Noisy motors were to be placed out of sight, and if possible, out of the operating room to minimize the sound generated during their use. Other dentists had devised ways to minimize the noise of an office or laboratory motor. William H. Taggart, inventor of the inlay process, suspended the motor in his office with a strong cord pulley to eliminate the vibration. The normal installation of a motor was to screw it to the floor. The floor became a sounding board that intensified the noise of the motor's vibration. E.M.S. Fernandez offered another explanation. He claimed that Taggart's arrangement was more silent due to the large size of the motor which could reach full speed and power with fewer vibrations. Without the motor having to strain, the vibration was less, and therefore, so was the sound produced by the motor. Fernandez expected to find quieter motors such as those containing ball bearings at the World's Columbian Exposition in Chicago in 1893.[121]

Allan insisted that equipment should not be moved around the floor, therefore he separated the driving wheel and standard of a dental engine from the foot control. The engine was operated by pressing on the control or treadle which was placed under the back of the chair.

The color of the spittoon was important to Allan who used a porcelain bowl decorated in red and gold instead of the usual nickel-plated one, which had to be polished to keep it shining brightly. Others entered the debate over the material of which to construct spittoons, which centered on glass, porcelain or polished metal. A.B. McVay of Streator, Illinois, claimed in 1908, that nickeled bowls were easily polished and did not stain or appear as soiled after use as did most glass spittoons.[122] To rinse the spittoon during use a hollow rim with many orifices conducted the water into the bowl. Suspended on a bracket the spittoon was pushed out of the way when not in use.

Allan's cabinet was not totally satisfactory, although it contained 81 compartments into which he placed instruments of many sizes and shapes. He insisted that many drawers were necessary to help his assistant organize all the instruments used in the course of practice. Bridge work and the use of electrical devices since the late 80s, required a cabinet with even more places to hold instruments. Allan challenged dental furniture manufacturers to provide more elaborate cabinets.

Henry Arthur King of New York City described his reception room in 1898, "the appointments of the reception room of the dentist of today should be particularly calculated to court forgetfulness, and selective of a dainty bit of bric-a-brac, pleasing pictures, standard periodicals, piano, large comfortable chairs with nothing in sight suggestive of the operating room, [which] makes waiting restful and not at all tiresome.'[123] In his basement laboratory King mounted a special lathe with two to four stones on a steel spindle for rapid grinding. Polishing wheel chucks, brushes, mounted disks and engine burs could be attached to the ends of the spindle.[124]

Location in a small, far-western city called forth the special mechanical abilities of the dentist to arrange access to his instruments in his office. C.J.B. Stephens of Great Falls, Montana described his second floor office including a reception room, two operating rooms (the second one was used by Dr. G.H. Chase, ("a first-class general practitioner"), laboratory, extracting room, retiring and storage rooms. Stephens' operating room, measuring 11-1/2 feet by 15 feet, contained "a suspension engine with water motor, controlled by a speed regulator and reversing attachment operated by the foot."[125]

In a wall cabinet he designed, Stephens suspended his appliances by springs taken from cut down window shade rollers. These rollers were fitted with metal trimming for winding the rollers and connected to cords which were attached to miniature lights, cauteries, pluggers, head-lights, etc. The system was operated by a switch and battery powered.

To use an instrument, Stephens threw the switch and brought the appliance to the chair. When finished with it, Stephens released it and the instrument wound itself under the tension of the roller into its position in the cabinet. The cabinet was closed by a sliding front door.

Stephens' ingenuity also extended to the gas supply which he built. Great Falls did not provide gas in 1897,

Board of Public Health Dental Clinic at 1008 Nicollet Avenue, Minneapolis, Minnesota, circa 1923. From Minnesota Historical Society.

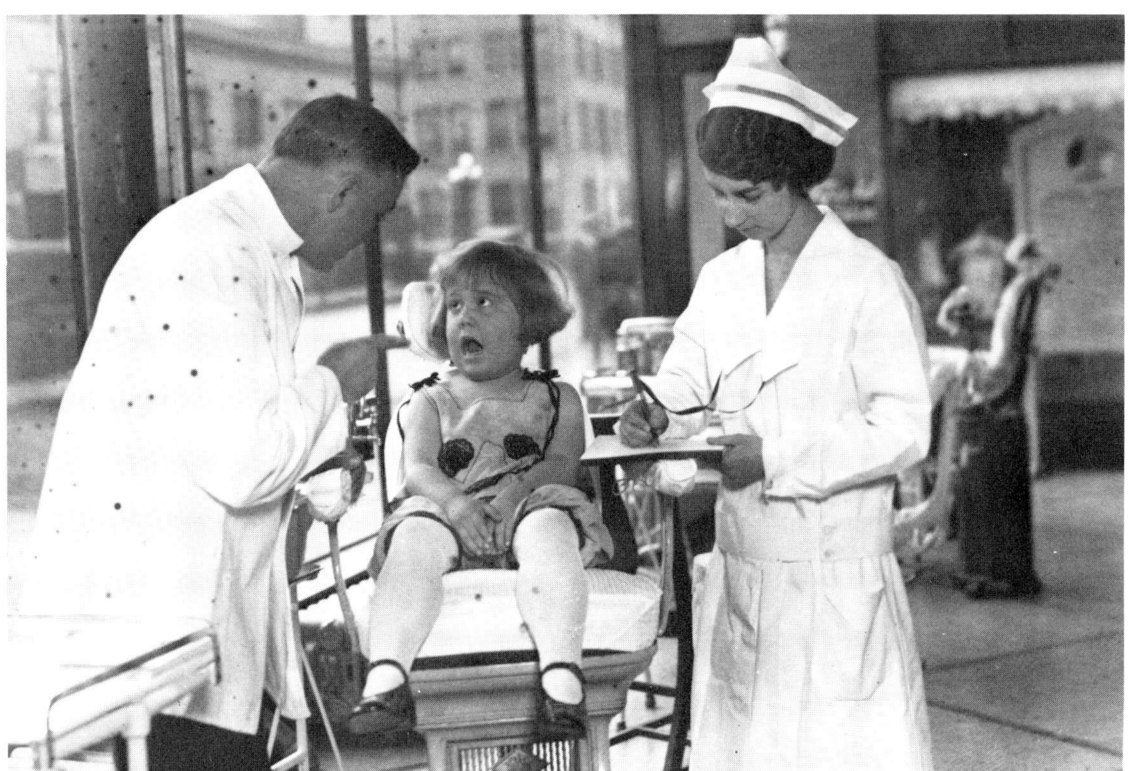

Child in dental chair in M.E. Jordon's office playing with ducks in the spittoon "duck-pond." Jordon catered to her patients by appealing to their sense of play. From *Operative Dentistry for Children* by M.E. Jordon, 1929, pg. 8.

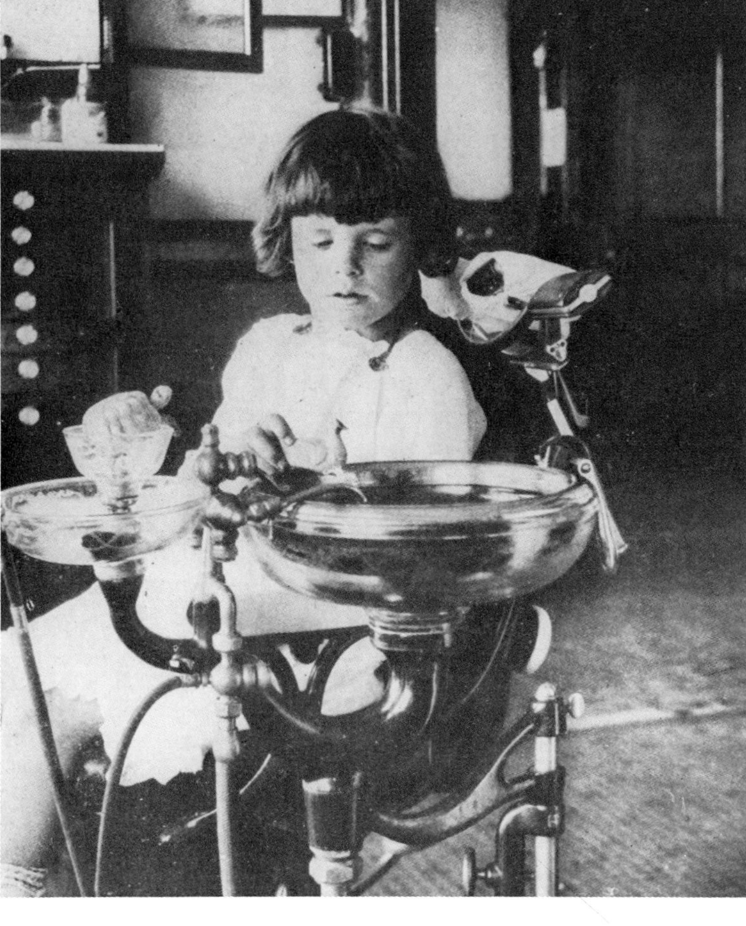

Office of M. Evangeline Jordon, specialist in children's dentistry in the early 20th century. The simplicity of the furnishings and smaller chair could better accommodate the child's body. From *Operative Dentistry For Children* by M.E. Jordon, 1929, pg. 169.

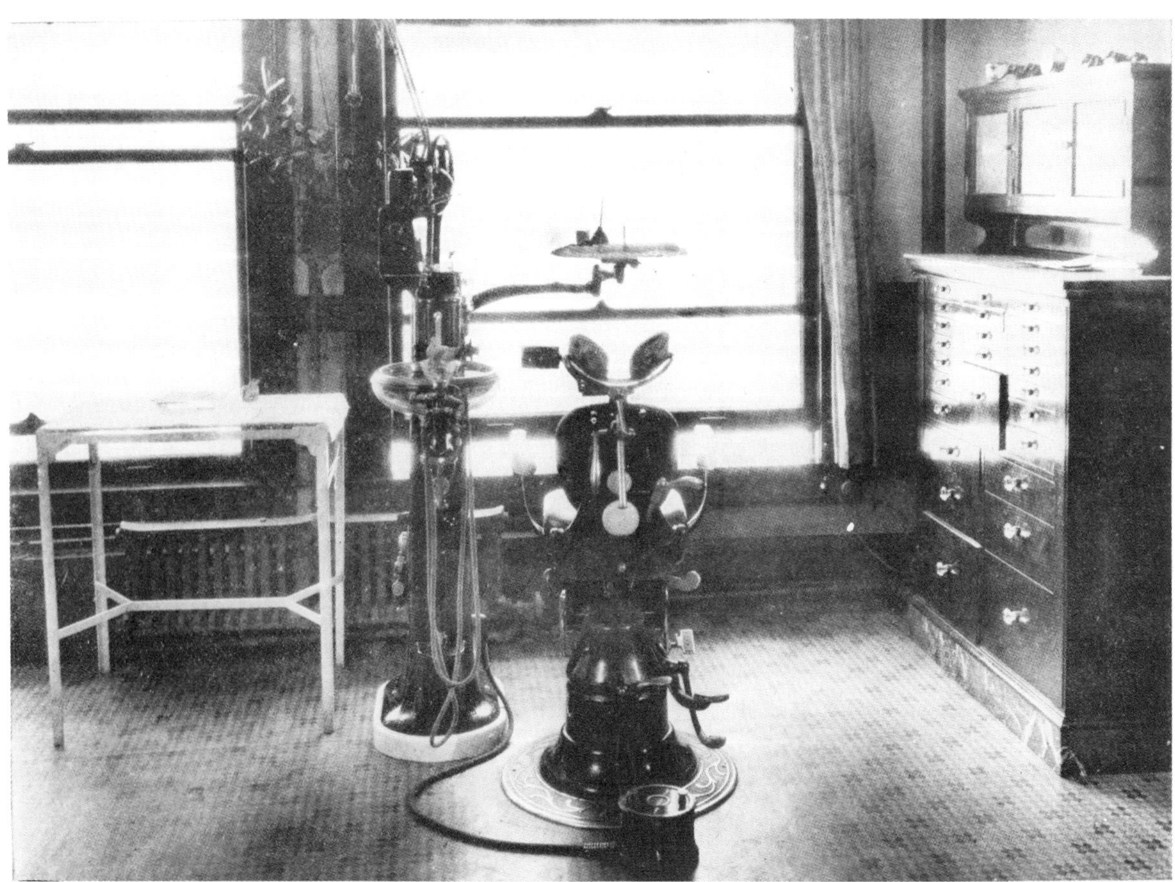

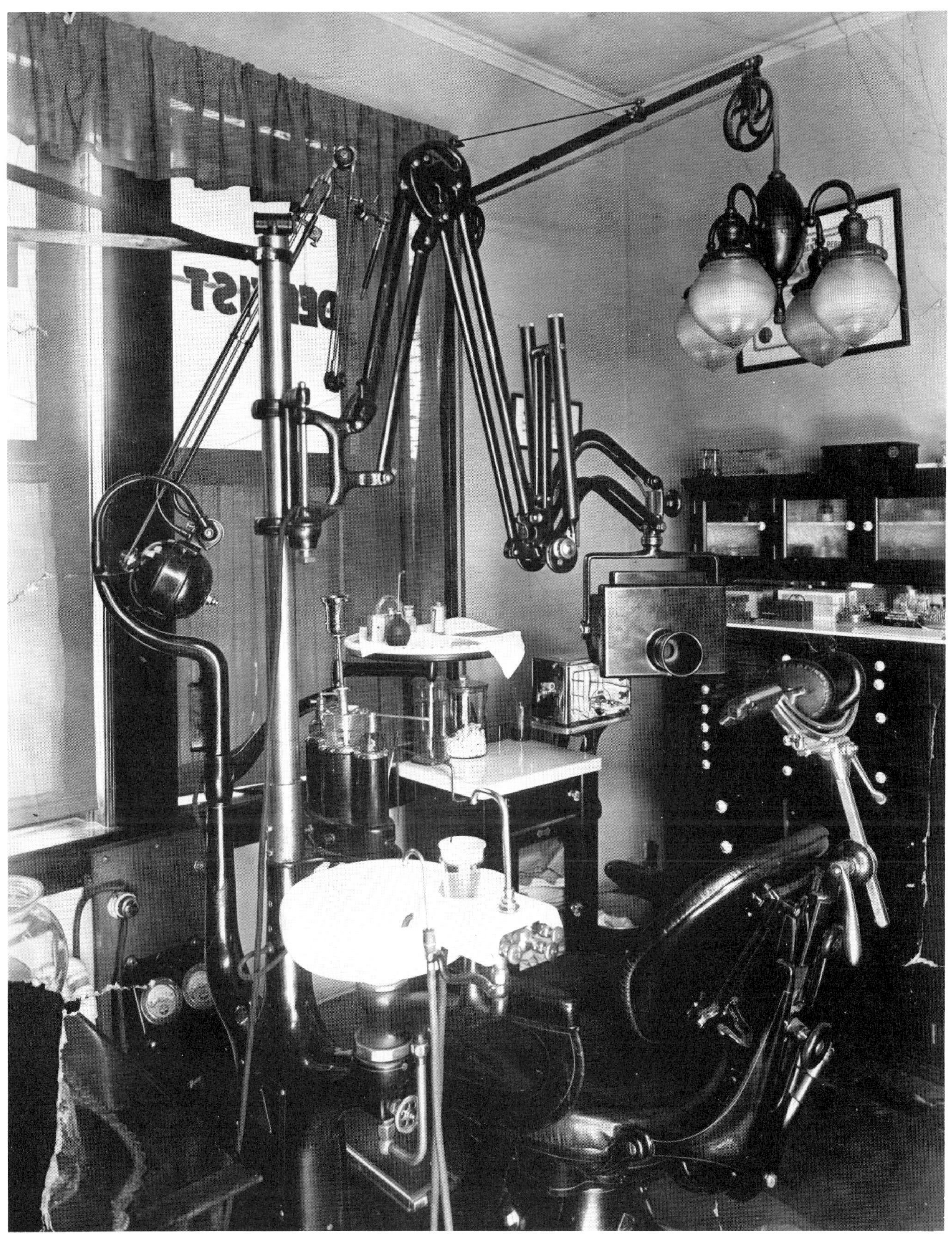

A cluttered office. This more fully furnished office enabled the dentist to serve the patient with a variety of techniques. However as equipment became more elaborate and more specialized, the office filled up with machines that could appear frightening and chaotic to the patient, therefore good design became imperative to make the best use of the space available. From General Electric X-Ray Department, circa 1930.

therefore, Stephens had a 100-gallon-capacity gasometer made. He linked the gas reservoir to a carburetor to manufacture gas. The gas was used to operate the blowpipe needed in the laboratory for soldering metals and making bridges.

There were numerous opportunities for noise control in the 19th century dental office. Stephens' contribution consisted of placing the anvil, used to swage false teeth, in a box with one end closed and the other open just wide enough to admit the 6 inch cube of iron which became the anvil. By filling the box with sawdust and placing the iron cube on top of the sawdust the ringing sound of the hammer striking the anvil was dampened.

Stephens echoed the views of Fleischman in 1850, and undermined the views of some of his contemporaries, that all dental instruments should be hidden from the patient. He believed

> that with the modern appliances and the advancement in operative dentistry, there is [not any] fear among the more intelligent class, that formerly existed. I do not hide my instruments, nor am I ashamed of their appearance, but have them in easy reach, every one in its place, and all are put to good use.[126]

Exposing dental equipment to the patient, led to the view that there be an open discussion of all dental procedures with the patient. Thomas Lewis Gilmer (1849-1931), over his half-century of practice, had adopted a forthright policy of "telling the patient everything which he thought should be withheld, because the patient might refuse to permit him to operate." Then he would ask if he should proceed and the patient would answer "whatever you think best testifying to the value of his approach and the tact with which he implemented it."[127] Not all patients were so confident of their dentists.

Economy of space and equipment was a prominent factor in setting up many 19th and 20th century American dental offices. Typical of the small-town dentist who could not afford to rent separate rooms was E.S. Fuller of Piqua, Ohio, who in 1898, divided a room measuring 18 feet by 24 feet into a waiting room, operating room and laboratory.[128] Two decades later a dental manufacturing company would argue that a good operatory could be constructed in a space measuring 22 feet by 26 feet.[129]

Fuller's equipment was mechanically powered since he could not afford electricity. A sewing machine, like a spinning wheel a century earlier, became the source of parts for Fuller, who was forced to make his own equipment. Fuller used old sewing machine parts to construct a foot-powered lathe, although he would have preferred to have had an electric motor. He described the non-electric mechanism as "A large pulley balance wheel operating a small pulley on a shaft above. A second pulley, larger, connecting with the lathe head. It gives a high rate of speed, is

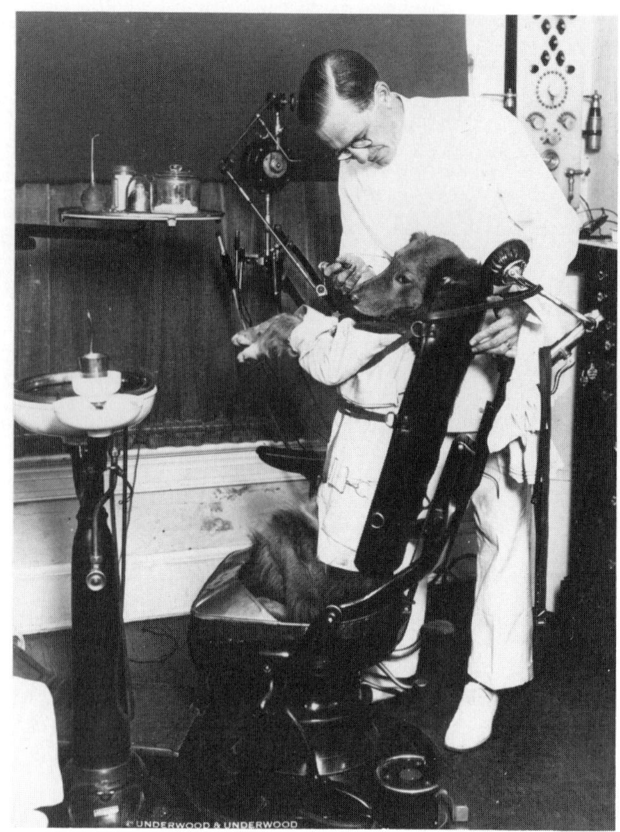

Unknown veterinary dentist circa 1930.

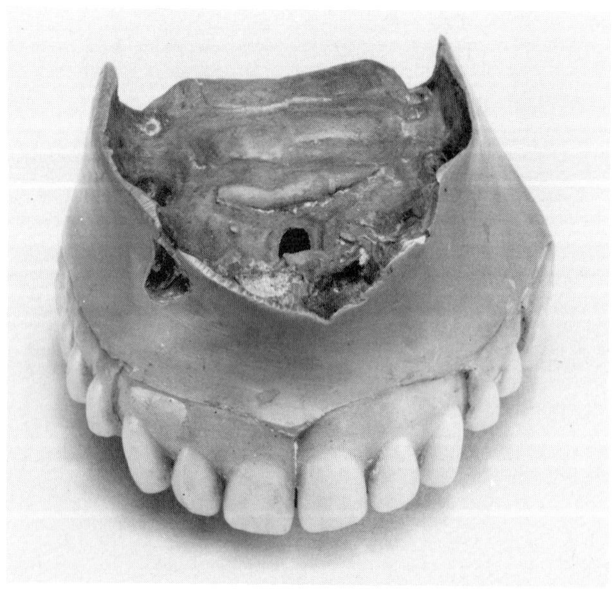

Veterinary dentistry engaged the talents of some dentists. Dr. Land, grandfather of Charles Lindbergh, made a set of artificial dentures for his dog. This set of teeth is in the National Museum of American History, Smithsonian Institution. Courtesy Smithsonian Institution.

WE TRADE!
Dental Work of All Kinds For
Any Kind of Country Produce-
Chickens. Eggs. Hogs. Cows. Horses. Mules
Hides. Tallow. Beeswax. or Anything of Value
NEW ART PAINLESS DENTIST

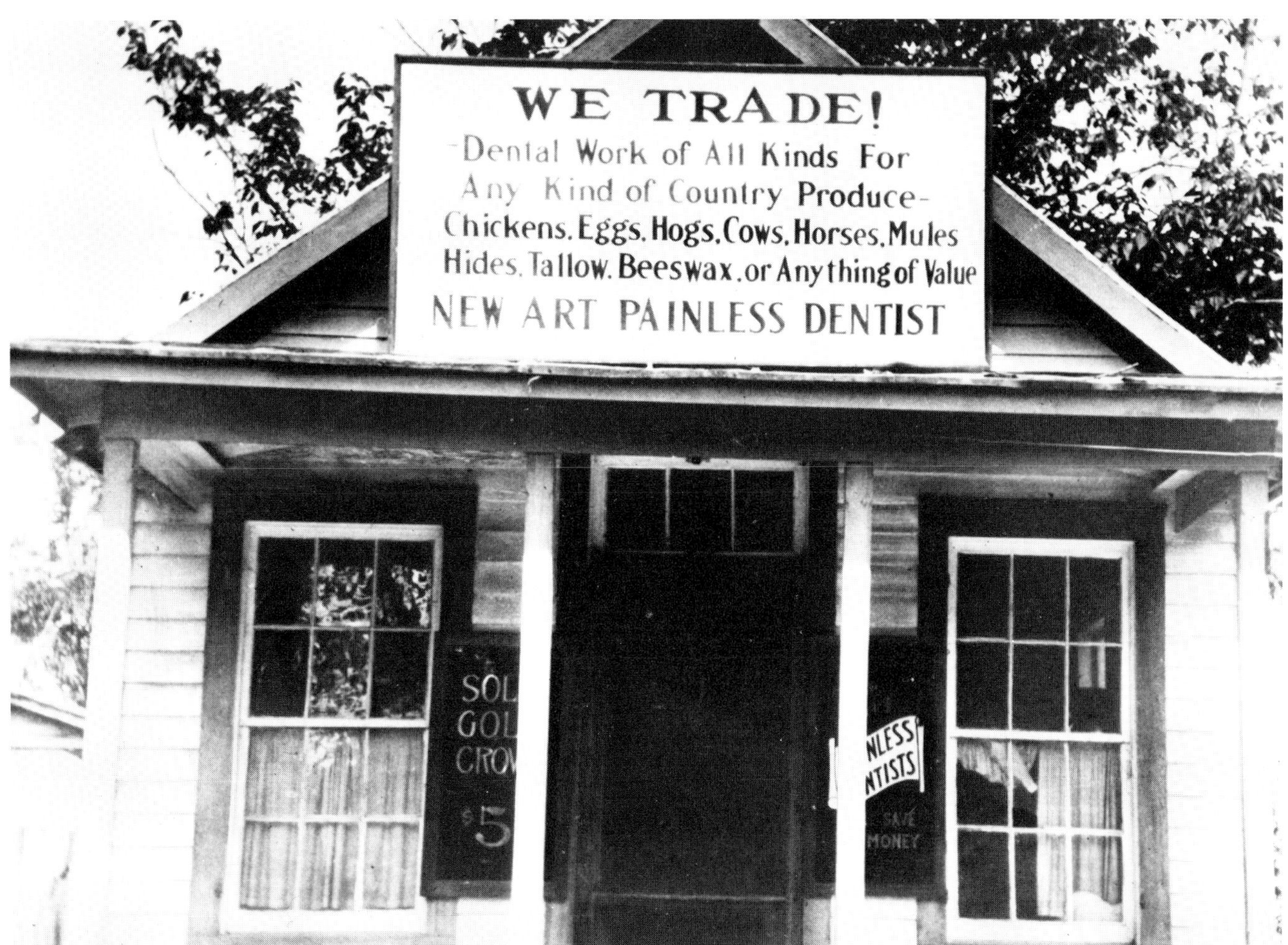

A dentist offers in-kind trade to attract patients during the Depression in rural Georgia. Note the signs, partially obscured on each side of the doorway, referring to solid gold crowns and painless dentistry, two of the major selling points of American dentistry well into the 20th century. Although they were much more difficult and laborious to insert, dentists always preferred gold fillings to amalgams. From Library of Congress.

steady and decidedly inexpensive."[130] Foot-powered engines did not lose their value entirely after electric engines became available. Occasionally foot power was used to do "rougher work." A.B. McVay in 1908 used a foot-powered engine to do the "rough" drilling to preserve his electric engine for the finer, delicate work by keeping it true and perfect, "for surely this has much to do with the comfort or discomfort of the patient."[131]

An electrically driven burring engine or engine for use with other hand-pieces made a major difference in the daily routine and health of the dentist. With electrical power the dentist "can distribute the weight of the body on both feet and maintain a steadiness of hand not possible when the engine is propelled by foot power."[132] With the replacement of the mechanical dental engine there were fewer instances of "dentist's leg" growing out of constantly pedaling a foot treadle to operate a dental drill.

Fuller made his vulcanizer and stand serve a triple function. He placed it near the door to use as a water heater. To function as a soldering stand he took out the bowl of the Lewis case heater that was inserted into it. Its normal function was to make hard rubber plates for artificial teeth.

In 1898 H.B. Hinman of Bucyrus, Ohio, a city of 7,000 population, worked in an office suite of three rooms: a laboratory, 15 feet by 17 feet, a combined waiting room and operating room, 19 feet square and a toilet room, 3-1/2 feet by 8 feet. Hinman was proud of his Columbia chair, Columbia electric engine and a Clark spittoon with a convenient saliva ejector.[133] The Columbia chair, which was displayed at the World's Columbian Exposition in 1893, was the first dental chair to use hydraulic pressure to raise and lower it.[134] A corrugated rubber floor around the dental chair made standing all day less tiring for the dentist's feet and leg muscles.

Hinman was also proud of his cabinet that was designed according to the plans of his friend, Dr. J.S. Cook of Marion, Ohio. The instrument drawers swung out so that everything could be reached from the operator's chair. Made from quartered oak with a beveled, French-plate mirror and felt-lined drawers, the cabinet cost Hinman $30 and served him as well as a cabinet that was advertised for $75.

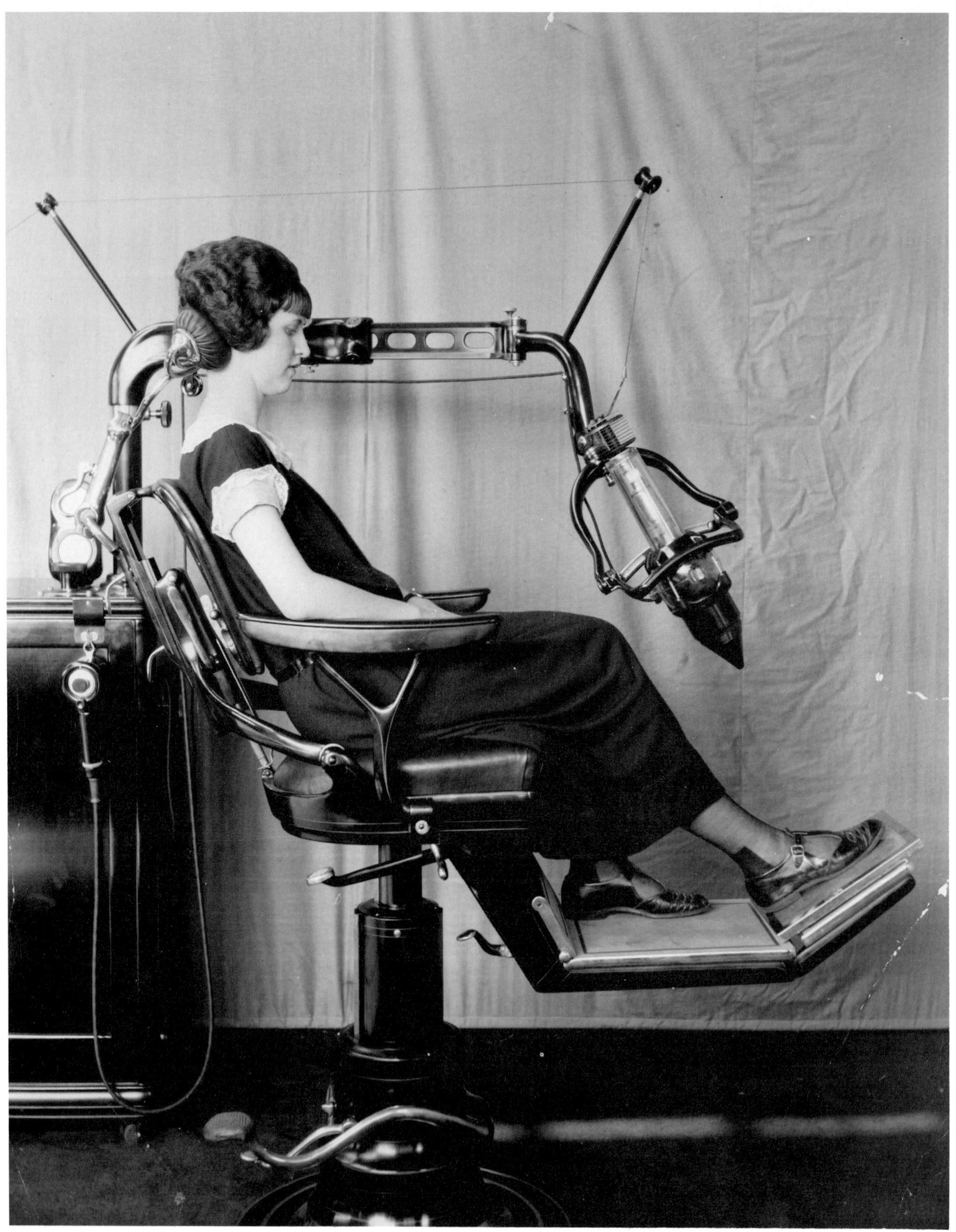

Photograph made by the Ritter Company modeling its X-ray unit beside one of its chairs in the 1930s. The predominance of women as patients in the photographs of this book is not an accident. Dentists frequently mentioned the fact that a majority of their patients were women and they arranged their offices and waiting rooms to please female expectations. From Ritter Dental Manufacturing Company, Rochester, New York.

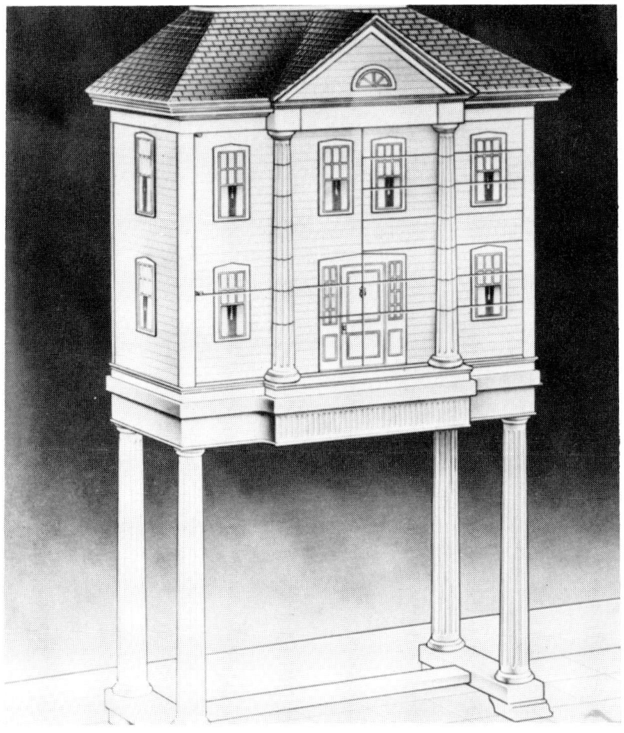

Dental cabinet in the shape of a dollhouse manufactured between 1930-33 by the American Cabinet Company. These unusual cabinets were used to entice the child into the dental office. The sections of the two columns in front of the house served as pulls to open the drawers. From American Cabinet Company Catalog.

Dr. Leonard Chapman of Chicago set up a dollhouse cabinet in his office in this period. He placed plaster animal figures on top of the cabinet and awarded gold stars to "good" patients. He also displayed his patient's artwork and posters of cartoon and nursery rhyme characters. From Richard and Dorothy Glenner, Chicago, Illinois.

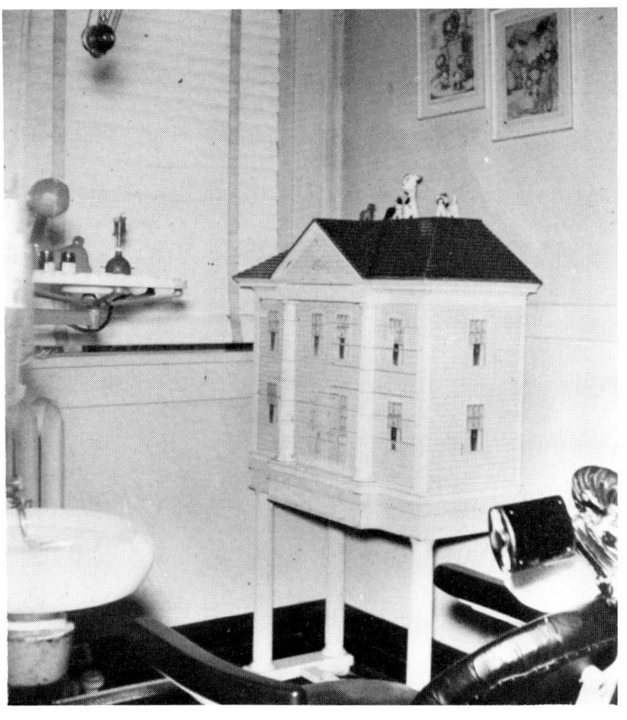

Hinman's patients were predominantly females who he accommodated by stocking the waiting room with illustrated magazines and providing a light and airy lavatory.

Dr. J. Allen Osmun's office, situated in Newark, New Jersey, displayed one of the more elaborate attempts to secure good, controllable light at all times of the day.[135] Several trials were required before the operating room was arranged suitably in 1898. The operatory was built out over an areaway and appeared to be an elongated, bay window measuring 11-1/2 feet long and 9 feet wide. The lower part of the walls were paneled mahogany wainscoting and the upper walls were covered with tapestry to reduce glare and eyestrain. The roof and ceiling was constructed of glass: a layer of white ondoyant in the ceiling covered by skylight glass installed in the roof. These two layers were separated by an air space of 3 feet. Osmun observed that a 4 or 5 foot space would have been even better for the purpose. Three ventilators leading from the air space supplied a constant stream of fresh air. A second ventilator on the roof, resting on brass plates, created a draught. Light green curtains or shades placed crosswise in the room between the ceiling and roof were pulled across the glass to block unnecessary light from entering the room.

Osmun also arranged a well-lighted laboratory which was 15 feet square beneath his operating room. Installed in the room were a half horsepower electric motor, an electric furnace for continuous gum work, compressed air for soldering, plate glass tables for plaster work and an open flue and bench for vulcanizing.

In 1899 F.P. Cronkhite distinguished between a well-supplied office and laboratory and an "aristocratic machine shop" as his friend, Dr. Root, described a heavily decorated office.[136] There was no point in putting expensive rugs on the floor and costly bric-a-brac around the room if patients were laborers who would not appreciate these items. However, all patients should be spared the sight of dental implements whenever possible. Economical, artificial light was supplied to Cronkhite's office by six incandescent lamps suspended over the chair and a 16-inch aluminum shade in front of the chair to bounce reflected light into the patient's mouth, and undoubtedly, eyes as well.

A mainstay in Cronkhite's office was a hand-piece connected to a Cleveland Champion air pump which provided air under pressure up to 35 pounds per square inch. With this instrument Cronkhite forced the air around the roots of teeth and under the gum margin to remove mucous and blood. His treatment for pyorrhoea included spraying air with drugs into infected pockets. Pressurized air was also used for drying before setting a crown and for cleaning out a root canal.

Cronkhite's two workbenches were made by the dental equipment manufacturers Ransom and Randolph. They were placed on either side of a cabinet with space on a flat surface for a vulcanizer. An additional furnace was used to melt and refine the stray chips of gold resulting during the manufacture of gold crowns and inlays. In his unostentatious office Cronkhite provided for his self-improvement. He occupied the time between appointments reading dental journals from the office library or in perfecting his mechanical techniques, rather than passing time in the waiting room chatting.

Eugene Maginnis of Chicago, an alumnus of Northwestern University Dental School, described his office for the Alumni journal. He furnished one of the most economical, but cleverly designed dental offices in 1908.[137] Exclusive of dental equipment, he spent $50 to furnish what he considered to be an office with a clean, pleasant atmosphere. In fact, Maginnis believed the operatory, which was 14 feet by 16 feet, was larger than necessary, but "not objectionable." Although the room was spare, each piece was located to maximize its effectiveness. A linoleum floor for ease of cleaning and for comfort while standing set the tone for the rest of the room. He selected standard operating and laboratory equipment, including a gas line piped throughout the entire length of the bench with connections for Bunsen burners, a stove, a blow-pipe and a light. The bracket table, used to hold instruments and supplies while working on a patient, was attached to the casing between the two windows and could be moved almost 180 degrees, as well as raised and lowered.

This Civilian Conservation Corps (CCC) photograph was taken in the 1930s. In this scene everyone is immaculate and gentle, while preparing the patient for treatment. The CCC, a "pet project" of Franklin D. Roosevelt, was the first of the New Deal relief agencies put in place in response to the crisis of the Depression. Of the 10,000 photographs taken between 1933 and 1942, when the program ended, about 2,000 are devoted to medical and dental subjects. See Pete Daniel, Mary A. Foresta, M. Stange and S. Stein, *Official Images New Deal Photography*, Smithsonian Institution Press, 1987, pg. 66, and John D. Stoeckle and George Abbott White, *Plain Pictures of Plain Doctoring*, MIT Press, 1985.

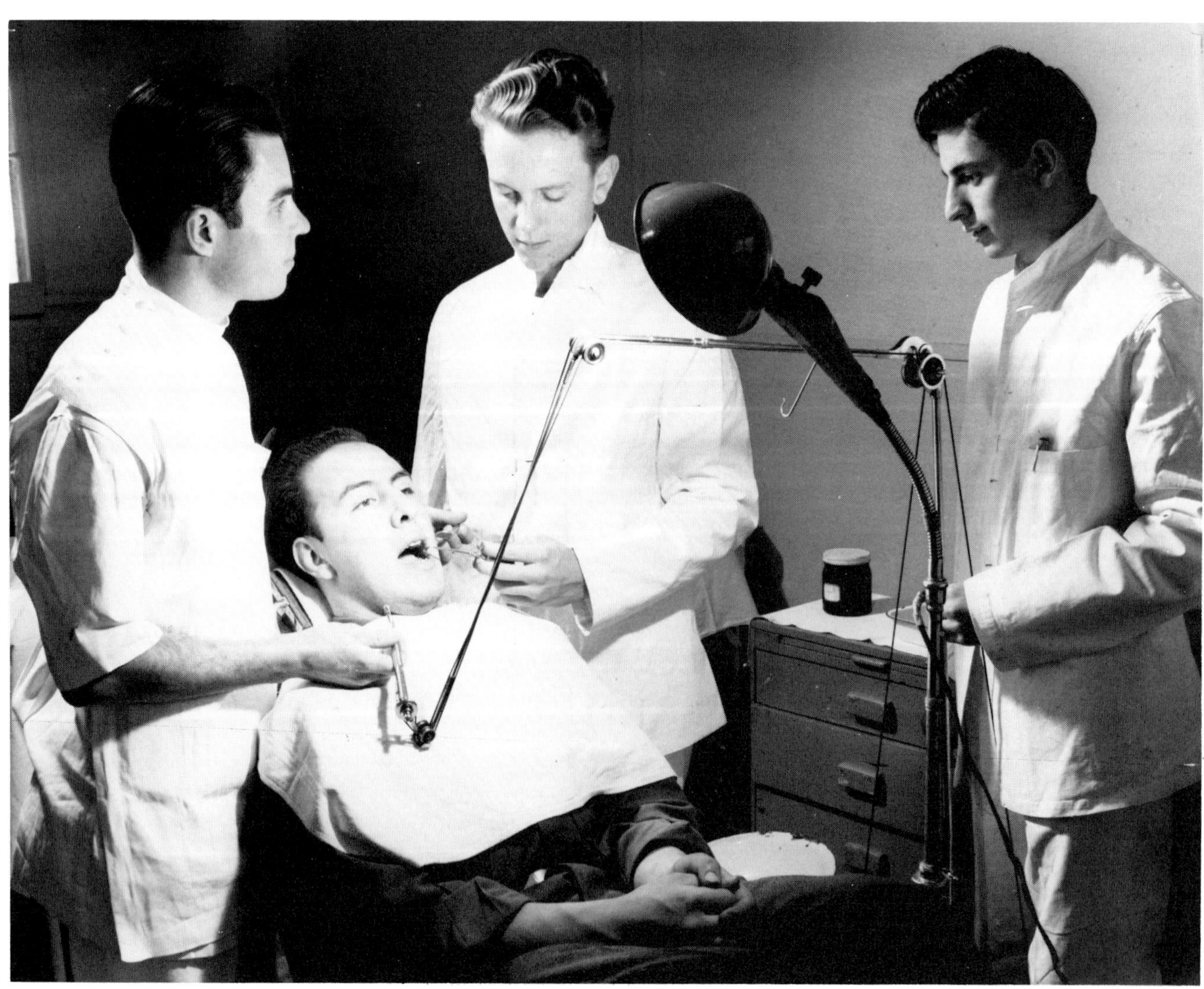

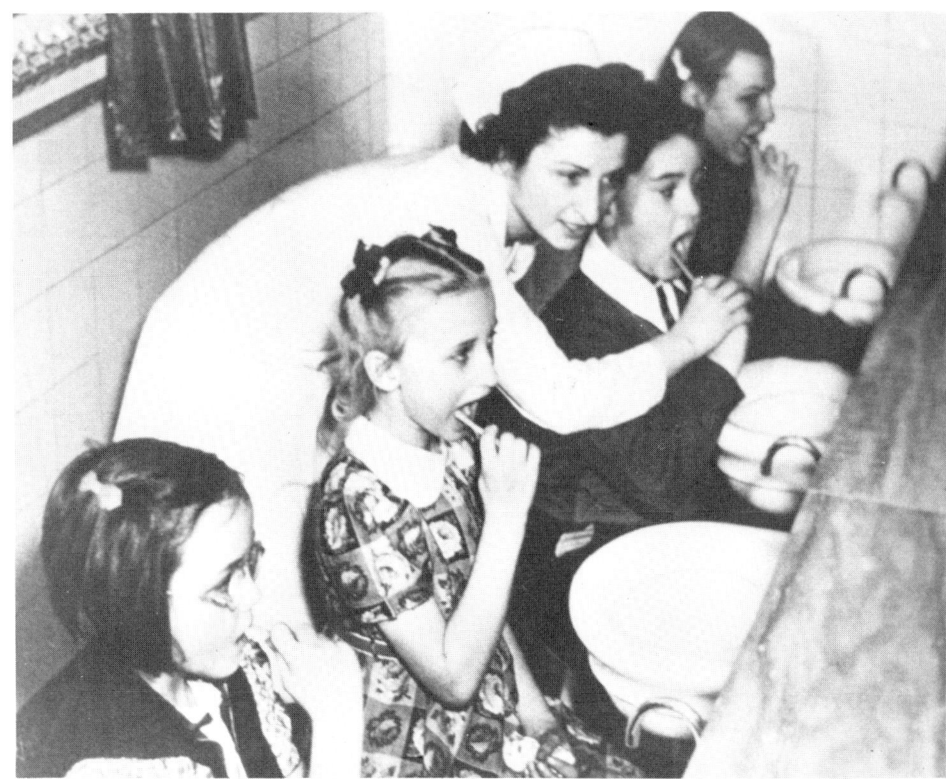

A dental hygienist at the Guggenheim Clinic in New York City teaches youngsters correct toothbrushing techniques, circa 1940. From Library of Congress.

Maginnis solved the lighting problem by having two very long windows rather than one large window in front of the dental chair. He could control the light by closing off one or a part of one window and letting light enter from its highest point, which he believed was essential for dentistry. In his office the light could come from a height of 8-1/2 feet. He enhanced the quality of the light by tinting the walls in a dark color "to correspond to the black box of a camera or of the human eye."[138]

Another low cost, and obviously, socially determined office belonged to T.M. Jamison of Okolona, Mississippi.[139] His practice was small and deliberately restricted due to racial prejudice. In 1898 he described his small office in a town of 2,500 people. However, only white people were eligible to become Jamison's patients. Therefore, Jamison refused to serve half the people who lived in Okolona, claiming that "I do not work for the 'dusky element.' " Jamison did not want to risk the boycott of white patients if he had treated the teeth of "Negroes." He furnished his two-room office with straw matting on the floor and a piece of oil cloth under the operating chair. A screen placed near the chair closed off a place used to deposit soiled garments and cloths.

Jamison employed an office boy but could not afford electrically driven engines or appliances. He worked only with mechanically operated appliances and without a fan. His philosophy toward his practice and office was straightforward:

> The country dentist cannot hope to enjoy the luxury of Oriental rugs, Turkish divans, and rich draperies, yet there are none of us so poor, or whose practice is so small, that he cannot provide a comfortable and inviting office and enjoy the distinction of being cleanly.[140]

In the same year a Chicago dentist, Edward S. Barber had to settle for an unusual-shaped office (7 feet 9 inches by 20 feet long) in order to get a more even or natural light into his operating room.[141] After practicing for two years in an office which faced south, Barber realized that in Chicago, a northern light would be more steady, and not produce as much glare and shadow as did the light entering from a southern exposure.

His office walls were decorated with burlap up to a height of 52 inches with a 1-inch border of mahogany rail. The upper wall was painted in a tinted color and the floor was covered with brown cork. Barber employed a revolving cabinet because it utilized space better than any other cabinet and provided ready access. Barber shared a common reception room with three other offices.

By placing the records of his patient's visits on a revolving file he was able to notify patients every six months that they were due for a dental check-up. All people whose names came up at the beginning of the month were sent notices to remind them to make an appointment for an examination.

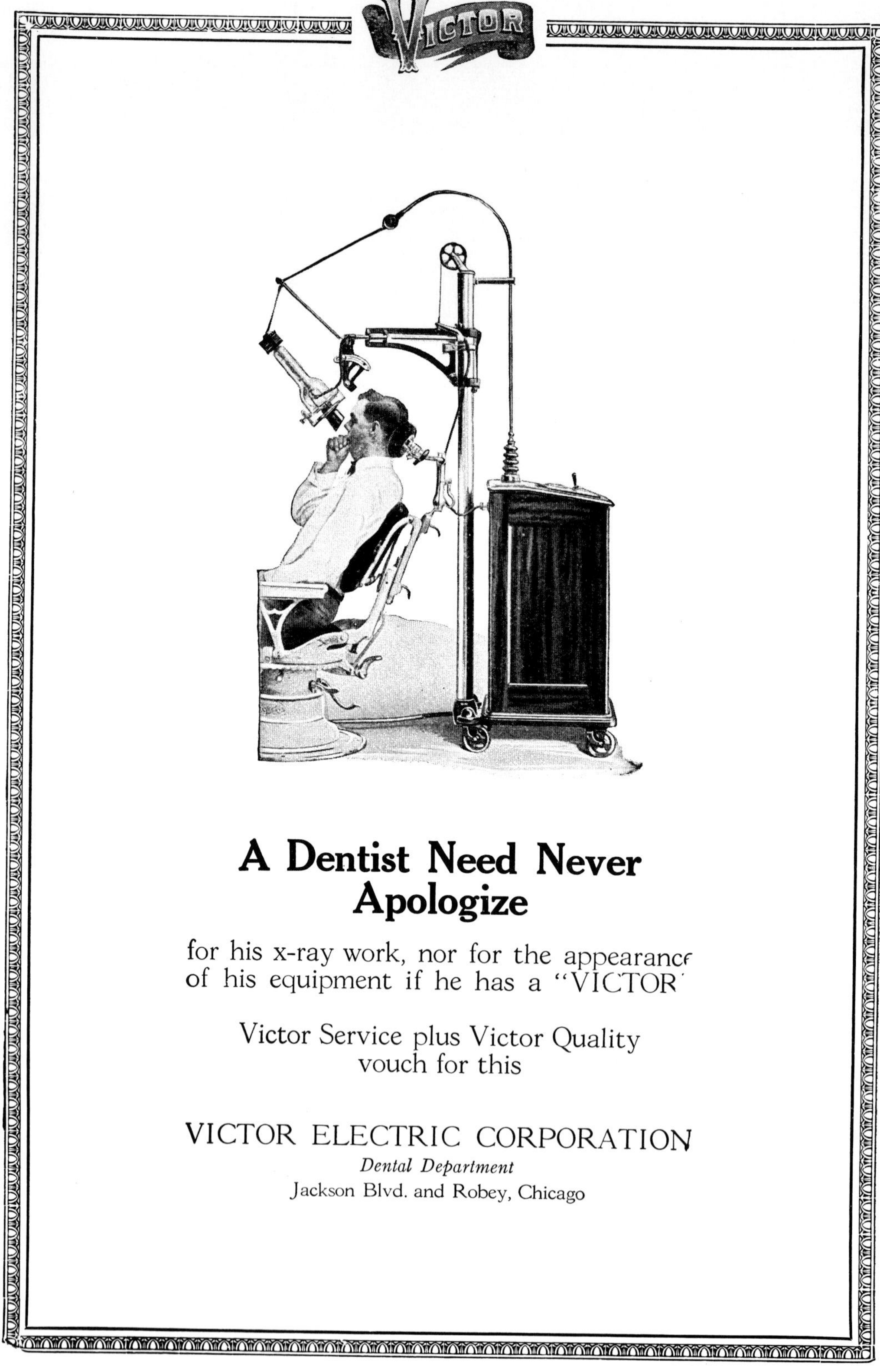

Advertisement alerting the dentist to the quality of X-ray equipment and its impact on his patients. From Victor Electric Corp. Catalog, 1919.

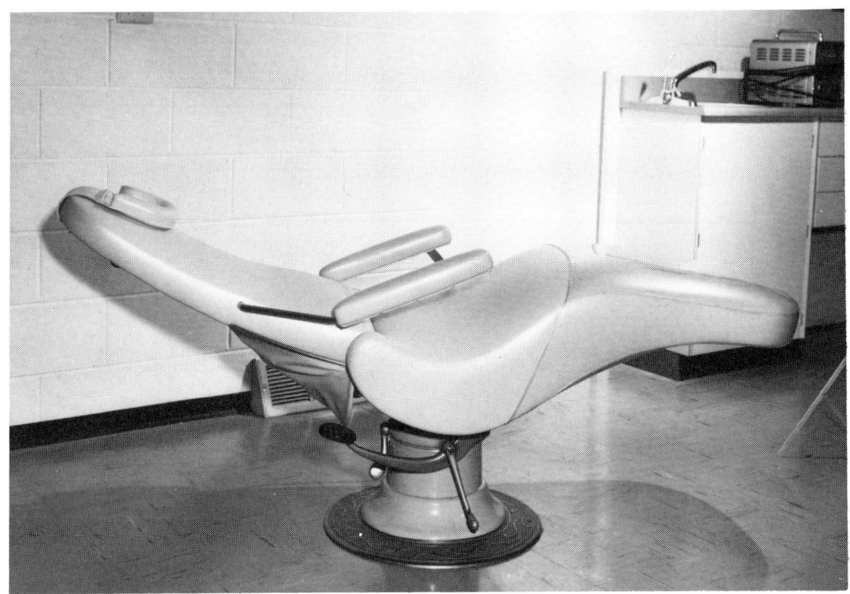

First reclining dental chair invented and built, in 1958, by John L. Naughton, Des Moines, Iowa. The chair revolutionized dentistry by introducing "sit-down" dentistry, now a standard operating practice within the profession. The chair is in the National Museum of American History, Smithsonian Institution, gift of the Den-Tal-Ez Company. It should be noted that the English dentist, Alfred Coleman, whose book *Manual of Dental Surgery* was revised by Thomas C. Stellwagen for American students in 1882, recommended that the young dentist sit down while doing gold fillings. In this position the novice would be able to remain steady and endure the long procedure. To work on the patient the dentist tipped back the Wilkerson chair in use at the time, one of the first dental chairs to allow this flexibility in position.

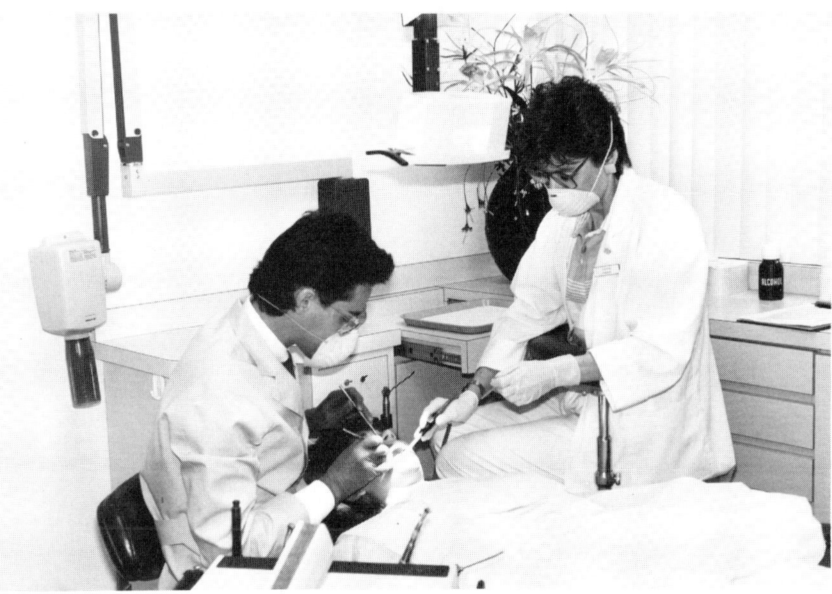

Present-day office of Robert M. Pick of Aurora, Illinois, a periodontist, who is pushing ahead the frontiers of modern dental technology by employing laser surgery in treating his patients for gum diseases. Pick and his assistant also wear gloves, masks, glasses, and lab coats in keeping with the totally clean office.

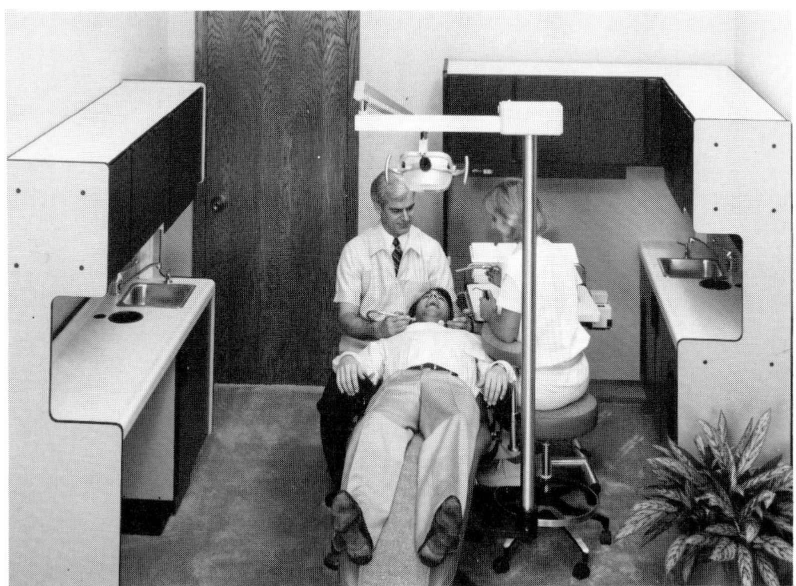

Total operatory system produced by ADEC of Newberg, Oregon in 1986. State of the art dental office by the leading American dental manufacturer in the 1980s. From ADEC.

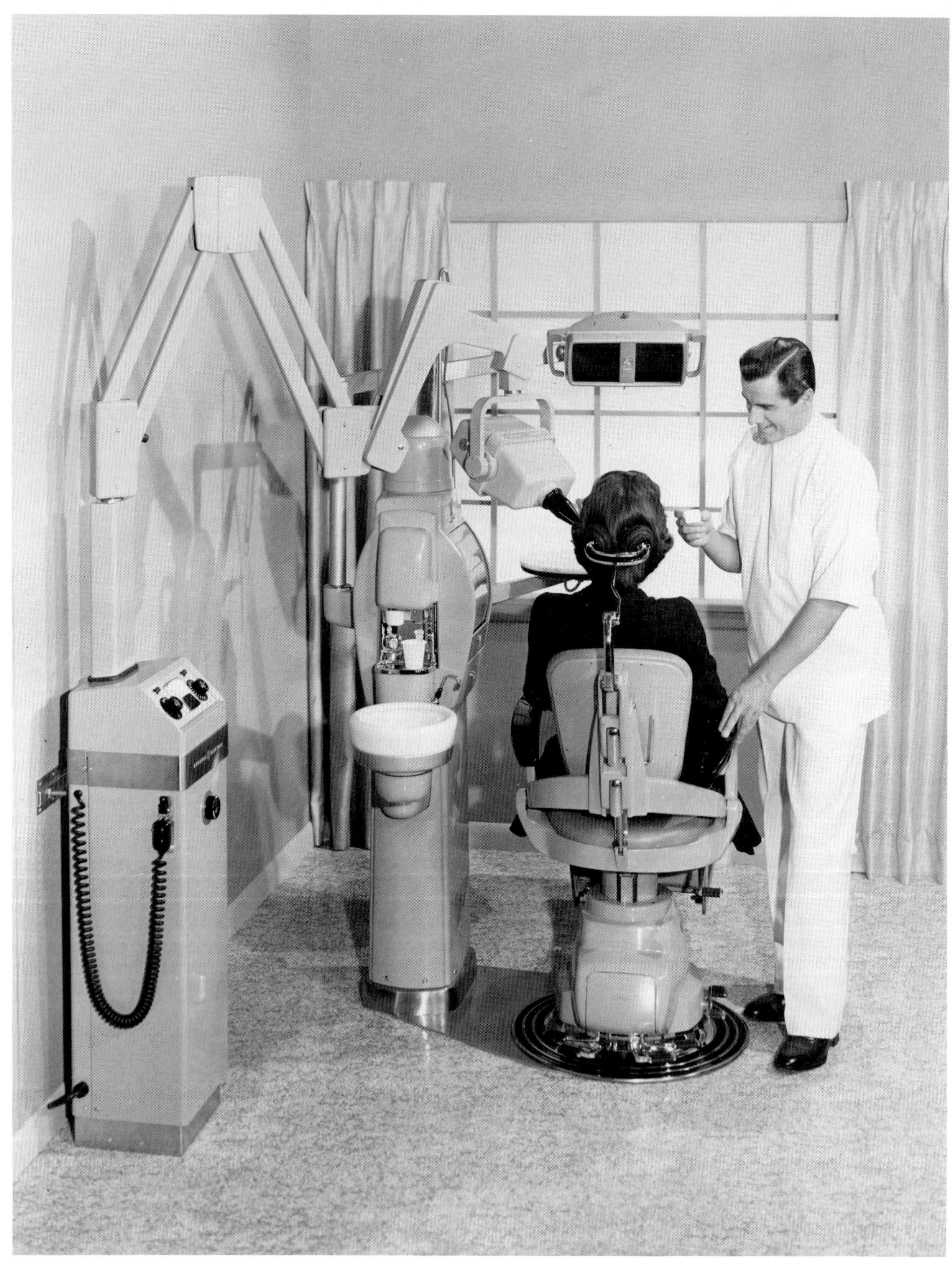

General Electric X-Ray 1960s office. This is a typical promotional photograph. From General Electric Company.

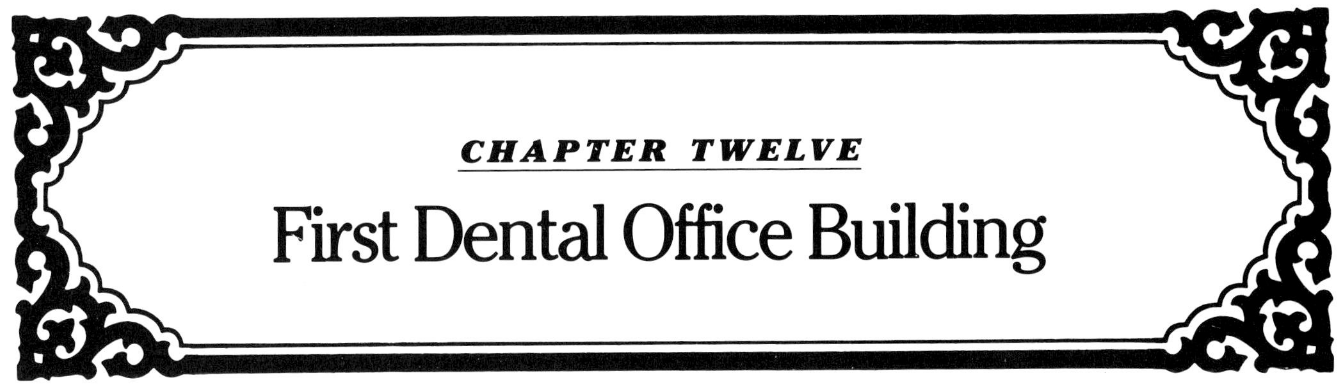

CHAPTER TWELVE

First Dental Office Building

The first building to be constructed entirely for the practice of dentistry was built by Alfred C. Fones (1869-1938) of Bridgeport, Connecticut in 1912.[142] Inspection of Fones' office inspired Ottolengui to resume the series on dental offices in *Items of Interest* in 1913, after he had discontinued it for lack of contributions. Fones, who was born in Bridgeport, graduated from the New York College of Dentistry in 1890 and practiced with his father, Civilian, until his death. Fones was elected president of the Bridgeport and Connecticut dental societies. He won several medals bestowed by the dental societies of New York State and Connecticut.[143]

Because of his contributions to preventive dentistry, and especially, in teaching dental health care to children, he is regarded as a pioneer in this field. His leadership helped to introduce dental hygiene into schools throughout the U.S. Fones, in 1900, offered preventive dental services to his patients and noted that their general and dental health was better than that of his father's patients, who were not offered these instructions and services. Fones' assistant, Irene Newman, was trained to give prophylactic care to patients, a profession which she practiced for 30 years. Several other dentists had employed nurses in their offices or were being assisted by their wives by this time, and generally, promoted the practice of preventive dentistry. Robin Adair of Atlanta, Georgia employed a dental nurse since 1909, whom he called "the first dental nurse in the South."[144] W. George Ebersole had employed a nurse since 1905 in his Cleveland practice.

Fones' most important achievement in dentistry, which changed and extended dental office practice, was his establishment of the first school for dental hygienists. All of the graduates obtained jobs in the local schools. Their function was "to provide an added service to school children, offering them prophylactic care, instruction in brushing and flossing, and education in nutrition and general hygiene."[145] Fones designed a space in his building to train hygienists. The first class graduated in June 1914, and by 1916 when the last class was graduated, 97 dental hygienists had been trained. The first graduate, Irene Newman, received license number one in Connecticut, the first state to issue a license to dental hygienists. Fones coined the term dental hygienist for his female colleague, a term he used to indicate that the hygienist provided preventive services in the dental office, which did not include the treatment of disease, a practice that was reserved for the dentist. Fones enlisted prominent physicians from Harvard, Yale, and the universities of Pennsylvania and Columbia, including E.S. Gaylord, M.L. Rhein, Rodrigues Ottolengui and T.P. Hyatt, to teach in his dental hygiene school. Offering their instruction without pay because they believed in the program, their lectures were compiled into the first dental hygiene textbook *Mouth Hygiene*, which was published in 1916. Edited by Fones, R.H. Strang and E.C. Kirk, the authors believed that "at least eighty per cent of dental diseases can be prevented by following a system of treatment and cleanliness."[146] When Fones' school closed, three dental schools opened programs for dental hygienists, a move which Fones applauded. Among the most successful was the second school, the Forsyth-Tufts Training School for Dental Hygienists established in 1916 in Boston.[147] Morale among the graduates of the dental hygiene programs was high enough by 1923 to result in the formation of the American Dental Hygienists' Association.

Dental hygiene as a term to convey the concept of caring for teeth to prevent decay was used since at least 1871 and grew out of an early oral hygiene movement. Before Fones, other dentists had suggested that women be employed to assist the dentist including N.W. Kingsley (1844), Thaddeus P. Hyatt of New York (1903), and Cyrus Mansfield Wright of Cincinnati, Ohio (1902). As noted above, Kells and Rhein were among those who employed women assistants, who they trained in their offices. Fones gave credit to Wright for visualizing the role of the dental hygienist. Wright designed a course for dental nurses which was given in 1910-11 in the Ohio College of Dental Surgery.[148] The course was dropped in 1914 and after opposition from dentists none of its graduates were permitted to practice. Two of the women continued their studies and became dentists.[149] F.W. Low of Buffalo, in 1902, advocated another approach to dental hygiene through the establishment of a new profession which he called odontocure. The role of the odontocurist was to clean and polish teeth, similar to the manicurist who cleaned the fingernails. The odontocurist, most likely a female, would bring an orange-wood stick and some pumice and possibly a flannel rag to the client at home on a biweekly basis. For cleaning the teeth and gums she could charge 50 cents.[150]

Fones built a suite of dental offices in a two-story structure, 80 feet long, that was designed in the pattern of a carriage house. On the first floor was a garage for four cars, with space for a lecture hall for the dental hygienist school, in addition to patient dressing rooms and a secretary's office. The school was equipped with 16 Diamond chairs loaned by S.S. White Dental Manufacturing Company. Each chair contained a worktable, cuspidor and manikin head. Sterilizers and supplies were provided for students to clean their instruments which they placed in a japanned locked box. The students were examined on their skills in selecting the instruments to remove pencil marks from the teeth of the manikin, which simulated removing tartar from human teeth. On the second floor were four operating rooms, two prophylactic rooms used by the dental assistants, a laboratory and a room that was used for both making and developing X-rays and as a lunchroom.[151]

The floors on the lower level were covered with red Welsh tiles. The waiting room provided a restful atmosphere decorated with paneled wood walls of American hazel wood finished in soft brown topped by a 2-1/2 inch wide ceiling border in caen stone. A carved mantle also was faced with caen stone. All floors on the second level were made of a grey composition called "Sanitas." Ottolengui believed that Fones' office was "the finest dental office in the world."

Dr. Fones' operating room gathered light through a large window facing the dental chair and a skylight. Foot stirrups were set in the floor for the dentist to rest his feet while working on a patient.

In the prophylactic rooms, furnished with white-enameled appliances and furniture, the nurses sterilized equipment and a dental chair accommodated a patient. The laboratory contained a chemical hood with a flue leading to the roof to release the gases and odors released by acids, soldering, casting or vulcanizing.

Ottolengui stressed that Fones was not a wealthy person. ". . . luxurious as it is, [the building] has been constructed and is managed on purely business principles. Everything is so systematized, invested capital, cost of maintenance and office charges are so harmonized, that Dr. Fones himself is practically rentfree, so much so that nearly all that he does himself is profit. Thus a wonderfully unique, absolutely aseptic, thoroughly professional dental establishment has been proven to be possible along purely business lines."[152]

Fones buildings were photographed by traveling photographers who captured the images of all commercial structures in many small towns at the end of the 19th century.

CHAPTER THIRTEEN

Floating Dental Offices

Dentists, as we have seen, have a long tradition of serving on seaworthy vessels beginning with Fauchard's experiences leading to dental innovations and extending to employment by the shipping industry to serve passengers and crews during their voyages. Percy C. Lowery (1885-1978) earned the money to set up his first office, as did many other young dentists, by working as a purser on the S.S. Huron during the summer after his graduation in 1910 from the University of Michigan School of Dentistry. He began to practice on October 4, 1910. Since he could not afford to rent a room, he slept in his waiting room. To greet his patients properly he had to rise early. He treated farmers, who were going to market, and therefore, arriving at the dental office unusually early. His income as a dentist during the year was inadequate, so the following summer, he resumed the purser position and hired a classmate, G.W. Fitzgerell to care for his patients in his absence. In the fall he continued his practice without further interruption. Lowery specialized in prosthetic dentistry and developed his practice to the point that he built a second office in 1914, and a decade later, designed a "palatial" office which was the "epitome of efficiency."[153]

The most ingenious water-born office was installed on a river boat by F.H. Houghton of Daytona, Florida at the turn of the century.[154] He and other itinerant dentists in this period continued to travel by a variety of methods including horse, buggy, and wagon trains to serve cowboys, logging camps and other groups of scattered American settlers. Before setting up his floating office Houghton had practiced for two decades during the winter months by rotating stops in the towns along the waterways of Florida. He was the only dentist who visited the area, in which thousands of people lived, therefore Houghton proposed the boat with a dental office as a solution to meet their dental care needs all year long. Having migrated from northern cities with established dentists, Houghton's patients were used to good dentistry, which Houghton proposed to deliver in a properly outfitted dental office.

In 1899 to serve his widely scattered patients he built a floating dental office which he piloted along the east coast of Florida. Named the "Dentos," the boat was 53 feet long, with a deck 20 feet wide and a capacity of 10 tons. The hull of the boat was made of cypress and the cabin of Georgia pine. The Dentos was furnished with the latest equipment.

The vibration of the water and wind on calm days did not disturb the dentist or patient having his teeth repaired while floating along the river. The patient was distracted by the palm trees and tropical plants growing along the shores. Houghton arranged to meet his patients by sending cards to them and by announcing the time of his stops through the local newspapers.

A houseboat served as a dental office in the 1970s in another locale. Ethel Groce, a medical missionary, lacking training in dentistry, treated people who spent their lives on small boats called junks and sampans along the coastal waters of Hong Kong. Her patients neglected their teeth until they became uncomfortably diseased. On her houseboat clinic she used an old forceps to extract the teeth of those who came to her when in pain.[155]

Meanwhile in another part of the world an American dentist joined a medical ship, the famous Project Hope. Charles B. Cartwright used his sabbatical to serve with the U.S.S. Hope in Natal, Rio Grande do Norte, Brazil during the summer of 1972. The S.S. Hope was a fully-equipped hospital ship, which was operated and paid for by voluntary personnel under the direction of Dr. William B. Walsh, to provide medical and dental services without charge to anyone. "The ship ha[d] a fully-equipped three-chair dental clinic and laboratory, as well as a small dental library and conference room." A fairly modern dental school in the city of Natal drew upon Cartwright's talents as a teacher.[156]

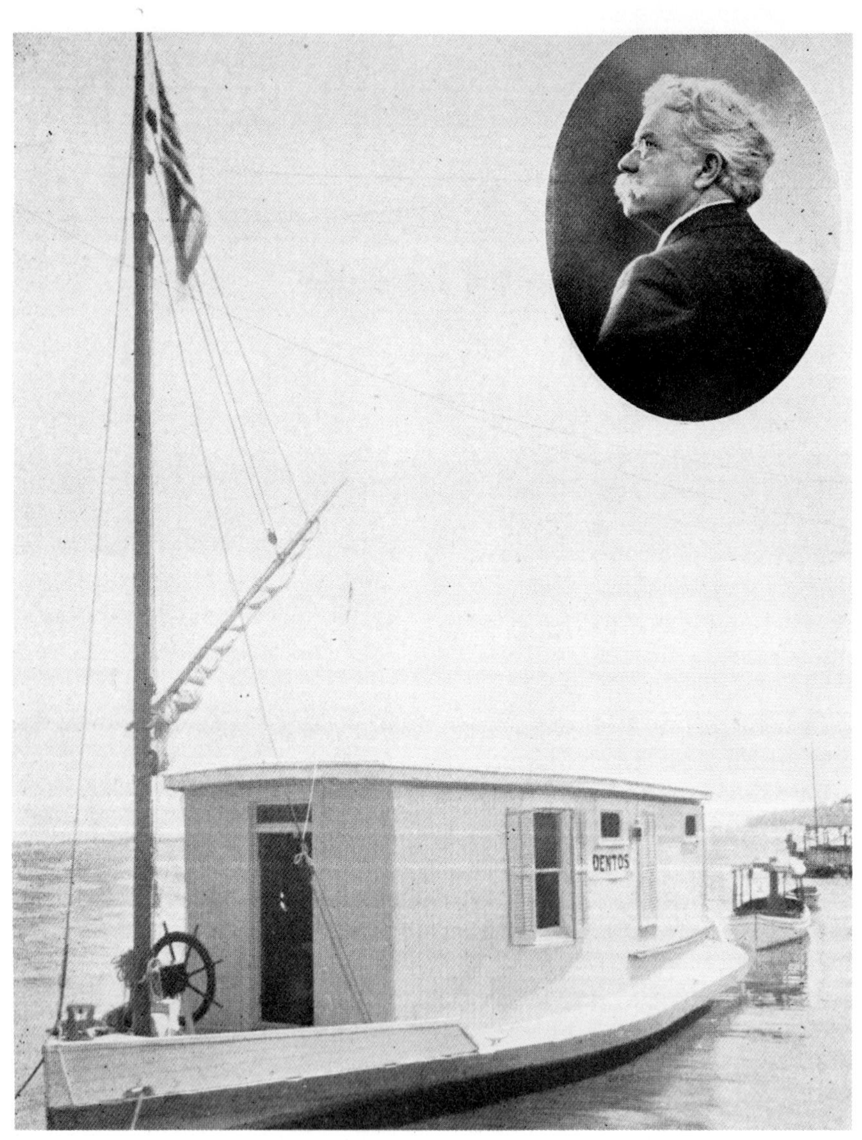

The dental office boat of F.H. Houghton, Daytona, Florida, in 1899. Houghton brought itinerant dentistry to a new level of comfort and adaptability by outfitting a houseboat with a dental office to accommodate his patients who lived along the waterways of Florida. He would announce his arrival in the newspapers or send a post card to his patients. From *Items of Interest*, Vol. 21.

CHAPTER FOURTEEN

Foreign Dental Offices

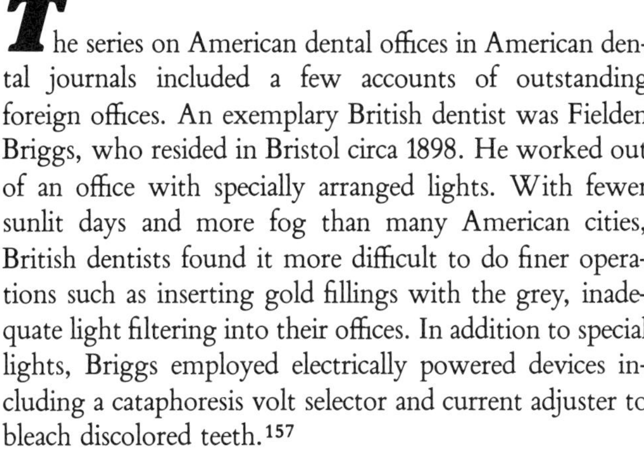

The series on American dental offices in American dental journals included a few accounts of outstanding foreign offices. An exemplary British dentist was Fielden Briggs, who resided in Bristol circa 1898. He worked out of an office with specially arranged lights. With fewer sunlit days and more fog than many American cities, British dentists found it more difficult to do finer operations such as inserting gold fillings with the grey, inadequate light filtering into their offices. In addition to special lights, Briggs employed electrically powered devices including a cataphoresis volt selector and current adjuster to bleach discolored teeth.[157]

Briggs was a gifted dentist and successful inventor. Among the instruments Briggs designed were a set of pluggers used to insert gold fillings. These pluggers were popular with dentists throughout the world. Briggs also designed and improved a more mundane but essential appliance, a self-emptying spittoon. Artistically shaped in the form of a clam shell it was attached to the wall by a bracket. Instead of pulling a plug to empty the water, the pipe was bent up so that when the water rose a certain distance in the shell it was automatically siphoned away.

Dentists working with precious metals lost some of their material during the process of making gold crowns, repairing teeth or removing loose fillings. Briggs developed a method to retrieve the lost metallic scraps. He installed an extra tank under the floor to collect the pieces of metal which were ejected into the spittoon by the patient. The amount of precious metal retrieved in a year was valuable. Dentists who placed an Oriental rug under the chair could retrieve enough gold to buy a better rug after a few years of use if they destroyed the rug and extracted the gold pieces which fell to the floor. Briggs was exemplary in other aspects of his profession. He was among the first generation of dentists to answer mail by dictation and to employ a secretary to transcribe his letters.

One foreign dental office was so attractive, simple and scientifically correct that a German author, George Randorf of Berlin, described it in 1897 for *Dental Items of Interest*.[158] The office was operated by Alexander Vasilovitch Fischer, dentist to the Girls' and Orphans Institute in Moscow, Russia. He practiced in a room painted white with brown linoleum on the floor. For antiseptic purposes he wore a white linen, tightly fitted outfit extending from head to toe. On the glass bracket table, which was removable for cleaning, he placed his instruments and materials for repairing teeth. Fischer commented to the author, who visited him in Moscow, that he was removing the last ornamental things from his office so that he could clean every item completely. Each patient wore a white apron tied around his/her neck while undergoing treatment. The simplicity, economy and cleanliness of Fischer's office was singled out to remind American dentists of their responsibilities to their profession and their patients.

Cephas Whitney of Kingston, Jamaica, B.W.I. designed a semi-circular laboratory bench in 1899. Placed to receive the light from the windows, he provided 10 feet of work space within his reach while seated, by revolving his stool from one end to the other of the bench.[159]

Robert Marcus of Frankfurt-on-Main, Germany provided two principal requirements in his office—good light and clean air. His office was situated in the business section of the city with a scenic view of the countryside. He was among those dentists who gave his patients a local anesthetic by mixing electricity and chemicals. He applied electricity, known as cataphoresis as part of his anesthetic procedure while working on sensitive dentin, during extractions or in treating the gum disease, "periostitis." A chemical solution was applied to the gum as well as the electrical apparatus.[160]

Frank R. Faber, who practiced in Constantinople, Turkey, enjoyed reading about other dental offices in Ottolengui's series, therefore, he reciprocated by sending in a description of his apartment house/office. It occupied a suite that had four facades, thus assuring a generous amount of light and air. Faber obviously most enjoyed decorating his Oriental reception room in the Moosharaben style. Walls covered in walnut panels placed over red paper and accented with red silk curtains reflected light in a harmonious pattern. Carved teakwood furniture from India was placed around "fine old" wool, Turkish carpets. Turkish and Persian tiles were gathered individually and put in place by craftsmen whose unpredictable work schedules added to Faber's burden in decorating this unusual dental reception room.

The operatory, in contrast, was so compact every instrument and device was within reach. The nitrous oxide apparatus stood under the wall clock to the left of the chair. Dentists in Constantinople had to stock artificial teeth since there were no suppliers in the city. Faber filed 15,000 teeth in a cabinet covered with a white cloth which became his "dental depot," a term used for suppliers of dental materials. Mirrors were inserted into the door panels to make the room appear larger and to please female patients. Since the city did not supply electricity, Faber employed an Edison-Leland battery to power his hand-piece.[161]

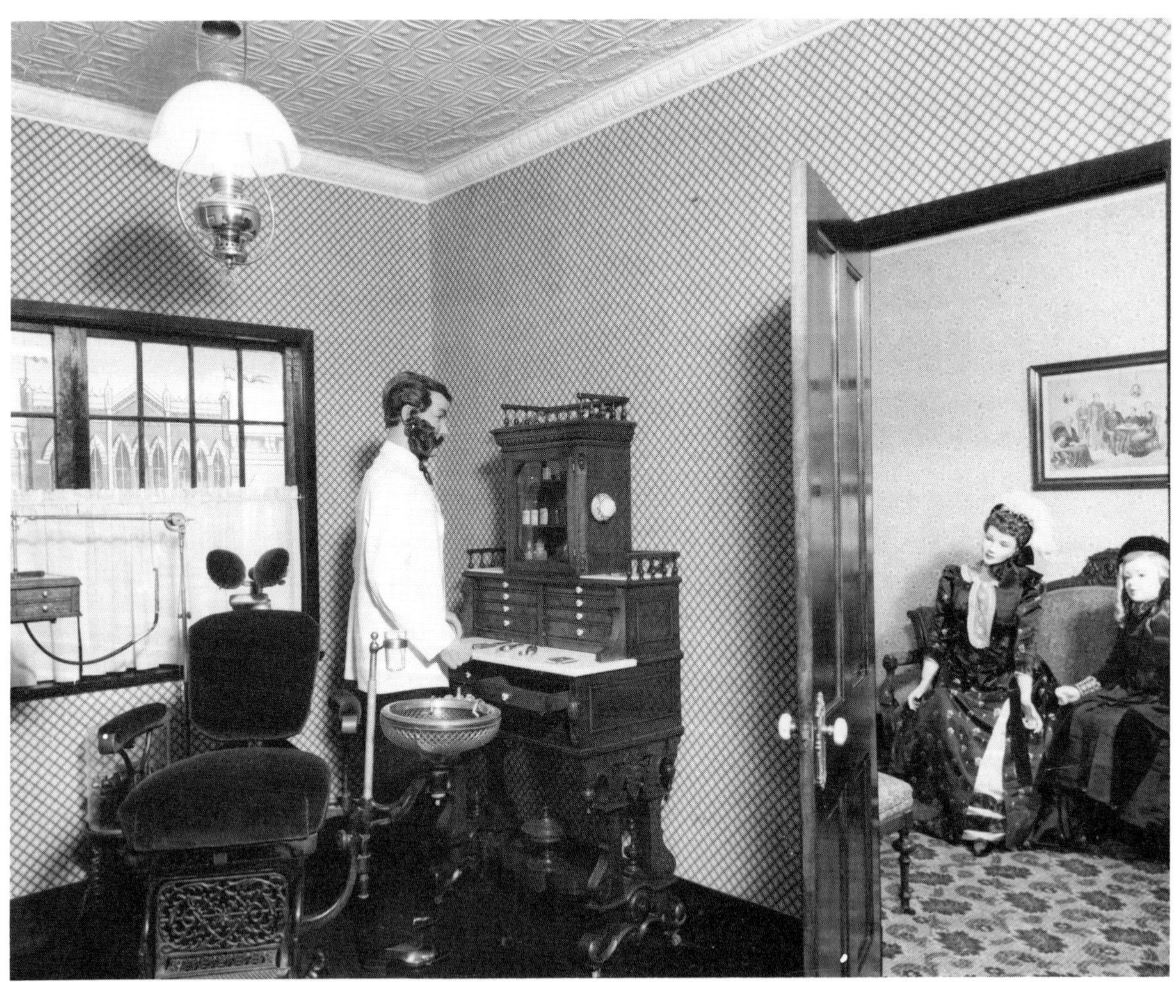

Exhibition of dental office which was first used by Joseph William Wassall in 1909, prominent Chicago dentist. Dr. Kermit F. Knudtzon, Chicago dentist, acquired Wassall's office from his estate and exhibited it next to his office until 1950 when he retired and donated Wassall's office to the Chicago Historical Society, which then exhibited the office until 1975. Presently it is on exhibition in the main waiting room of the Loyola University School of Dentistry in Chicago to help celebrate its centenary in 1988. Loyola took over the Chicago College of Dentistry in the 1920s. The dentist stands in front of the Archer cabinet, which appears to be the only example of this early and interesting cabinet on public view. From Chicago Historical Society.

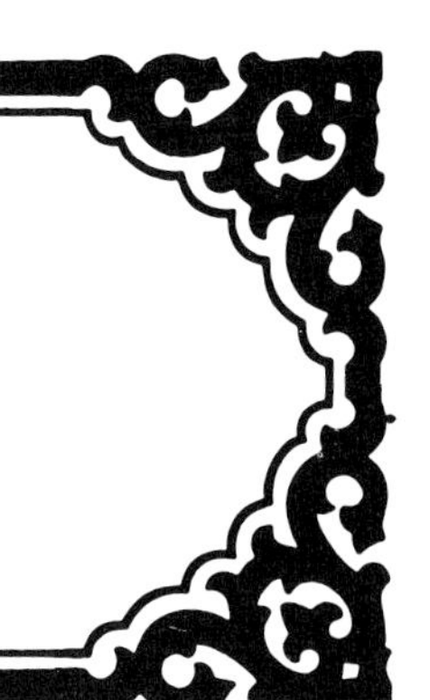

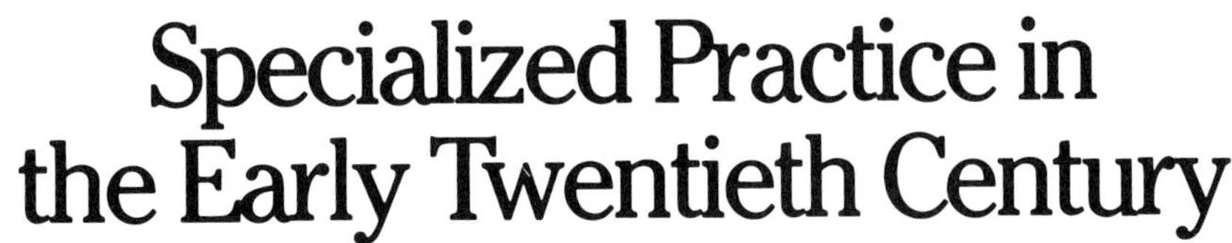

CHAPTER FIFTEEN

Specialized Practice in the Early Twentieth Century

After the first World War a few American dentists' offices began to include features common to other business and professional offices. An example of the new, large, efficient and specialized dental office and practice is that of Dr. George B. Winter of St. Louis, a popular exodontist, who worked in a suite of 22 rooms.[162] Described in 1913 and 1920 this large office consisted of two reception rooms, a secretary's office, an administration room, a private office and library, two X-ray rooms, a developing darkroom, a bacteriology and pathology laboratory, a sterilizing department, four operating rooms, four rest rooms, a linen room, a nurses' dressing room, a storage room for gas cylinders, and a research department. All operating room windows were made of translucent glass. This elaborate space, furnished with the latest devices and backed up with a useful record system, provided opportunities for Winter to run his office as an efficient business and to provide patients with a greater range of services.

Walls, floors and ceilings were painted or tiled in shades of white. The room for extracting teeth was bare and small (9 feet by 10 feet) with a white tile floor and marble baseboard. White was chosen so that any blood which settled in the room would be easily seen and could be removed to prevent the spread of infection. Winter recommended the Morrison chair or the older Archer chair in which the patient would be held more securely when anesthetized or resisting treatment.[163] Rooms in which patients were treated were fitted with call buttons so that patients could summon an attendant if they felt uncomfortable while waiting in the dental chair. Winter preferred that his cabinet be constructed out of wood because the wooden drawers would fit together tighter and keep out dust better than looser fitting metals.[164]

To equip this type of elaborately furnished office, dental supply firms such as Frank S. Betz of Chicago sold complete sets of furniture. For the waiting room Betz advertised in 1916 a 12-piece set for $75. The set included a rolltop sanitary desk, office chair, clock stand, hall clock, settee, arm rocker, armchair, ladies' rocker, straight chair, library table, reading lamp and genuine Axminster rug.[165] Larger office sets included wall mirrors, screens, leather wastebaskets and assorted chairs.

In the bacteriology and pathology laboratories mouth secretions were analyzed. The operating rooms were supplied with anesthetics that were piped into the area. Equipment was sterilized in a glistening room furnished with a high-pressure steam unit and two autoclaves. Instruments were laid out and their placement memorized so that the dentist could find the piece needed without taking his eyes off the tooth he was treating.[166] Two carts-on-wheels, supplied with shelves and a drawer, contained sterilized equipment packed in sterile envelopes, and were ready to be rolled into an operating room for immediate use. Winter collected data on his patients and classified it for application to other patients and for his publications.

As a specialist, Winter received patients referred by other dentists and took X-rays of patients for dental colleagues.

A few dental offices were run by women who were highly successful dentists in this period. A female dentist without peer, Minnie Evangeline Jordon (1865-1952) opened an office in the early 20th century.[167] Born in Illinois and raised in Rochester, Minnesota, and Los Angeles, she began her career as an elementary school teacher and worked as a dental assistant during the summer in California. Her interest aroused, she enrolled in the School of Dentistry at the University of California and graduated in 1898. Although she began her practice as a general dentist, by 1909 she had restricted her patients to children under 16, a dental specialty which she launched in the U.S.

Courses were taught on children's dentistry as early as 1897 when John Hurty at the Indiana Dental College taught a course on dentistry for children.[168] However, dentists did not specialize in children's dentistry until the 20th century. Rodrigues Ottolengui, who edited the series on dental offices discussed above, promoted the work of the first children's dentist, Evangeline Jordon, whom he met in San Francisco in 1915. He praised her paper delivered at the dental congress held in conjunction with the Panama Pacific World's Fair. Jordon discussed children's dentistry, a practice which later was named pedodontia.

Jordon published her experiences and ideas about treating children's dental diseases, and especially, preventive dental techniques in a series of articles in *Dental Items of Interest*, which appeared over a decade and a half. These articles were collected into a volume and published in 1925.[169] The book was reprinted in 1925, 1927 and 1929. She urged that children be instructed as early as possible, and certainly, by the time they entered kindergarten, on how to brush their teeth, and then, to make sure they could clean their teeth properly, they were to be observed while using a toothbrush. She summed up her philosophy toward the prevention of children's dental disease: "Rid the country of the deadly candy shop and grocery store, get most of our living from the vegetable garden and the family cow, and apply the teachings of oral hygiene."[170]

In her office she provided toys and other items to amuse and distract her young patients from worrying about the treatment of their teeth. She favored American Indian items such as a Navaho rug on the floor and as a wall covering. She decorated the walls with Indian baskets and weapons. Jordon chose Mission-style waiting room furniture to harmonize with the Indian artifacts. She used the unusual Indian items to spark discussion with young children who were waiting or while they were being worked on in the dental chair. She counseled dentists to choose office furnishings and decorations which would appeal to children such as Chinese, Japanese or other exotic artifacts. Jordon chose an S.S. White children's chair with porcelain arms and knobs, but replaced the hard porcelain headrest with a softer one covered in leather and gauze. While they sat in the chair her patients played with celluloid animals which they could float in the spittoon before it had been used. To explain the parts of the tooth and disease processes to the child she used imaginative drawings. She represented a tooth as a little house occupied with a little sister named Miss Nerve and little brothers named Artery and Vein.[171]

In the course of drilling and filling teeth, Jordon told stories and recited poetry which she had memorized in college in her studies to prepare her to teach in an elementary school. Her most successful story for children under age five was "A Little Red Hen" adapted to their experiences in California. In this version of the juvenile classic, written to inspire children with the value of laboring for their livelihood, the hen does all the work from planting, weeding, harvesting and grinding corn to making it into a cake, which she then enjoys all by herself, since all her requests for help in preparing the corn and making it into a cake had been refused.[172]

Jordan helped organize the American Association of Women Dentists (1928) which originated in 1921 as The Federation of American Women Dentists with Jordon as its first president.

Maud Muller Tanner continued Jordan's pioneering work in children's dentistry by becoming the first dentist to fit a child with artificial teeth in 1920. She also published the first book designed to educate children about the cure and prevention of dental diseases.[173]

In this period the Forsyth Infirmary in Boston was launched. It became an important private children's dental institution. This first philanthropic institution in the world devoted to dental care, education and research was funded by a $2 million donation from the Forsyth family, who were manufacturers of vulcanized rubber products.[174] The Infirmary, dedicated in 1914, in association with the Tufts and Harvard dental schools, not only provided dental treatment but carried out a preventive dentistry program.[175]

Women dentists did not restrict their practices to children. Some, such as Daisy Zachary Maguire (1880-1977) of North Carolina, had an unusually long career in a traditional dental practice.[176] She learned some of her first lessons in dentistry from her father and soon put her knowledge into practice. While her father was busy with a patient, Daisy, at age six, borrowed one of her father's forceps and extracted her cousin's loose tooth. After her father's death in 1898, she spent a year in Anderson, South Carolina as an apprentice to Dr. A.C. Strickland. Like her father, she became an itinerant dentist traveling through North and South Carolina and Georgia by horse and buggy. She carried a headrest to clamp on an available chair in which she seated her patients. Welcomed into the homes of her patients wherever she went, she lodged with patients along her route. In 1902 she married a cabinet maker, Wayne McGuire, who assisted her in the office until she received a telegram warning her not to practice dentistry without a degree. To obtain a license as a dentist she enrolled in an Atlanta dental school and graduated with honors in 1908, the only woman in a class of 64 men. Four years later her husband obtained his dental degree from Southern Dental School and they embarked upon a joint practice that would last 69 years. They set up an office with two chairs and units in one room. Each one served his or her own patients. Still practicing at the age of 96 (Wayne was 93) the couple spawned four other dentists among their three daughters and a son-in-law.

CHAPTER SIXTEEN

Military Dentistry through World War I

Dentists were incorporated into the American military forces after the Spanish American War. One reason for this delay in dentistry becoming an integral part of the military forces was its expense. Dental care was often more expensive than medical care, especially since gold was the preferred material used by dentists to repair teeth until well into the 20th century and tooth decay was rampant due to improper care. It was also less obvious which dental care was essential and which was cosmetic or even provoked by a desire to avoid military service. Supplying the Army and Navy with food, clothing and arms, in addition to care of the wounded, had first call on the always limited budget. The need for a dental corps within each military branch was proven by experiences in wars throughout the 19th century.

From the time of the Revolutionary War only one country made provisions for dental services for its armies and navies. The French Navy required that their surgeons have dental training, whereas the Continental and British armies made no special provisions for dental care of their troops.[177] Dental care was accepted as a part of medical care in the services. Physicians were expected to treat emergency dental problems, but could not provide extensive tooth repair or prosthetic dentistry. Although dentists were commissioned in the military services at the beginning of the 20th century, military physicians retained authority over dentists until after WWII.[178]

A French surgeon-dentist, Jean Pierre Le Mayeur, following the example of Pierre Fauchard, learned dentistry, and then, brought his skill to the colonies. Some of Le Mayeur's earliest opportunities to practice dentistry in America arose in Providence, Rhode Island when he served the French and Continental forces in 1781-82. Local civilian dentists also provided care to the soldiers under contract. George Washington, the most famous dental patient of the Revolution, was treated by Le Mayeur and seven other dentists and had several dentures made by his last dentist, John Greenwood of New York.[179]

The lack of organized military dentistry in the first half of the 19th century, in part, grew out of unorganized civilian dentistry. After the founding of the first dental school in 1839 and the American Dental Association in 1859, efforts to appoint official military dentists increased. In 1859 at the first convention of the American Dental Association the need for dentists to serve in the Army and Navy was discussed with no results.[180] This lack of action soon proved costly to the country during the Civil War. The demand for dental care was so extensive during the war that both armies in desperation arranged for civilian dentists to care for the soldiers on the battlefield or in the hospital. Before enlisting in the armies, physicians of both sides inspected the teeth as part of the general physical examination. Good strong front teeth were essential for tearing open the cartridges of powder used to load rifles just before firing them. Once in the service the soldiers received minimal dental care in an emergency.

The Confederate Army created a better dental system which could be considered a nascent dental corps. With an army of 600,000 men to care for, Dr. S.P. Moore, surgeon general of the Confederate States Army, brought dentists into the Army. He drew from a pool of 1,000 Southern dentists (there were 4,500 Northern dentists at the time). Ten percent of dentists had received a formal education. Their function was to examine each soldier admitted to the hospital. The Confederate Army dentist assisted by an attendant, worked in a room supplied with good light, hot and cold water, and soap. A carpenter made the dental chair to the dentist's specifications. Dentists used their own instruments with the materials supplied by the hospital. There was only one manufacturer of gold foil and dental materials in the South, which was Brown and Hope of Atlanta. With or without a supply of dental gold, Confederate soldiers were the least able to pay for gold fillings.

The first officially assigned dentist to a Richmond Hospital was W. Leigh Burton, who began to serve in March of 1864. Each day he treated fractures of the bones of the face, as well as putting in 20 to 30 fillings, extracting 15 to 29 teeth and removing tartar *ad libitum*.[181]

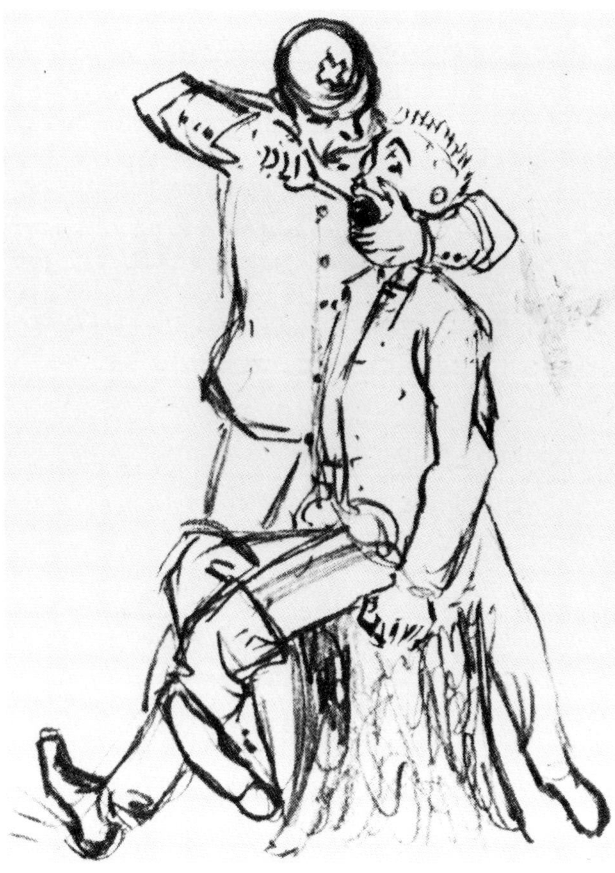

The demand for dental care by soldiers from both sides of the Mason-Dixon line was so great that charlatans grew wealthy by treating the troops. An impromptu, al fresco, tooth extraction caught Charles Reed's eye. Extraction by a military surgeon. From Library of Congress.

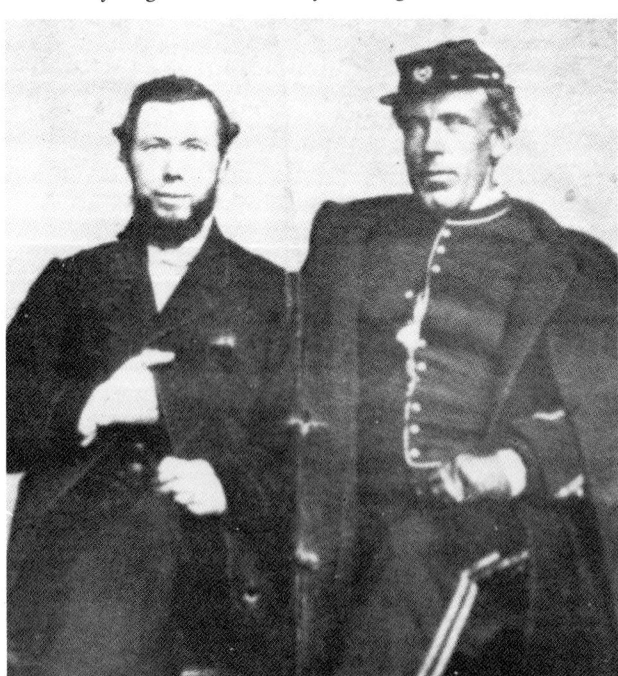

A civilian contract dentist with his commanding officer. This unidentified picture (carte de visite) was found inside a military dental kit. From Gordon Dammann, Lena, Illinois.

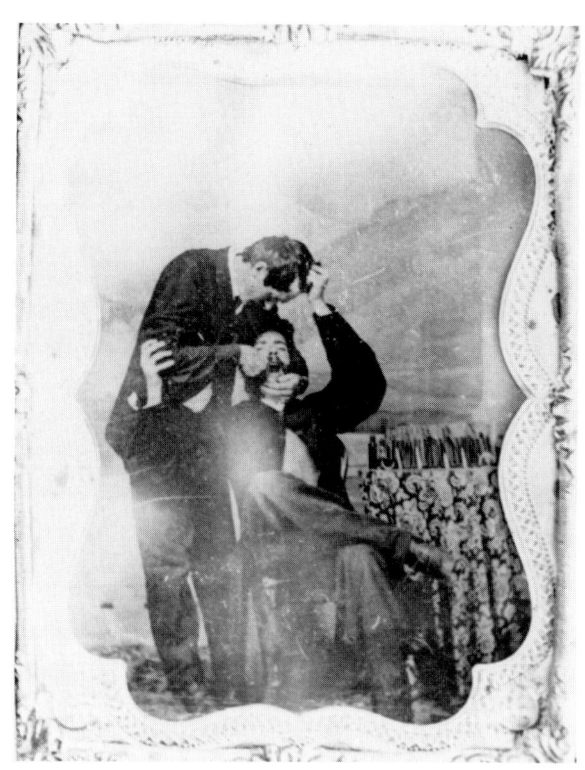

Posed tin-type of a Civil War era dentist extracting a tooth from a not-so-cooperative patient. In the closeup, notice the supply of extraction forceps and elevators in the case on the table. From Gordon Dammann, Lena, Illinois.

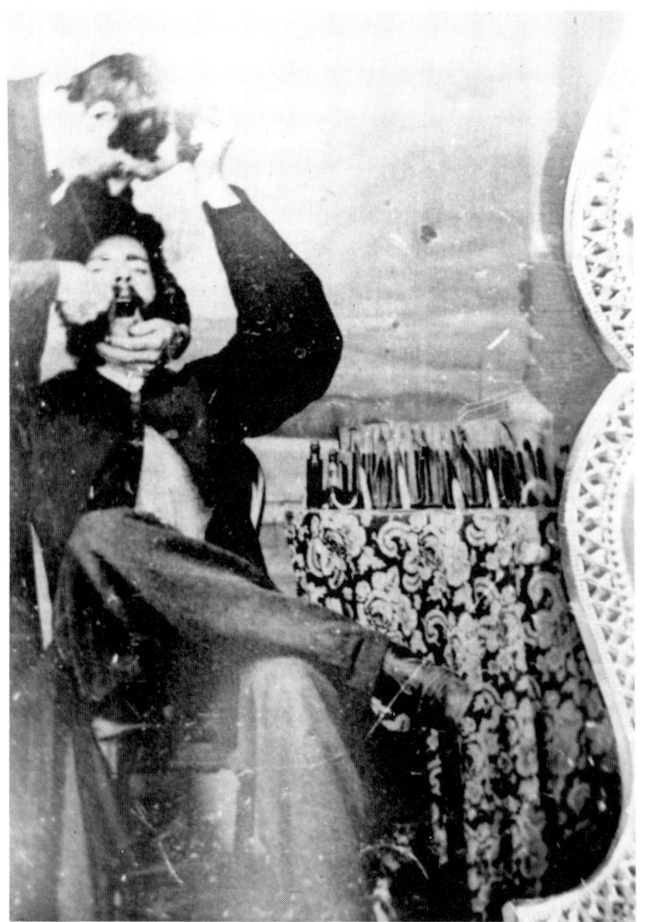

The Union Army could provide only emergency dental care (extracting teeth and lancing inflamed gums) for which it hired civilian dentists on contract. The lack of a dental corps within the Army led to episodes of excessive demand for local dentists. When General Sherman's army of 100,000 men entered Savannah in 1864, every dentist was called upon to treat dental emergencies. Many patients suffered broken teeth and fractured jaws from treatment by unskilled operators using crude equipment. One local dentist estimated that 100 dentists could have worked for six months on these troops.[182] Grim as the experiences of poor dental care were in both armies in the War Between the States, it remained until after the Spanish-American War at the end of the century before an Army Dental Corps was created.

After the Civil War the first Army dentist was appointed to treat cadets at West Point on April 4, 1872. He was an enlisted emigré at London, who joined the Army in 1856 at age 20. Hospital Steward William Saunders, whose dental education is unknown, but most likely he learned dentistry from a preceptor, had been assisting at operations, carrying out ward duties and serving as undertaker and dentist since his arrival at the school in 1858.[183] The first officer was appointed to serve as a dentist in the Navy at the U.S. Naval Academy in 1873. Thomas O. Walton, D.D.S., graduate of the Baltimore College of Dental Surgery in 1856, was appointed acting assistant surgeon as a volunteer officer to serve in the medical department. When Walton was discharged in 1879 the surgeon general first mentioned that a dental examination was included as part of the physical examination for entrance into the Navy.[184] Official histories of the Army and Navy dental corps provide the details of the important stages in the development of military dentistry including the interplay of proposals, legislation and battlefield experience, and their subsequent impact on civilian dentistry. Only a sample of the major events are discussed below for the important issues they raised in the practice of military dentistry.

On February 2, 1901 Congress passed a law creating a corps of 30 contract dentists for the Army to be attached to the medical corps but without military rank.[185] "The passage of this law gave the United States Army the first military dental corps ever attached to any army in the history of the world, and was the first opportunity given the common soldier to obtain dental service as a part of his medical attention."[186]

In March 1911 dental surgeons were commissioned as lieutenants, although a limit was set of one dentist per 1,000 enlisted men or a maximum of 60 dentists. Next year the Navy Dental Corps was created, and the following year a Navy Dental Reserve Corps, from which the active corps was appointed. Thus, the Navy was the last to obtain a dental corps, but the first to have a reserve dental corps to draw upon for active duty.[187]

The first opportunity for foreign service of the legislated dental corps came in 1901 during the Spanish-American War in the Philippine Islands where 60,000 American men were on duty. Five dentists, who had served for at least a year prior to the Act of 1901, were sent abroad and soon were joined by 11 dentists who qualified through

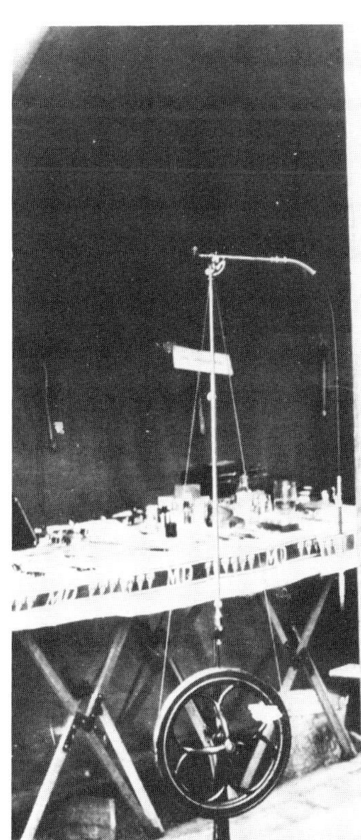
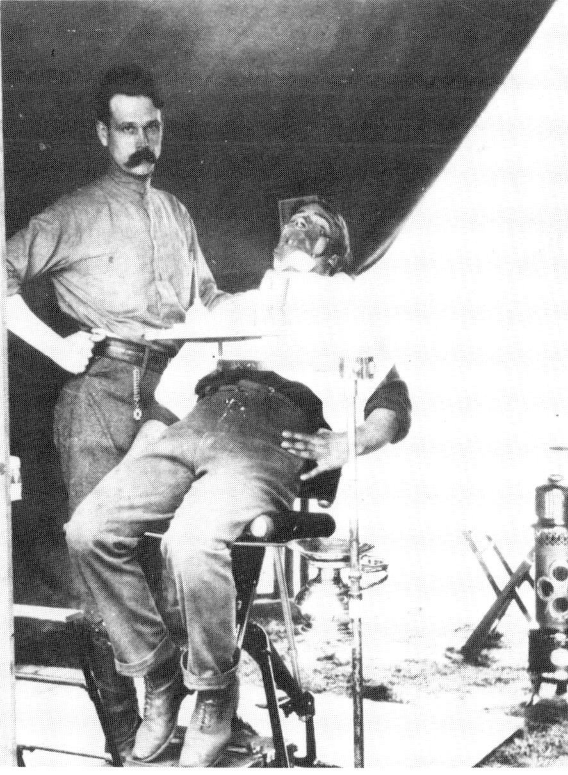

Unidentified photo, probably taken in Philippines, circa 1901-03. U.S. Army dentist working in a field tent. The Army Dental Corps was created on February 2, 1901.

examination.[188] Of these 17 Army dentists, only 10 had the necessary instrument outfits and some of these were incomplete. Experience proved that the most efficient method of employing the few dentists was to make them itinerant by sending them to stations, rather than sending soldiers to the dentist located at one central station. Before peace was declared on July 4, 1902 the number of Army stations in the islands was 140, which were reduced to less than 50 by 1904.[189]

During the hostilities in the Philippines the dentist and his equipment was escorted by armed men. The field equipment was packed in four chests and two crates. Included in Chest No. 1 were the operating dental instruments and appliances. In Chest No. 2 were placed supplies. The dental engine occupied a third chest. In a separate crate were packed the chair and equipment.

For those soldiers who needed prosthetic dentistry as a result of losing teeth on duty, two dental base stations with laboratories were established, one to serve the northern Philippines and the other in the south. Dental offices were also placed in hospitals and officer's quarters where the best light was available. Occasionally monasteries and churches were used for the dentist's office. Those dentists forced to use tents set up in the field discovered that this temporary office was the worst for dentistry. Exposed to the humid air, instruments soon rusted, and lacking adequate light the dentist could not see the teeth well.[190]

The burden of protecting instruments from the ravages of climate was shifted to suppliers. Special packing provided a solution. Root-canal cleansers, broaches, drills, explorers, separating files, Keeber saw-blades, flexible probes, burs, etc., corroded with rust after only a few weeks in storage in Manila. To prevent future shipments of such instruments from rusting and becoming useless, manufacturers sealed larger instruments in wax paper or rolled them in albolene and then placed them in corked phials. By using these methods of rust prevention, extra work was created for the dental corps in unwrapping and preparing the instruments for use on the patient.

By 1903 the Navy employed hospital stewards who were trained and experienced in dentistry. They worked at the Newport, Rhode Island station, on the U.S.S. Columbia and at the naval station on the island of Guam. The U.S.S. Solace employed a hospital steward until 1910 when he was replaced by Dr. E.E. Harris, the first graduate dentist to enlist in the Navy in 1904. The Solace also carried the first dental officer, H.E. Harvery, who served from 1913 to 1915. Acting Assistant Dental Surgeon James L. Brown became the first dental officer ordered to an overseas base when he reported to the naval station on Guam in 1913.[191]

Motor car equipped for dentistry which was outfitted by the Preparedness League of American Dentists in WWI but never sent to Europe. The organizer of this project was Dr. S. Marshall Weaver of Cleveland. From Walter Reed Army Record Photographs.

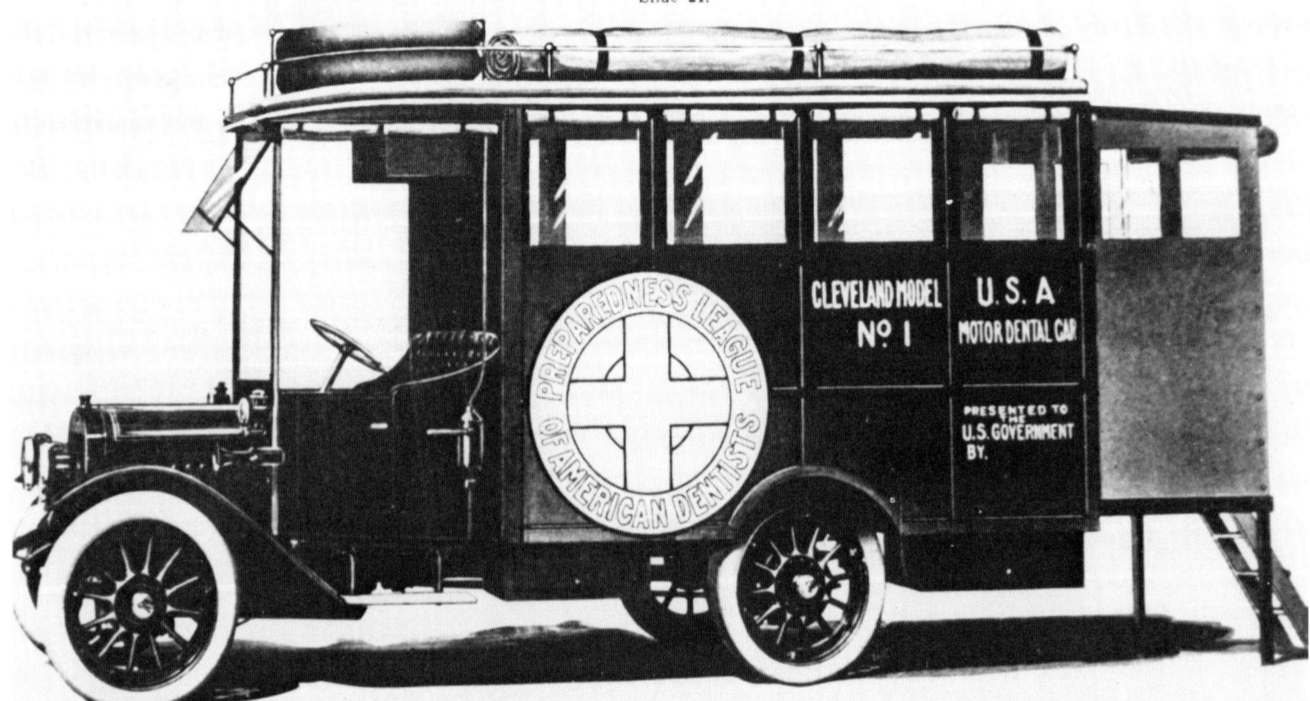

Car that has been designed and standardized by the Ambulance Committee of the Preparedness League of American Dentists, and accepted by the Wa Department, three of which are under construction and will be tried out in the various cantonments with the idea of testing out efficiency of equipment before being sent overseas.

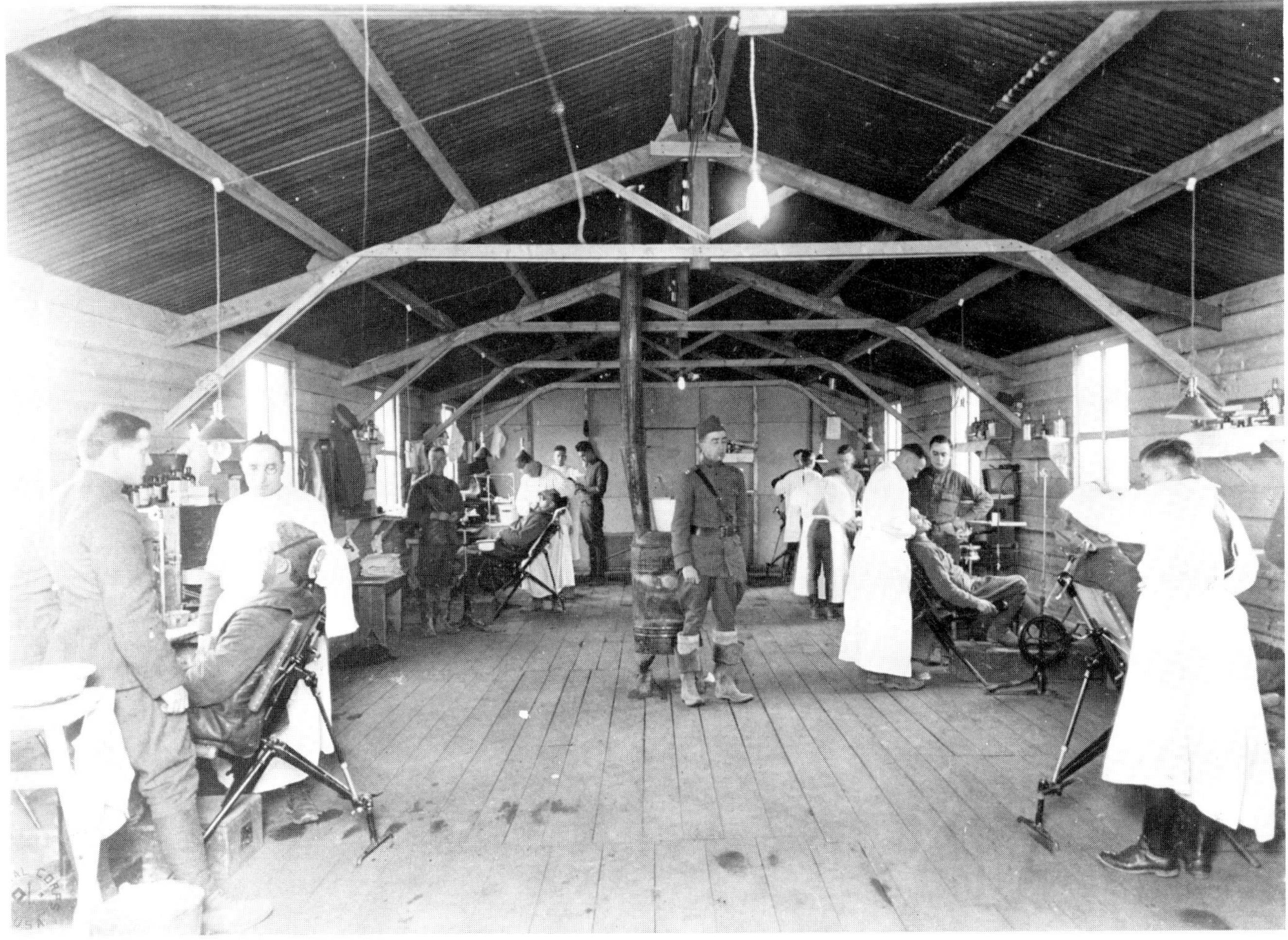

The Dental Department at Camp Hospital #85, Montiore de Bretagne, France. From National Library of Medicine, Neg. No. 79-294.

Army dental service required special training which many of the 4,000 dental officers who were called to duty in WWI had not received. Some benefited from the training they received from the Preparedness League of American Dentists formed in 1916. Its original purpose was to provide free dental service to men who wanted to enlist in the Army or would be drafted. Nearly 1,700 dentists, under the sponsorship of the Preparedness League, provided one million procedures at no cost to their patients during WWI.[192] The League also sponsored study clubs for those dentists who expected to enter the Army. A selected number of dental schools were mobilized by the federal government and students inducted into the Students Army Training Corps (SATC). Special courses to prepare the dentist for service in the Army were given at Washington University, St. Louis; Northwestern University, Chicago; and the University of Pennsylvania in Philadelphia. The government paid for each student, who, upon graduation, entered the Army. In addition to new courses, dental students practiced Army rituals such as waking up to reveille and marching to meals, and prepared for life in the war zone by digging trenches on the lawns of the colleges.[193] In March 1918, a field service school was established at Camp Greenleaf, Fort Oglethorpe, Georgia, for the instruction of dental officers and their enlisted assistants. In November 1918, at the time the war ended, 1,200 dentists had completed studies in Georgia.

After war was declared on April 6, 1917 the first contingent of Army dental corpsmen arrived in France that spring; 13 of the reserve corps had joined the Army Hospital Service and were on loan to England. Twenty-six dentists were sent as part of the regular dental corps which became part of the American Expeditionary Forces. French and English dental equipment was scarce, therefore most dental equipment and supplies were shipped from the U.S. Thirty-five Navy dental officers were on duty when war was declared and by the end of the war 500 Navy dentists were serving.[194]

For the troops going to Europe regular dental service on the transport ships began in late 1919 after the war had ended. The surgeon general intended to outfit future ships with dental offices, however, after WWI, this project was forgotten.

At first Army dentists were instructed to replace teeth only if they were lost in the line of duty. In March 1918 arrangements were made to replace teeth required for proper chewing, no matter what the cause of their loss. To meet this demand for more service a dental field laboratory, weighing over 200 pounds was issued to each Army division. By the end of the war 13,000 soldiers in France had received artificial teeth, a modest achievement when compared to the number of cases (35,657) treated in one month, (October 1944) in WWII. By the end of 1917, 140,852 standard operations (drilling, filling and extracting) and at the end of 1918, 544,516 operations were reported.[195] As military dentistry increased and dental records were collected, a second important function evolved: the identification of severely disfigured servicemen who were killed in battle.

Equipment for making artificial teeth, at first, was furnished to base hospitals, evacuation hospitals and large clinics. No prosthetic facilities were provided in the combat divisions and men in those commands who needed dental replacements had to be sent to a hospital or to one of the large clinics in the communications zone. It was soon apparent that there was urgent need for prosthetic equipment within combat zones to avoid unnecessary evacuation of personnel. Anyone sent to a base hospital for construction of dentures might be lost to his organization for as long as a man hospitalized with a moderately serious wound. The fact that a soldier could leave the combat zone for any type of prosthetic treatment encouraged the willful destruction of dental appliances and increased the demand for replacements which could not be considered essential. In one instance the strength of a company was seriously reduced due to absences for construction of dental appliances.[196]

The hurried and often inferior conditions of practicing dentistry in war zones led dentists to reflect on the impact of their methods on their patients. Believing that it was difficult to preserve the aesthetic quality of teeth on the battlefield, dentists worried that soldiers who suffered unsatisfactory or disfiguring dental treatment would be reluctant to receive dental care after they returned to civilian life. The reputation of the dentist was at stake from hasty, hurried treatment forced on him by operating with limited equipment in a war zone. Lt. K.F. Smith of Camp Grant, Illinois claimed in 1919 after his experiences in WWI, that it was possible to save teeth and practice good dentistry in the armed services with the consequence that two million servicemen would be pleased with their dental care and return for more after they were discharged.[197]

Before the war 80 percent of the U.S. population (20 million) did not visit a dentist except in an emergency.[198] Dentists such as Edwin N. Kent of Boston ascribed this lack of dental care to its cost and lack of education about caring for the teeth. Since they were educated in the military service, returning veterans were expected to be ambassadors of good dental hygiene to their families and communities. S.W. Foster of Atlanta, Georgia calculated that dentistry had been advanced by a quarter century as a result of experience in WWI.[199]

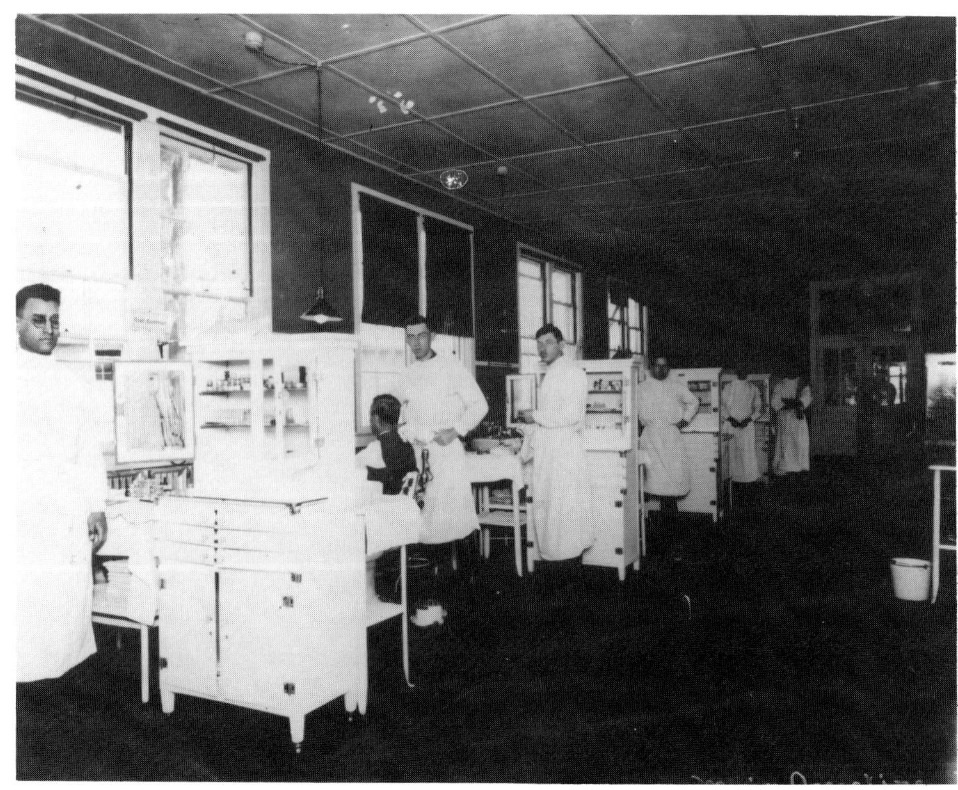

Main operating room of the dental clinic at Walter Reed General Hospital. Prior to WWI it was decided to use only portable equipment in the Zone of Interior, as well as overseas. By the fall of 1917 it was apparent that dentists could not operate as effectively with equipment which had been designed for portability. They preferred the chairs and units used in civilian practice. From National Library of Medicine, Neg. No. 79-308.

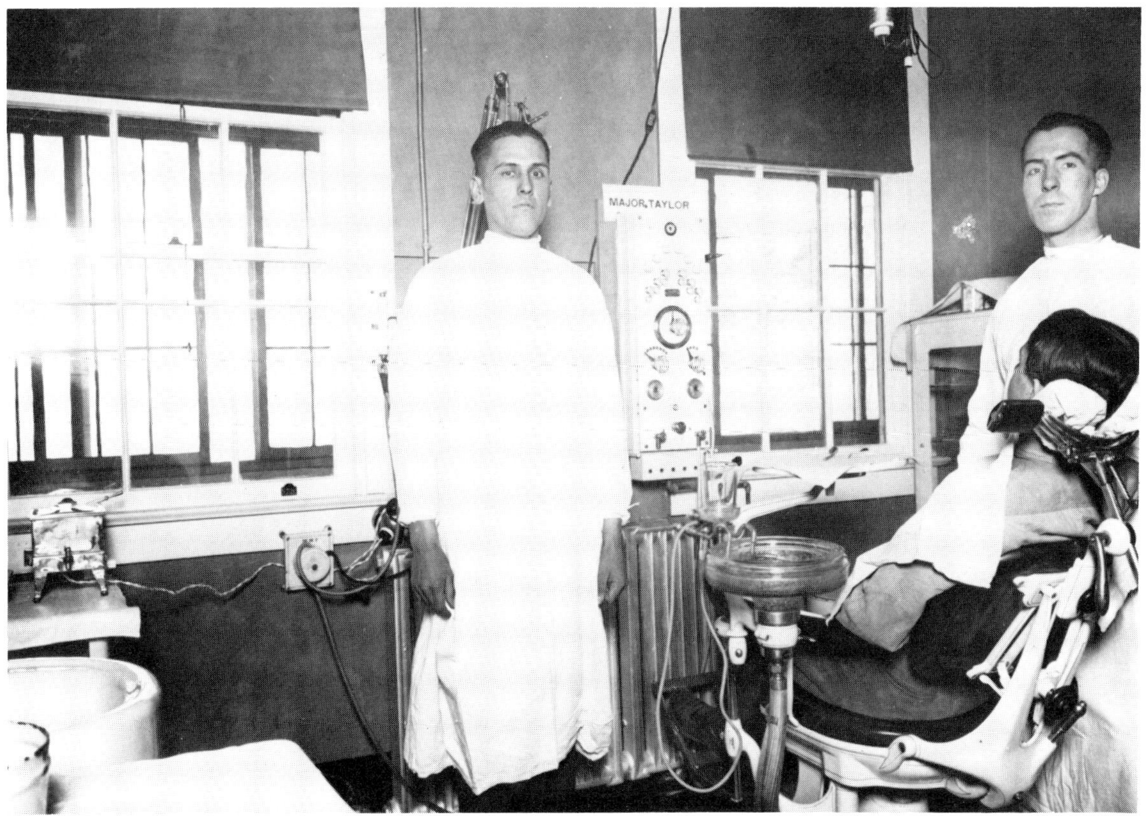

Examination room in the Dental Clinic at Walter Reed General Hospital. Electric sterilizer on the left and electric panel to the right of the attendant in the center reveal the state of the art of military dental facilities during WWI. From National Library of Medicine, Neg. No. 79-311.

Dentistry is performed outside, rather than in the tent to take advantage of daylight. The boiling water serves to sterilize instruments. The dentists used foot-pedal drills under these circumstances during WWI.

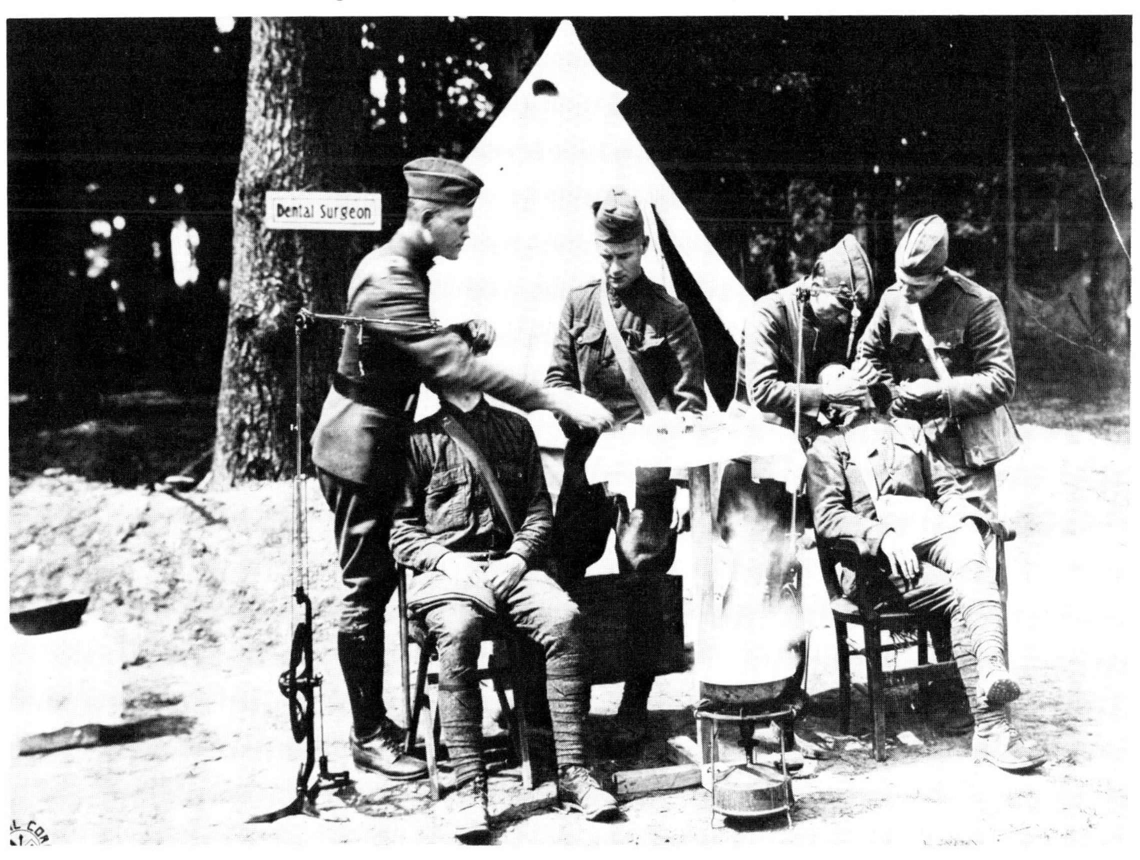

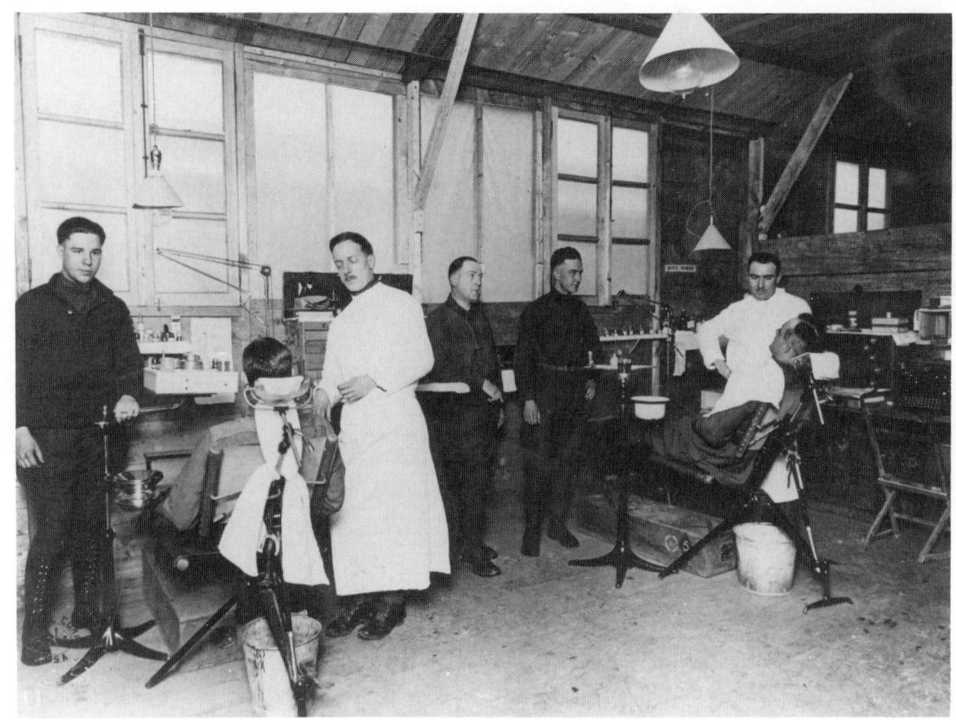

Capt. J.L. Smelltzer in the dental room of Camp Hospital #9 Chateauvillian, France, December 27, 1918. The dentist is using portable dental equipment. Dental equipment, even in its portable form, weighed 775 pounds, which made it difficult to move and sometimes had to be abandoned during an evacuation. The dentist worked in a permanent space as this wooden building testifies. This was possible because it was never more than 20 miles to the rear hospitals. Hospitals were stationary, since the combat lines varied very little. It was possible to bring troops back behind the lines for treatment and rest.

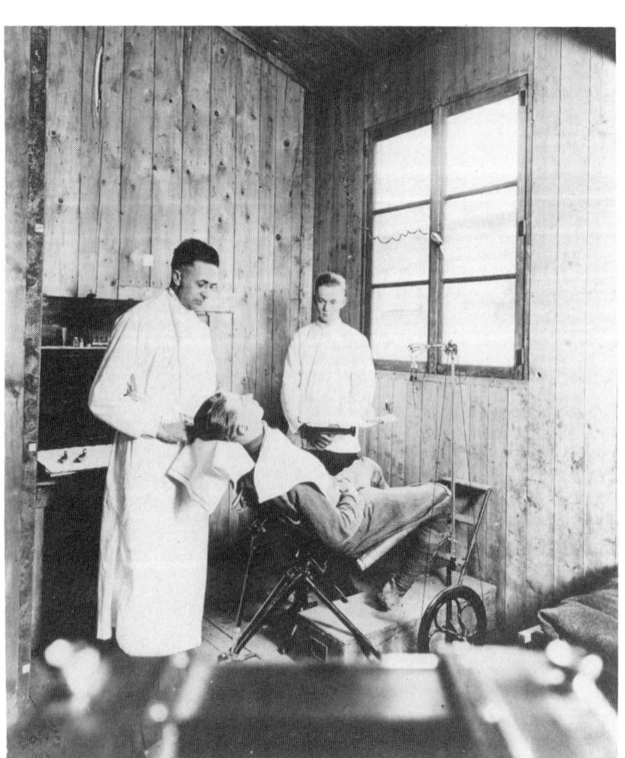

Dentistry continued after the Armistice was declared in 1919 at Camp Hospital #50, Tonnerre, France. Portable equipment was used in this clinic. A bucket beneath the dental chair is used to empty the spittoon attached to the bracket table on the left side of the chair. From National Library of Medicine, Neg. No. 79-269.

In this setting the military dentist has running water and electricity to run his drill. WWI photograph.

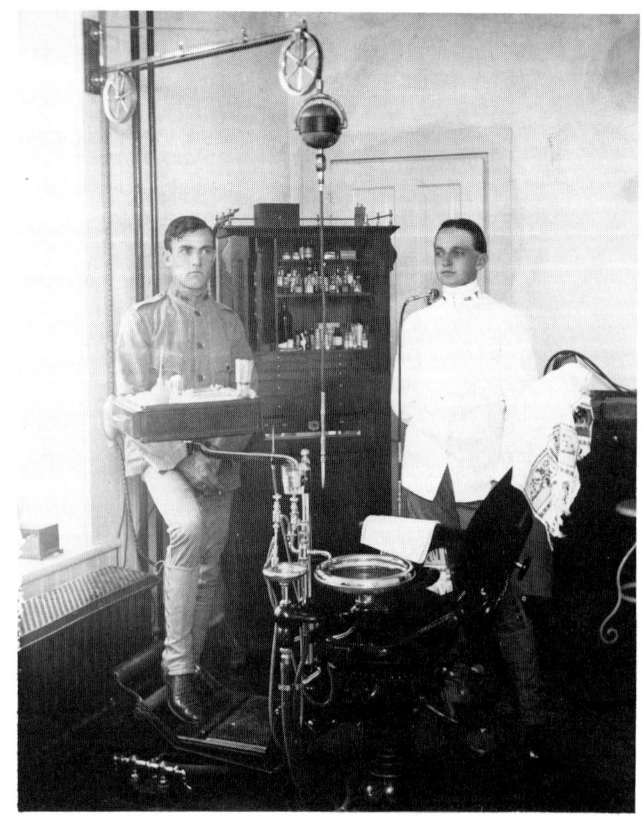

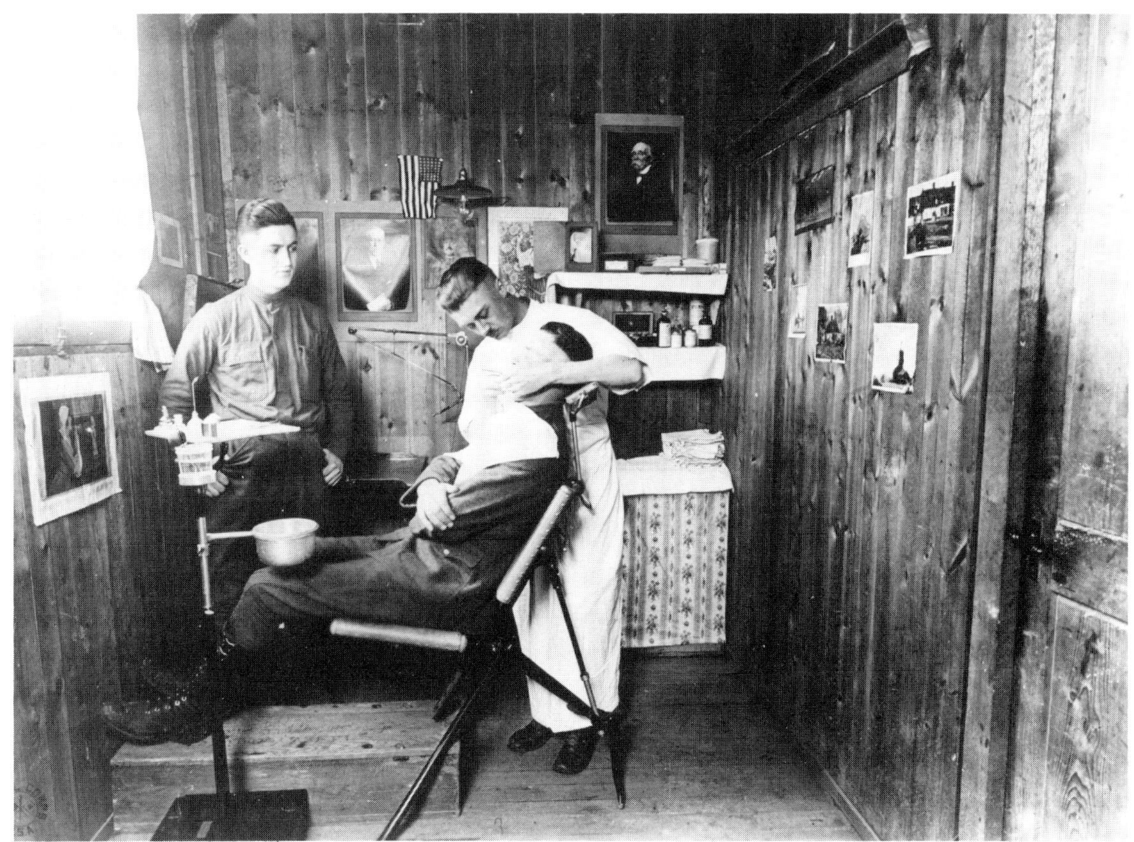

Camp Hospital #10 dental room in Prauthoy, France, January 1919. The portable dental chair folded down into the box upon which the patient rests his feet. From National Library of Medicine, Neg. No. 70-233.

Dental Clinic, Kerhnon, France, 1919. Soldiers are treated *en masse* in this clinic rigged up with portable dental equipment. From National Library of Medicine, Neg. No. 79-220.

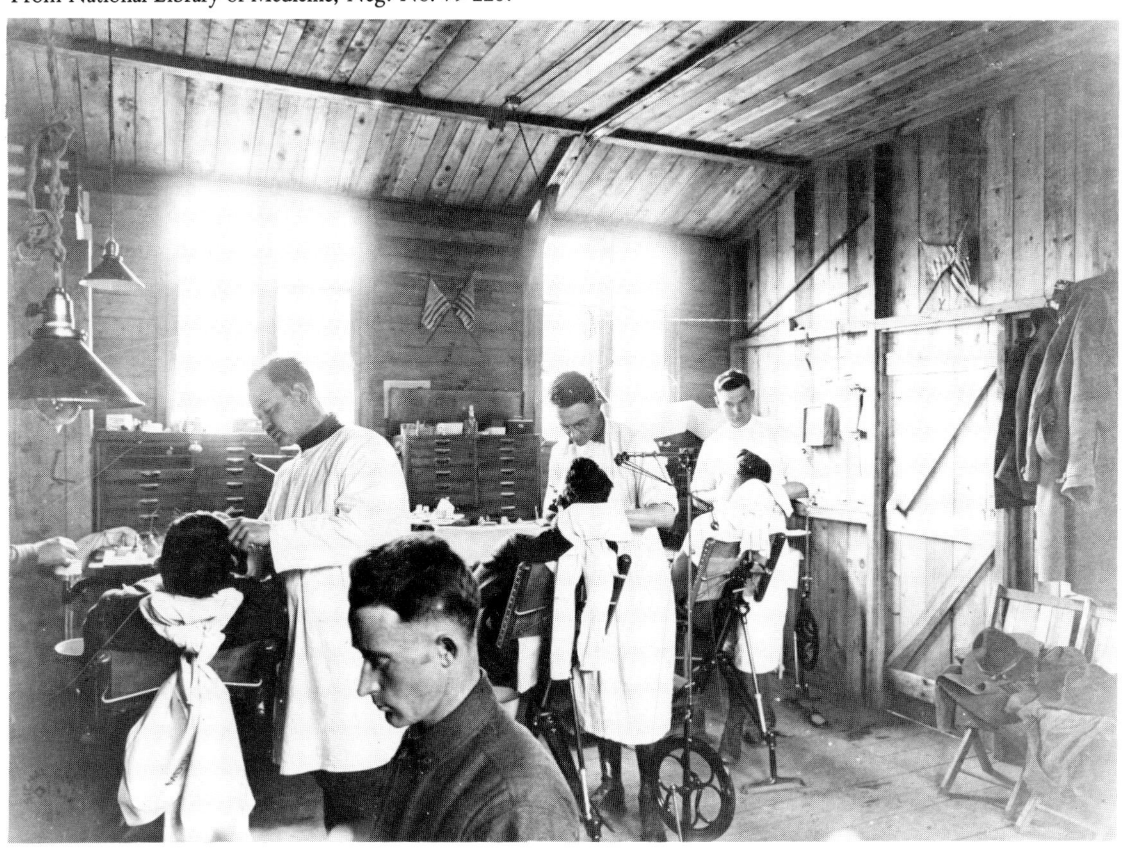

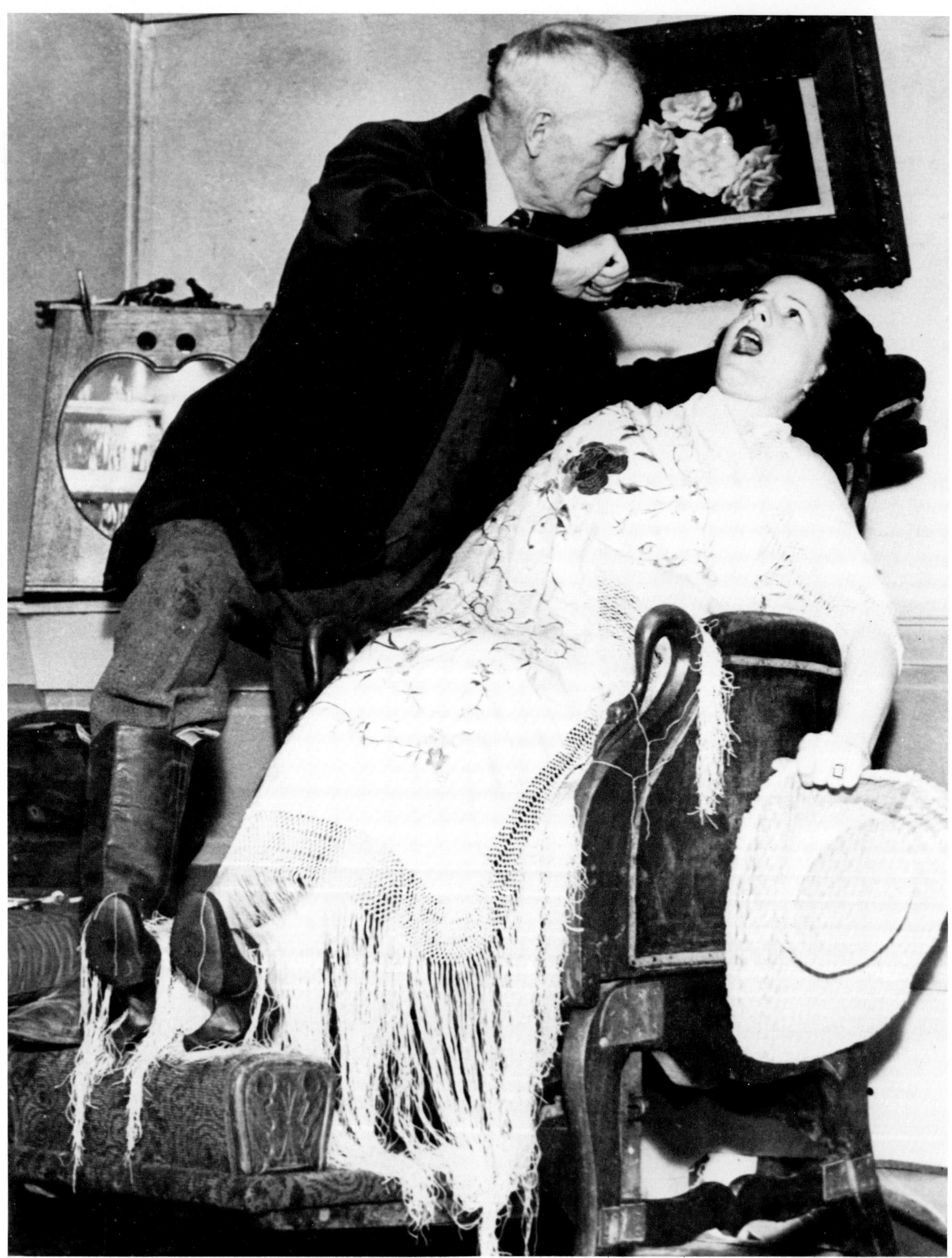

Scene from an early movie depicting a dentist at work before the turn of the century. Patient is seated in an Archer Dental Chair, which was manufactured in the 1860s and 1870s. The dentist is about to extract a tooth using a tooth key. Since it was before "The Age Of Sterility," the dentist is dressed in street clothes.

CHAPTER SEVENTEEN

Factors leading to Changes in Twentieth Century Offices

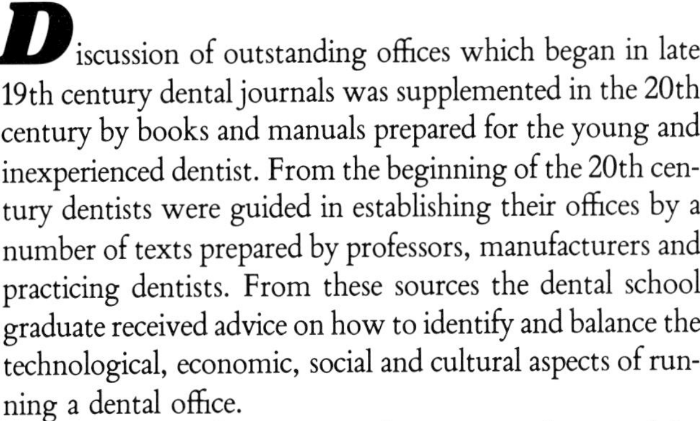

Discussion of outstanding offices which began in late 19th century dental journals was supplemented in the 20th century by books and manuals prepared for the young and inexperienced dentist. From the beginning of the 20th century dentists were guided in establishing their offices by a number of texts prepared by professors, manufacturers and practicing dentists. From these sources the dental school graduate received advice on how to identify and balance the technological, economic, social and cultural aspects of running a dental office.

Professors of dentistry such as C.N. Johnson of the Chicago College of Dental Surgery, in 1904, alerted the new dentist to the major factors he must consider in setting up his office. Johnson addressed the following topics: selecting and arranging an office, purchasing equipment, seeking and managing patients, keeping records of procedures done and fees charged and paid, employing an assistant, and contributing to the community in which the dentist lived. Johnson recognized the immense value of the dental assistant. He endorsed the broad scope of the dental assistant as described by Emma J. McCaw, a dental assistant, in her book on the functions of her profession. Johnson summarized the role of the assistant in his introduction: "The Assistant has taken from practitioners much of the detail and drudgery of his daily task and has left him free to concentrate on the science and technical problems of his practice, and in this she has added most materially to his efficiency and the output of his service."[200]

The most important objectives of the new dentist should be to find a locus in a congenial community, to make his presence known by his skillful care of his first patients, however not through advertisements, and to understand the social and cultural conventions of his patients. Dentists without an awareness of their community's cultural and ethnic heritage were given some broad guidelines. In the manual *Ritter Practice Building Suggestions*, published in 1924, the dentist read about the people who were most likely to be good patients. The Ritter Dental Manufacturing Company explained their views of the differences between American and other ethnic groups in their acceptance of professional dentistry. "Generally speaking, native-born Americans respond in greater measure to the teachings of dentistry than the other nationalities. Therefore, if the Americans and those of 'favorable foreign extraction', plus minors of foreigners above twelve years of age, are in the majority, then such a population should be favorably looked upon" as a source of patients.[201] When serving patients of other national heritages, the dentist was warned to be prepared to treat many more people at lower fees in order to earn a respectable income.

Along with advice on dental assistants and selecting patients, there were innumerable suggestions for equipping a new office. Dental offices that were described in the professional and advertising literature were often exceptional and too expensive for many young dentists. This promotional literature does not reflect the majority of offices used by the ordinary American dentist. From the information gathered in interviews with a dozen dentists who practiced in the 1920s, 30s and later, we have obtained information on how some of these less costly and more eclectic offices were arranged. The physical characteristics these offices share are location in one room, usually on the second floor over another business, a small waiting room, and a small closet-sized laboratory. The one chair office was equipped at a modest cost with furnishings, instruments and appliances purchased from retired dentists or their widows. Dr. Max Chubin, graduate of the Chicago College of Dental Surgery (Loyola College) in 1934, told us that he would read the obituaries, and upon finding a deceased dentist, contacted his widow and offered to purchase his office equipment. He located enough equipment to begin practice in the early 30s for an investment of $400. This office, located over a tire shop, obtained compressed air by tapping into the shop's supply through a copper tube. When the shop was closed in the evening the air was not available to the dentist.[202]

Important as the equipment and location of the dental office was, there were other compelling reasons for patients to see their dentists on a regular schedule. At the time when sterility in office procedures required sparkling new, white furniture and special disinfecting equipment a doctrine of disease linking the teeth to the welfare of other bodily organs and general health was pressed into the public consciousness. This was the focal theory of disease. While other organs could be the source of a focal infection the teeth were accepted as a major site which could be effectively treated and cured. The focal theory of disease came in a period when only 12 percent of the American population attended the dentist regularly and boosted the number of people who began to see the dentist.

The dental manufacturer realized the new sales pitch that could be made out of the discovery that dental health had an important effect on general health. The Ritter Dental Manufacturing Company published in 1920 a small book entitled *When is a Dentist a Success?*. Its theme was that the World War advanced the dental profession because it helped to bring the effects of tooth neglect on general health prominently before the public. As a result many were "averse to continuing their former role of walking poison factories—culture tubes for flourishing colonies of pus germs. Even little children in many progressive schools . . . knew the significance of the tooth-brush drill."[203] The dentist also gained in the perpetual rivalry with the physician, whom he criticized for advising patients to have their teeth removed to improve their health. Now the dentist could reverse his role and step into the physician's domain by claiming to improve general health and free the patient from other diseases by having the teeth cleansed and repaired.[204]

Patients were impressed with the conceptual basis for removing infective agents from their teeth, which superficially was reinforced by the newly sanitized dental office. The office became the tooth hospital and re-emphasized the link between surgeon and dentist—both worked in a sterile and antiseptic environment to treat life-threatening and serious diseases. However the dentist excelled by holding the key to other intractable diseases, by offering a cure through care of the teeth. In the new role of health conservation the esteem for the dentist rose. This led to patient tolerance of the new austerity in the office, stemming from more equipment and the emphasis on cleaning the teeth and preserving the gums.

Ritter spelled out some of the methods the dentist could use to capitalize on the new passion for implicating unhealthy teeth with serious diseases including rheumatism, arthritis, digestive complaints, etc. The text illustrated four cardinal principles for the dentist to adopt in practice: business psychology, business ethics, business systems and environment. Within the context of business psychology the dentist was urged to explain to patients the value of dental care for the preservation of their health. The dentist's services were to be placed as the focal point of good health. "In a word [the dentist] must talk health, not dentistry."[205] Business ethics implied that the dentist appear professional by the way he arranged his office and the clothes he wore. No longer would a white coat or sleeve protectors provide an adequate professional image. He must wear a gown and keep his hands manicured. To match his immaculate appearance the office must be clean and free of offensive odors caused by antiseptic solutions such as iodoform, carbolic acid and other cleaning agents. Ritter recommended preparing a glass jar half full of alcohol with a pinch of Diamond Dye to color it; then add ammonium carbonate (Squibbs Cube) until almost full. To this mixture one teaspoon of oil of lavender or oil of violet and a teaspoon of ammonia was added. The sealed jar was to be opened each morning to clear the air in the office before patients arrived.[206]

The business system and environment were tied to selecting the proper assistance and office equipment. These led directly to the reason for the book—to sell office equipment to the young dentist and the established dentist who wished to upgrade his practice. Office efficiency is vitally important to the dentist "who more than any other professional man, has nothing to sell but his time and his services."[207]

Two pieces of equipment were crucial in diagnosing focal infection. The X-ray machine, which most dentists used by this time, became essential in the detection of pockets of infection beneath the gums. X-ray film was only of value to the dentist who could interpret the shadows of infection, but the second device, a transilluminator, could be used to demonstrate to the patient as well, the specific areas of disease. By inserting the cool diagnostic lamp into the mouth and standing the patient in a corner lined with mirrors the dentist could point out the differences in the amount and color of the light passing through the tissues when damaged by, or free of, infection.[208]

Maurice Bremner, a dentist who practiced in the first half of the 20th century and who wrote an historical account of American dentistry in 1939, claims that changes in several techniques that improved patient care resulted in a loss of income for the dentist. These techniques included accurately fitted gold inlays introduced by William H. Taggart in 1907, and treatment of root canals under aseptic control. Both procedures were more exacting, and therefore, more time consuming than other procedures, which meant the dentist spent more time with a patient, although there was no mechanism for charging for the increased labor in treating a patient, unless he charged for his services on an hourly basis which was not considered ethical for a dentist.[209] Dentists who could not afford to purchase the special equipment invented by Taggart required for casting sometimes devised another method for the purpose. Max

Chubin put an inlay ring over a Bunsen burner and after the wax had burned out of it, he turned it over and put a piece of gold over the opening, and heated it. He used a foot bellows to oxygenate the torch. He placed a wet blotter on top of the gold in a plastic bowl. The rising steam forced the gold into the inlay.[21]__

Perhaps the greatest challenge American dentists faced in this period was the recession of 1929. While many wealthy people, who had been among their most faithful source of patients, lost money and could not afford their usual dental care, the poor often could not obtain even minimal treatment.[211] Dentists in big cities such as Chicago displayed ingenuity in attracting patients from the small pool of those able to afford dental care. Dr. Leonard Chapman, who loved children, installed in one of his two operatories in 1930, a dental cabinet in the shape of a doll house to entertain those children who became his patients. Doll house dental cabinets were sold by the American Cabinet Company for a few years between 1930 and 1933 and never manufactured again. On top of his cabinet or on his table Chapman placed a plaster Popeye statue. On the walls in the operating room he hung pictures of Humpty Dumpty and other children's story characters, as well as those created for him by his young satisfied patients.

The children were never shown the dental instruments which he kept wrapped in a towel. The instruments were renamed according to their use, i.e. "decay bugs" were removed with a "shovel," after the tooth was explored with a "toothpick." To amuse the children before he worked on their teeth he placed two cotton balls on the engine belt, turned on the engine and when the drill ran, the balls chased each other around the belt. He improved his waiting room by adding low-cost, but high-quality magazines, such as *National Geographic* to educate and amuse patients. During a period when he had few patients he kept a careful watch over those who came for treatment, and even, cleaned the mat outside the entrance to his office each evening, so that he could tell if anyone had arrived in the period before he returned the next day. Dentists in this period earned $100 per month, which was a sufficient income to live on, but their standard of living was reduced just as it had been for the rest of American society.[212]

Dental equipment manufacturers also learned to surmount the economic limitations faced by the dental profession and changed their tactics to sell more dental units. Since the number of new dentists did not increase sufficiently and many dentists used previously owned equipment, the American manufacturer advertised dental chairs and equipment on the basis that a good dentist would make more money if he purchased a second chair and could accommodate at least two patients at the same time. By arranging his work so that he could move quickly between two chairs, the dentist was expected to double his income. Due to the lack of patients and the extra energy required to work so rapidly, this strategy did not work out for many of those who purchased the second chair. The extra chair had another use. It accommodated an unexpected patient who arrived with an emergency dental problem. It would have been embarrassing for all to ask a patient in the chair to step out while the unexpected patient was treated, therefore, the second chair served a good purpose even when not anticipated to be in regular use.[213]

The dentist's economic difficulties in the '30s did not uniformly lead to more consideration for patients. James McManus, leader of the Connecticut State Dental Association had observed decades earlier in 1907 that "Everything in the modern dental office is of the kind that attracts wealthy people."[214] McManus' views continued to be shared by many dentists of his generation and their followers, who opposed efforts to provide free dental care to those who could not afford to have their teeth treated. Dentists who wished to organize clinics to serve the poor were challenged on the basis that the clinic was the first step in "socialized practice." Previously dental clinics were associated with dental schools. For instance, in 1910, four-fifths of the free dental care in Massachusetts was provided by the Tufts Dental School located in Boston.[215] However, clinic directors believed a clinic was the only alternative to socialized dentistry. By insuring that only those patients who could not afford a private dentist were treated in the clinic, all dentists were protected. There was even the expectation that those who would become economically independent would seek private dental care in the future. An editorial in the *Philadelphia Record* in 1938 evaluated the American dentist's services to the public:

"The dentists of America aren't doing half the job they should. They admit it. They point out that seventy percent of the people in the United States are not receiving adequate dental care. The dentists are tilting at cavities with tooth picks."[216]

Dental clinics survived the opposition of dentists in private practice and are an integral part of modern dental practice. The history of their introduction, development and effectiveness merits careful analysis in another essay.

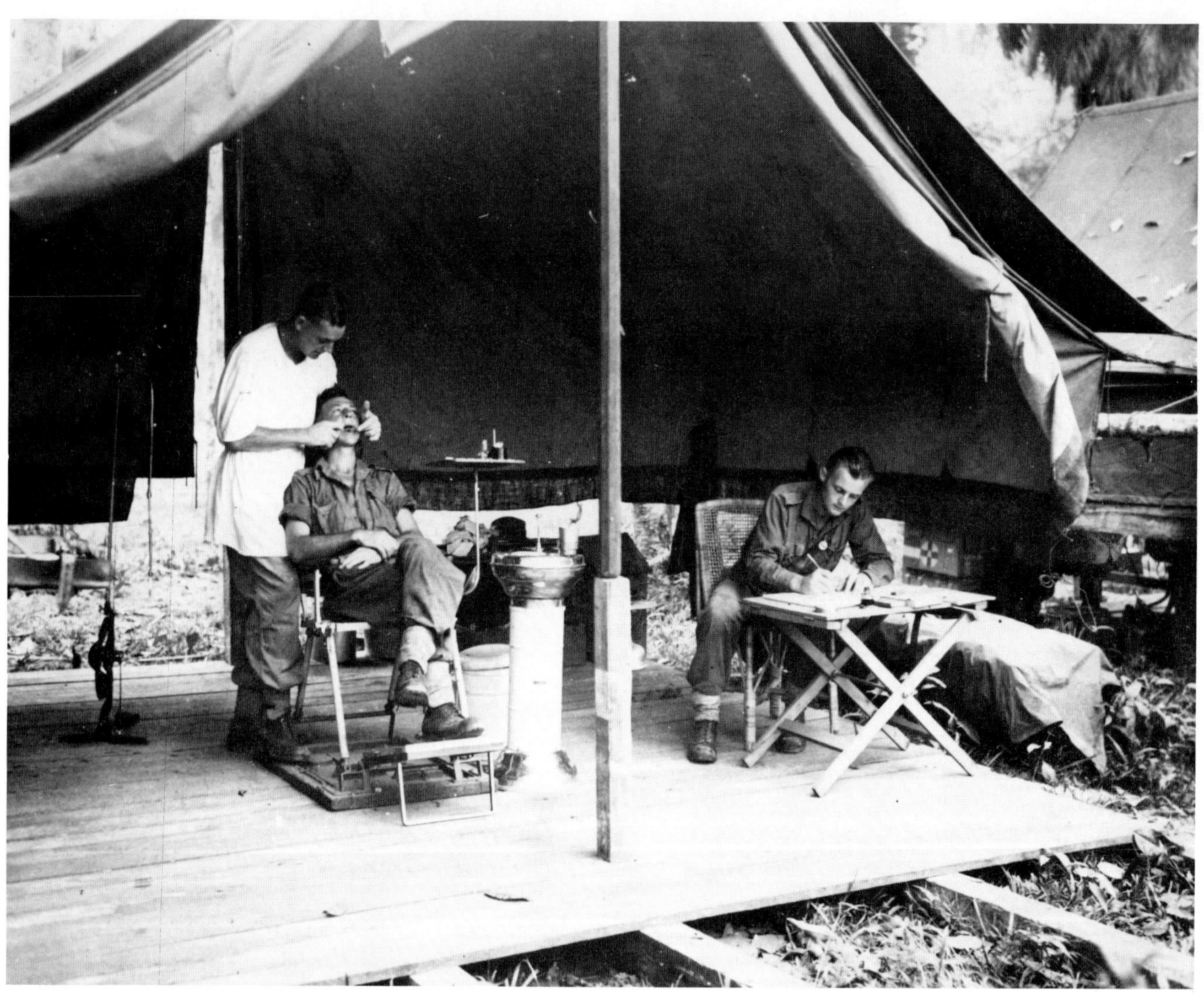

Dentistry in the jungle of the Pacific without electricity or plumbing during WWII. From Otis Historical Archives, AFIP.

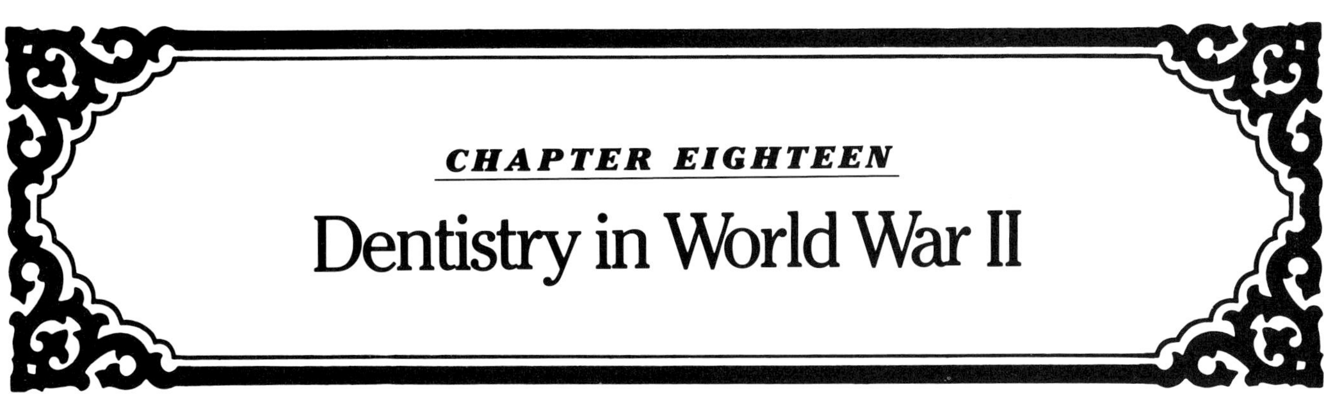

CHAPTER EIGHTEEN

Dentistry in World War II

In the decade before WWI the average American citizen had received inadequate dental care[217] which had important consequences for the Army Dental Corps program. Private dentists through the Preparedness League, who served so well in WWI by treating the teeth of those about to join the military forces, were not reactivated in WWII. By this time dentists believed that the federal government should bear the expense and provide dental care for all military personnel.[218] The lack of dental care for many Americans was brought into sharp focus by the condition of the teeth of one-quarter of the soldiers who required emergency dental treatment immediately after joining the military services.[219] It was soon evident that to neglect routine dental care of servicemen led to many dental emergencies which overtaxed the dental corps.[220] Dental care became even more critical when less rigid requirements for dental health permitted more recruits to enter the Army.

In 1940 the American Dental Association estimated that 267,000 dentists or a ratio of one dentist to 463 people (a quota that was many times greater than could be obtained) were required to treat the American population. In 1938, there were 5,197 officers enrolled in the Army Dental Reserve.[221] Most of them had not seen duty outside their private practices except for a few who had been enrolled in the Civilian Conservation Corps. During the war the armed forces inducted 15,000 dentists, almost a third of all American dentists, which left the civilian population with even less adequate dental resources.[222]

In WWI and WWII the dental corps functioned under the supervision of physicians and surgeons. During combat emergencies dentists were called upon to assist the medical corps, and in other instances, could be assigned to administrative duties. The employment of dentists for other than dental purposes during WWI, when more rigid dental standards were maintained among inductees, did not tax the dental program as it did in the second World War, when the need for dentists to work full time on treating soldiers was essential. Exacerbating the shortage of dentists and equipment during WWII was a new pool of patients that resulted from lowering dental requirements for induction.

All military, without regard to rank, and at the government's expense, were eligible for dental care. No soldier could refuse dental care if it appeared that untreated teeth could lead to disablement and unfitness for active duty.[223] A policy was adopted to bring each soldier up to a standard of dental health, so that he would not be incapacitated by dental disease. Dental care was extended in the Army to civilian dependents, which was obtained at the expense of providing less care, or not completing a procedure, before the soldier went into combat. The pressure to treat civilians was applied by military supervisors, who did not understand the time and effort involved in dental procedures, which created problems for the dentist. The Navy prevented such dilemmas from arising by not permitting any civilian to receive treatment from a military dentist.[224]

The number of soldiers treated for dental disease increased to the extent that 845,000 dentures were made for soldiers on active duty between 1942-45, compared to 13,140 during WWI.[225] An average of 109 dentures, 32 denture repairs, and eight bridges were completed each year per 1,000 soldiers.[226] During the war 2,566,000 dentures were constructed for military personnel. Since 38 percent of all patients received two appliances, 1,860,000 patients were given dentures. Soldiers, who witnessed the loss and destruction of millions of dollars of military equipment accepted little responsibility for the care of their new dentures and were cavalier in taking care of them.[227] Fifteen percent of all military personnel wore prosthetic devices. During mobilization the need for prosthetic service increased out of all proportion to the increase in strength of the Army.[228] Enlisting the laboratory technicians needed to produce these teeth required ingenuity, since in 1942 there was a total of 12,000 trained dental technicians in the U.S. and many of them were ineligible for military service. The Army set up training programs for technicians. Nine schools were in operation in 1943 with over 5,000 students enrolled.[229]

To remedy the lack of dental technicians in the Navy, in 1947, the Navy appointed Alfred W. Chandler, who had joined the Naval Dental Corps in 1917, as assistant chief of the Navy Bureau and head of the dental division. He established the first Navy schools for dental technicians at Bethesda, Maryland, and later, at Great Lakes, Illinois and San Diego, California.[230]

Shortages in manpower were matched in equipment shortages. The much greater need for office equipment is reflected in the fact that in 1940, civilian dentists purchased 2,000 units and 2,500 chairs, whereas, in 1943, the Army alone needed 5,500 units and 5,000 chairs. Manufacturers of chairs and units increased their production from 50 to 300 percent to meet this demand. Supplies were curtailed by the reduction of shipments from European countries. Prior to WWII American industry produced 60 to 70 percent of the 33 million burs used each year, with the remainder coming from Europe.[231] Extending the life of equipment was crucial. Therefore, to conserve and repair dental equipment, 180 enlisted men were sent to dental manufacturing plants for intensive two-week courses.[232] Experience in the second World War proved that in an emergency in which millions of men and thousands of dentists were mobilized, the amount of dental equipment and supplies far exceeds peacetime needs.[233]

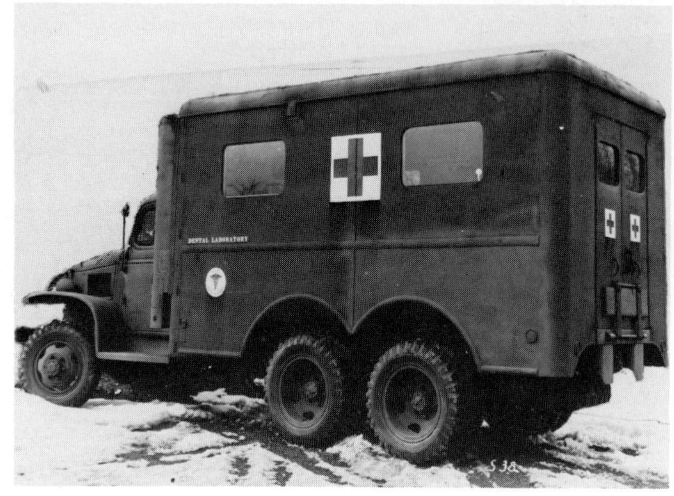

Mobile Army Dental Laboratory vehicle used in WWII. For information on the dental operating truck see George F. Jeffcott, *United States Army Dental Service in WW II*, 1955. From Otis Historical Archives, AFIP.

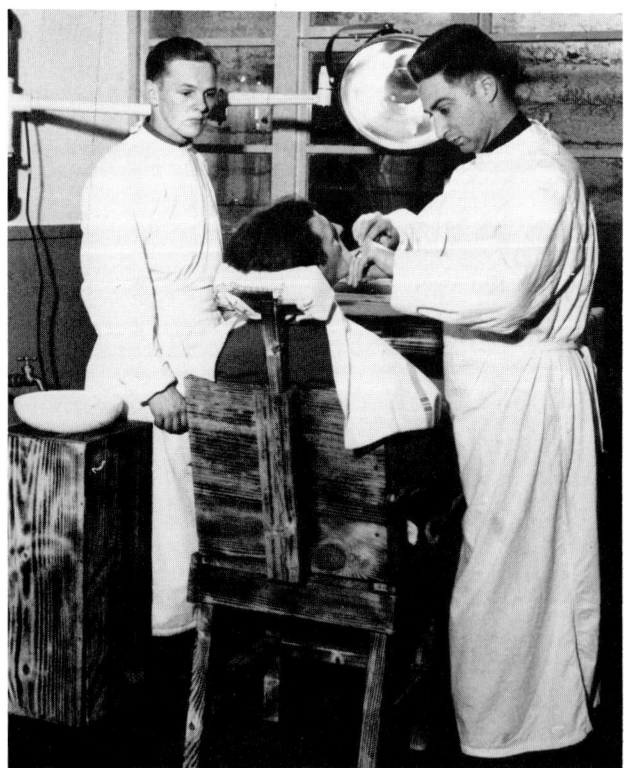

U.S. Army station in Iceland. First Lt. William Fishman attending a patient in 1942. All the equipment is modern except the chair which is made of old lumber. From Otis Historical Archives, AFIP.

The training of the dentist determined the type of equipment he would use. The Army supplied dental foot engines to dentists in the field, but young dentists who had never used them before refused to peddle them. They either employed an assistant to do the "footwork," who was then lost for other duties, or had the shop devise a means of mechanizing the foot engine. The efforts to avoid using the foot engine used personnel and supplies which led authorities to make electricity available to dentists to run their engines, since electricity was being supplied for other purposes.[234]

Dental assistants and hygienists were even more difficult to enlist in the military, therefore 2,909 civilian assistants and 500 civilian dental hygienists were on military duty during the war.[235]

Dental services became so important to WWII soldiers that inability to get dental replacements in 1943 became the number one gripe of those who wrote letters to family and friends. This information was discovered in a review of censored letters ordered by General Eisenhower.[236]

The experiences of dentists in WWII had an impact on rehabilitation medicine. Military dentists used, and extended for use on other parts of the body, several new materials. To control the cost of dentures military dentists fitted dentures made from acrylic. When artificial eyes also were needed, several dentists assisted in the development of acrylic artificial eyes to replace the glass eyes no longer available from European makers. Another material, tantalum, used in dental bridges, was adapted for use in constructing metal plates to replace the missing bone of the skull.[237]

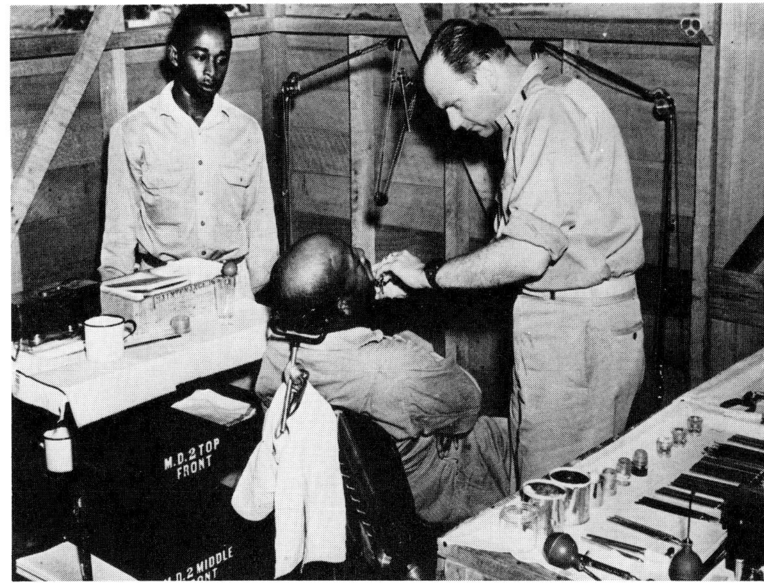

Dentist examining the teeth of a master sergeant during WWII. From Otis Historical Archives, AFIP.

Dentistry in the jungle, New Georgia Island, 1943. The dental assistant pedals the engine for the dentist. The dental officer is using the M.D. Chest No. 60, which contained a portable dental chair, foot-powered dental engine, sterilizer, instruments and supplies. These chests were shipped with dental officers all over the world. From Otis Historical Archives, AFIP.

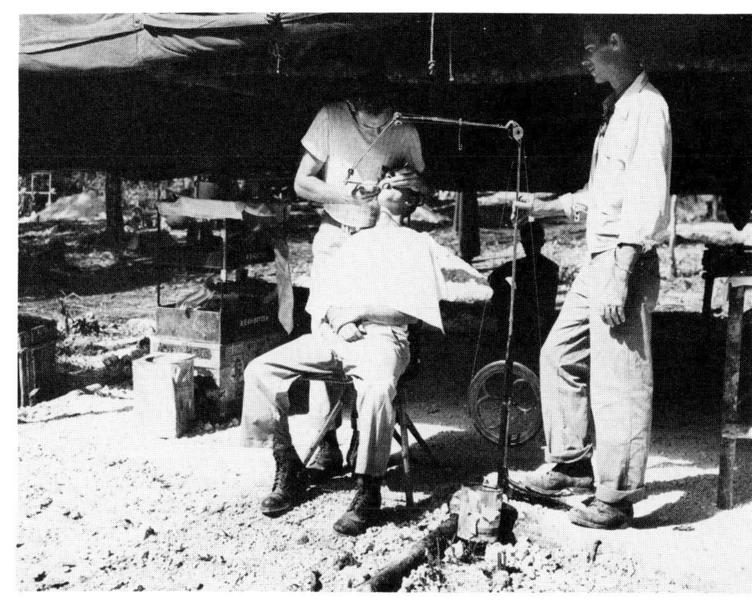

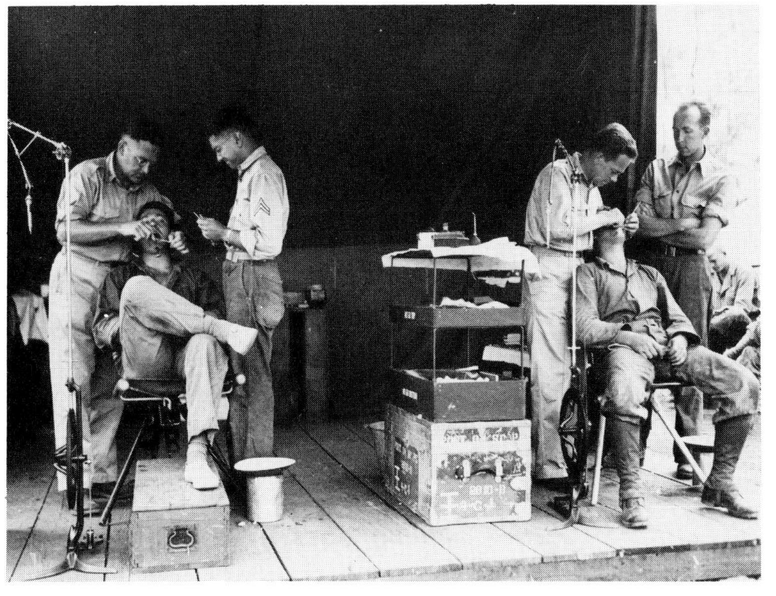

Capt. J.P. Mackinnon and Lt. Clifford S. Johnson treating patients in the dental tent, 185th Infantry in Rockampton, Australia, 1942. The dentists are using M.D. Chest No. 60. From Otis Historical Archives, AFIP.

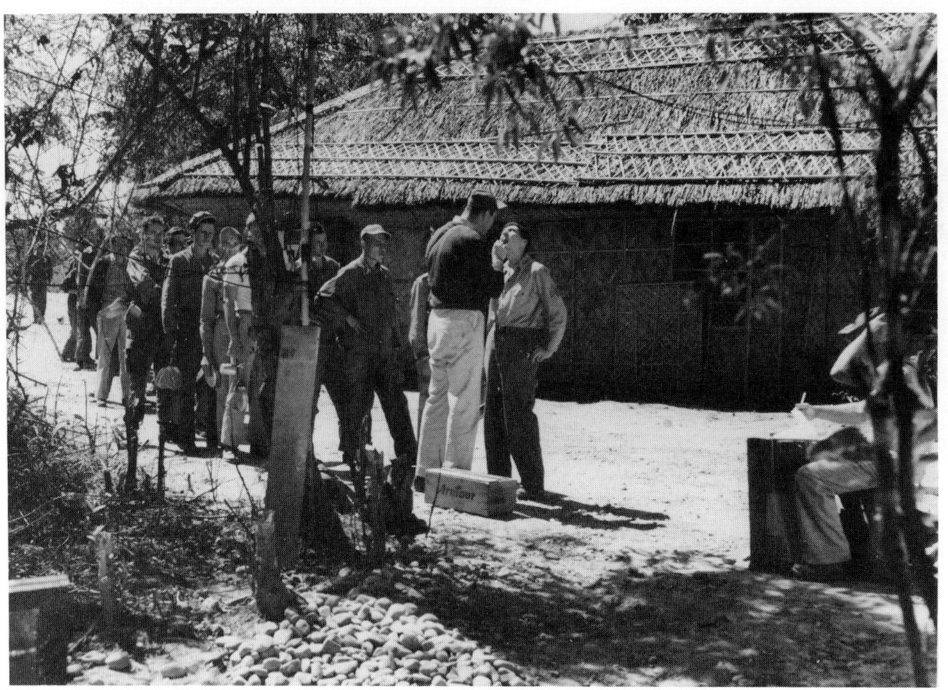

A continuous check of all 1st Air Commando Force personnel was made by the dental officer. Here he waylays the men as they stand in the chow line at the Hailakandi (India) base, WWII. From Smithsonian Institution, Neg. No. 67636AC

In War Theatre #22 Saipan, Marianas Island. Electricity in this remote place made it convenient for this dentist to run a drill to clean out a cavity in 1944. From U.S. Army Air Force.

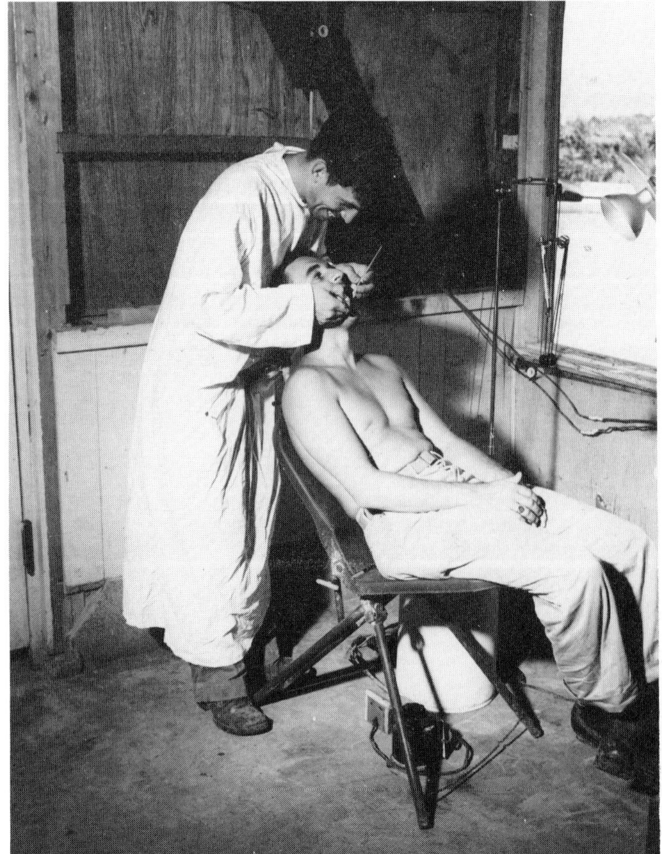

Capt. Sanford S. Golden, Cleveland, Ohio, 1945, works with a drill powered from a jeep battery and hooked up to a starter and two starter buttons. The system provided two speeds and avoided pedaling the drill by foot power. From Otis Historical Archives, AFIP.

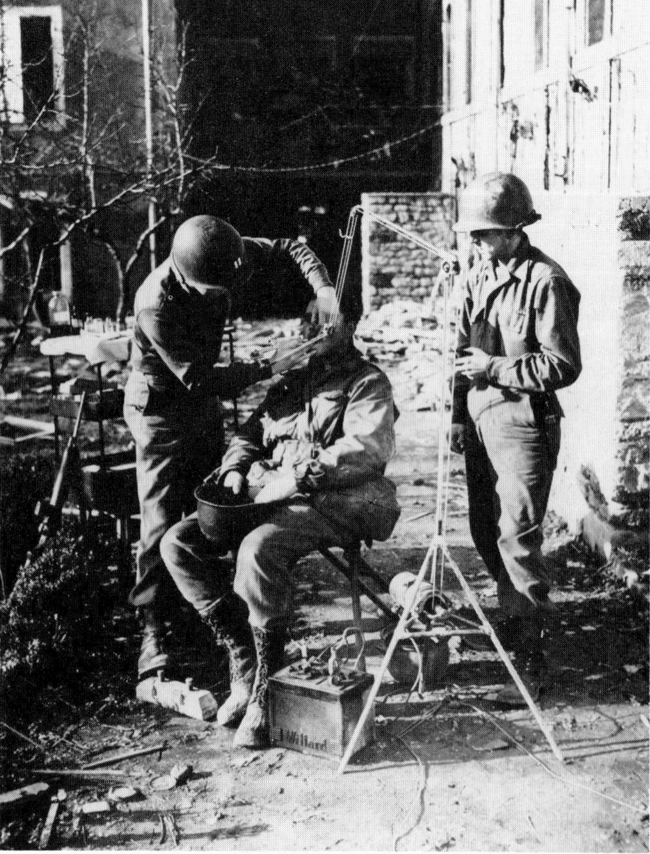

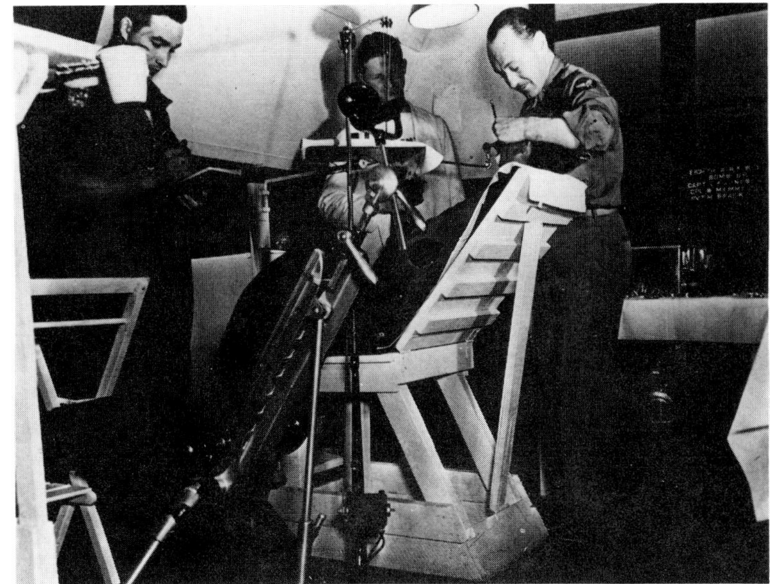

Cpl. W. Manny and Pvt. M. Spack, dental technicians, assisting Capt. L.F. Jones at an Army Air Force Station of the 8th Air Force, England. Chair is improved and dental engine is electrically powered. From Smithsonian Institution, Neg. No. 62678.

At Hailakandi, India, the dental officer maintained an outdoor clinic, using a grass awning for sunshade. Here he gives dental treatment to one of the men of the 1st Air Commando Force. From Smithsonian Institution, Neg. No. 67655AC.

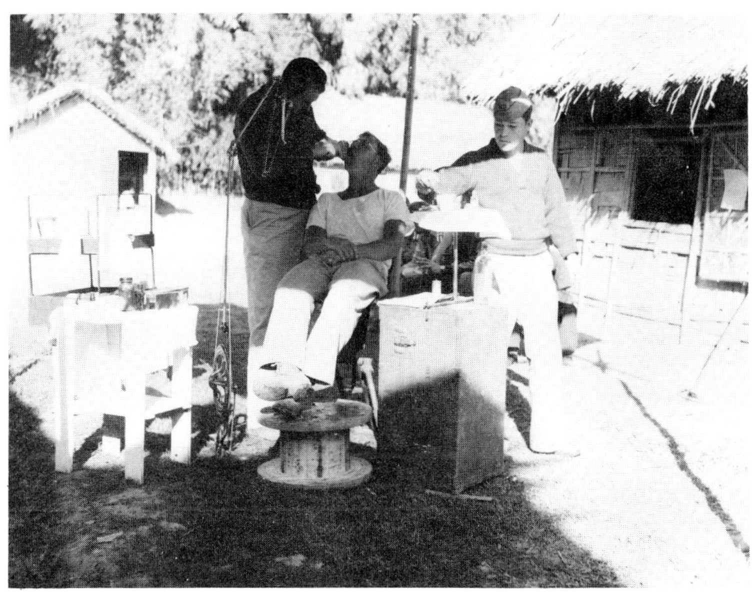

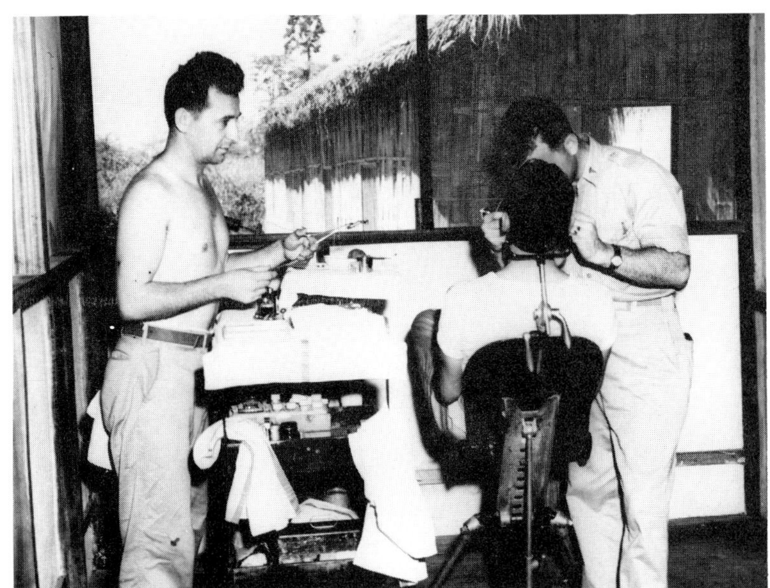

At the dispensary of the 3rd Ferrying Squadron, 1st Ferrying Group, dental attention is given to one of the men based at Chabua, Assan, India, July 1943. From Smithsonian Institution, Neg. No. 68802AC.

Dental technicians working on plaster teeth in the Central Dental Laboratory during WWII. From Otis Historical Archives, AFIP.

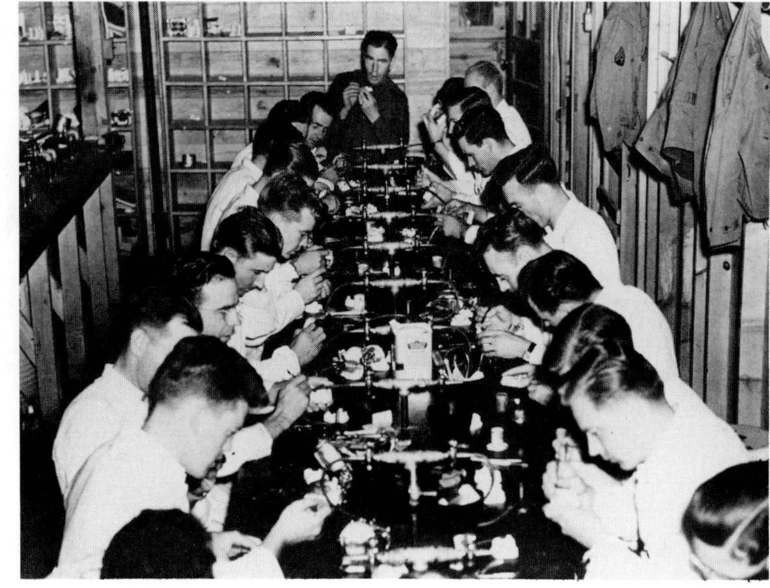

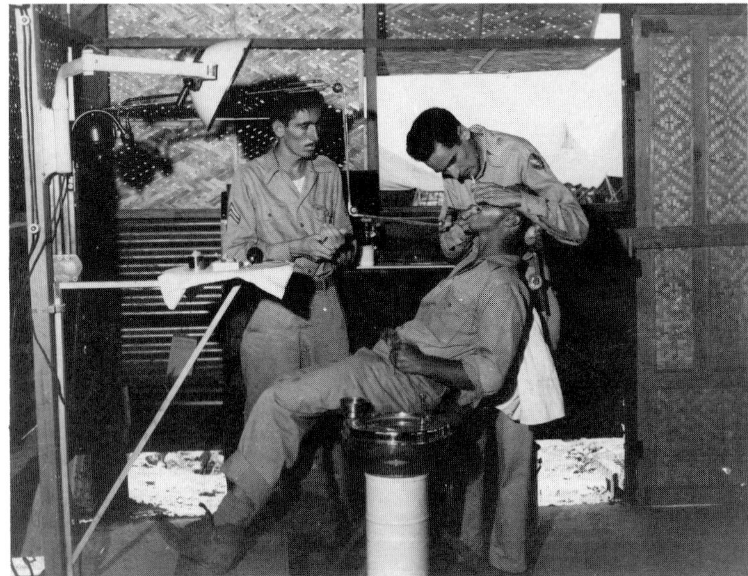

Dental treatment is given a GI in the dental clinic of the 22nd Replacement Depot of Manila, Luzon, Philippine Islands. This section is equipped for all types of dental work, including surgery and prosthetics, July 1945. From Smithsonian Institution, Neg. No. 69695AC.

Haven Class Hospital ship operatories. Hospital ships carried full base dental equipment including prosthetic and X-ray facilities. Larger ships employed an oral surgeon as well as an exodontist, WWII. From Navy Medical Command Archives.

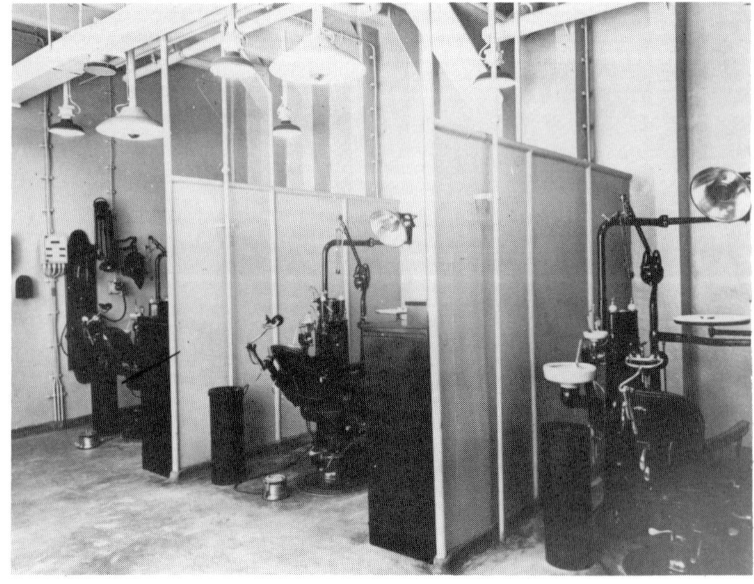

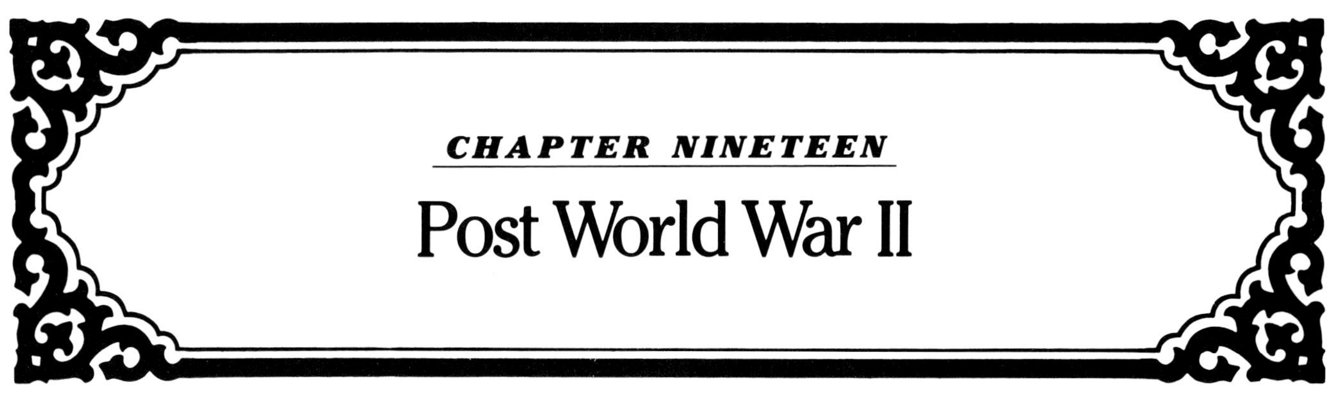

CHAPTER NINETEEN

Post World War II

The second World War changed the economic expectations for manufacturers, as it did for the professions and businesses. Dentists who remained out of the services had been in demand and those who returned from the war experienced little competition in setting up a private practice. At first equipment was difficult to locate and supplies were short. American dentists enjoyed a new prosperity. Between 1939 and 1953 the gross income for dentists increased over 157 percent or over $1 billion per year.[238]

Undoubtedly the most dramatic change in the dental office resulted from the introduction in the 1950s of high-or ultra-speed hand-pieces. This technological event deserves greater scrutiny. While industry had used high rotational speeds for years, the dentist did not adopt higher speeds until late in the 1930s when he realized that diamond cutting tools performed better at speeds higher than 1,000 to 2,000 rpm, the speed at which his instruments ran. Dentists were reluctant to use higher speed hand-pieces because of the fear of lack of control.[239] Actually there is no less control of the hand-piece at higher speeds. In fact there is a specific advantage over the lower speed hand-piece. Because the torque is less than it is at lower speeds, the hand-piece may be used with less pressure. There is no evidence to show that dentists used any higher speed than 4,000 rpm in their hand-pieces before 1946.

Beginning in the 1950s a variety of high-speed belts and gear-driven hand-pieces and contra-angles were developed. Motors on older units were converted to increase their speeds by rewiring the motor armature and shunting out the motor resistors. Speed was also increased on the older units by converting the idler pulley to a ball bearing type, varying the slack in the engine belt and installing high-speed pulley transmissions.

The dentist became aware of the potential of high-speed hand-pieces when several dentists realized that the procedure of cutting tooth enamel could be vastly improved because of a discovery made in carrying out an assignment for the Royal Australian Air Force. John Walsh reported in the *New Zealand Dental Journal* of 1949 that "higher rotational speeds [of hand-pieces] produced vibrational frequencies that were more acceptable to patients than those produced at conventional speeds."[240] Although Walsh's publication was largely unnoticed in the U.S., his discovery was confirmed by Ingraham and Tanner, who reported to the American dental community in the *Journal of the American Dental Association*, in 1953, that they also observed that both the patients and operator experienced less tension when the speed increased to over 6,000 rpm.[241] How were these discoveries made and why did the dental equipment manufacturers respond by producing high-speed hand-pieces and auxiliary equipment in the mid-50s? The sequence of events in the design and invention of the high-speed hand-piece is based on published sources, which one of the inventors has challenged, but until new publications appear we must rely on them.

Several British historians of dentistry described the sequence of events which led to Walsh's discovery of the effectiveness of the high-speed hand-piece. The idea for the high-speed drill came to Walsh in 1945 while he was testing the hearing of discharged airmen in Melbourne. It was generally known that the conductivity of teeth and bone to sound "was the major contributing factor to the unpleasantness of the dental drill."[242]

Malvin Ring described Walsh's experiences that led him to patent a high-speed dental hand-piece.

> Using the tuning forks of various frequencies which were being used in the hearing tests, [Walsh] decided to test the upper limits of the vibration sense of bone which he had detected at frequencies below about 100 Hz in idle experiments on his own teeth. He discovered that the maximum unpleasantness of vibration sensation occurred about middle C, 256 Hz, and that frequencies two octaves higher, 1,024 Hz, were not perceived as vibrations at all. This crucial discovery led Walsh to suppose that higher speeds of rotation of the dental drill would alleviate the patient discomfort which he had now traced to vibration as well as sound.[243]

Walsh's work, through a provisional patent and letters to colleagues, was communicated to American researchers, who were experimenting with high-speed hand-pieces driven by water rather than air. Robert Nelsen was the inventor and leader of the U.S. project to produce a high-speed hand-piece carried out at the National Bureau of Standards. The project was funded by the American Dental Association. Nelsen decided that a water-driven turbine would achieve not only a high speed but a sustained high running speed, limited only by the fluid drive to 75,000 rpm. In fact Nelsen and his associates perfected and reported on a hydraulically powered turbine, contra-angle piece with a speed of 61,000 rpm in 1953. This was the first clinically operating turbine hand-piece. The first commercial-model, hydraulic-powered turbine hand-piece was subsequently manufactured by the Bowen Company and called a Turbojet. The speed was soon surpassed by the gear-driven, Page-Chayes hand-piece introduced in 1956. In the meantime, J.V. Borden who worked with Nelsen at the Bureau of Standards utilized the turbine concept and produced an air-driven turbine hand-piece for commercial use. The Dentists' Supply Company manufactured it. It was sold under the name Airotor in 1957, and became the first commercially useful, air-driven, ultra high-speed hand-piece.[244]

The evolution of hand-pieces with increased speeds were summarized by Harold C. Kirkpatrick of the University of Pennsylvania Dental School in his classic text first published in 1959. Fitzpatrick listed the speeds obtainable with the best equipment according to his assessment in the following table

Date	**Base Speed**	**Max. Speed**
1939-43	500 (rpm)	4,000 (rpm)
1944-46	500	10,000
1946-50	500	25,000
1950-55	500	45,000
Date	**Base Speed**	**Ultra Speed**
1955-56	500	200,000
1956-58	500	300,000
1959	500	1,000,000[245]

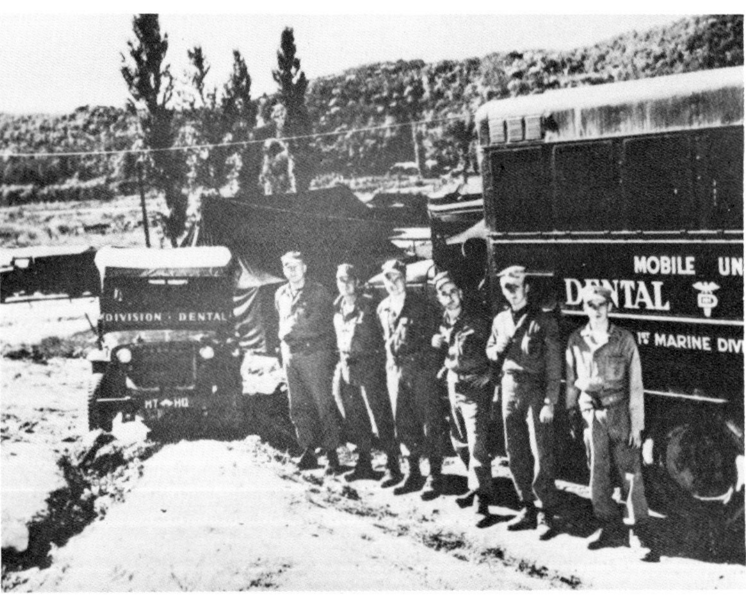

In the Korean War, the Marine Corps provided "front line" dentistry for their troops when they changed their basic combat mission from amphibious to defensive land warfare. This dentistry was provided by either mobile dental units or in Quonset huts. The mobile dental units were utilized to bring dental treatment to small stations, usually in remote areas. From Mobile Dental Unit, 1st Marine Division, Korea.

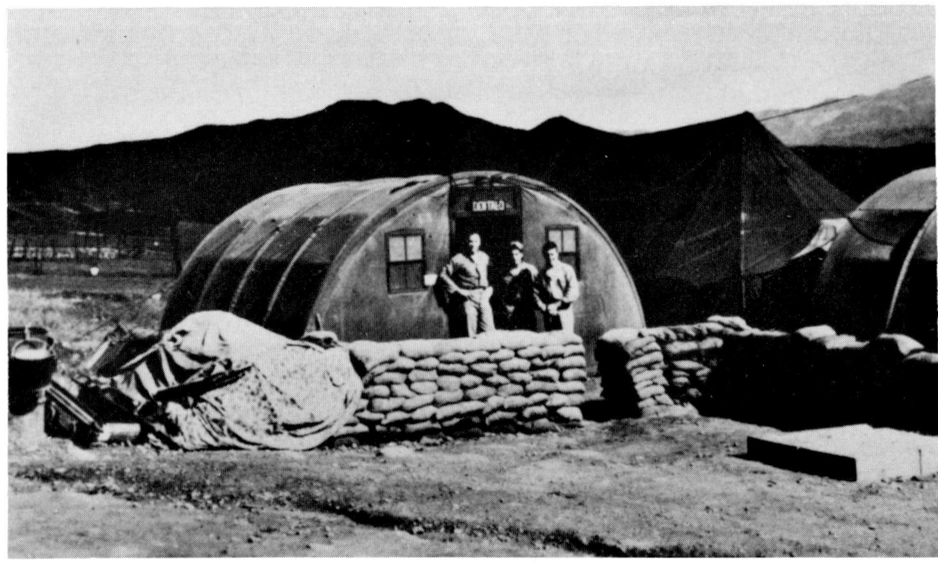

U.S. Marine Regimental Dental Office, Korea, October 1952.

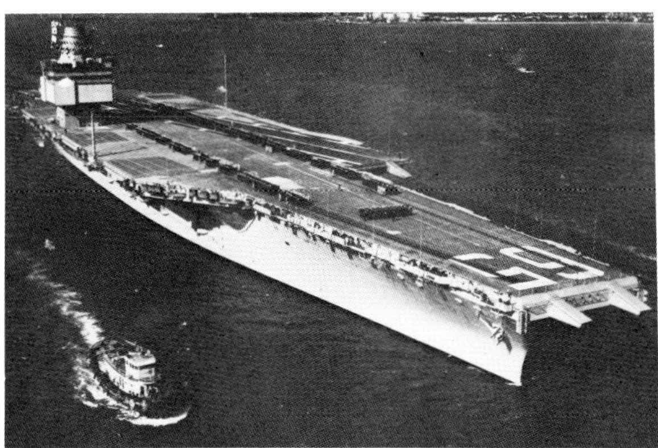

U.S.S. Enterprise. First nuclear-powered carrier commissioned, November 25, 1961.

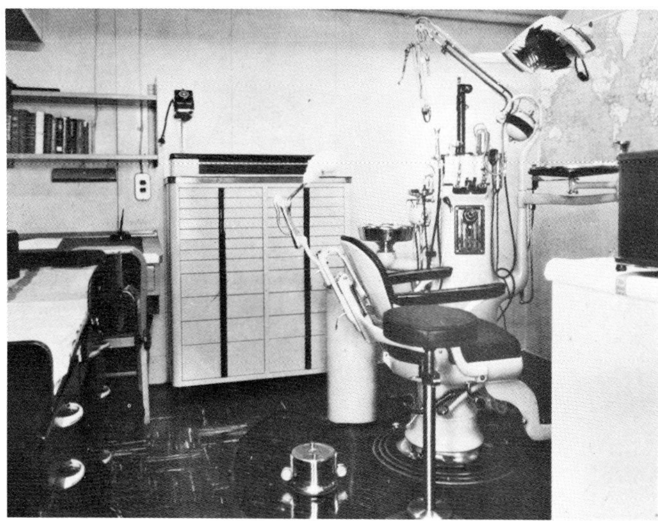

One of six operating rooms on the U.S.S. Enterprise, 1961. These dental operatories were equipped for stand-up dentistry. The units were too high to properly adjust this equipment for sit-down dentistry which was coming into practice at this time.

Lt. Col. Jack Rice, graduate of Ohio State College of Dentistry in 1959, at his workbench. His distinguished career, beginning in the year of his graduation and ending 30 years later with his retirement, and award of the Legion of Merit Medal, demonstrates the amazing versatility of the American dentist. Serving at bases throughout the world, he participated in a variety of socially beneficial programs, as well as providing excellent dental care to all he served. He received a commendation in 1976 for his suggestion that dental acrylic be used to repair radar illumination tubes. His advice was taken at a saving to the military of millions of dollars in equipment. From Jack Rice.

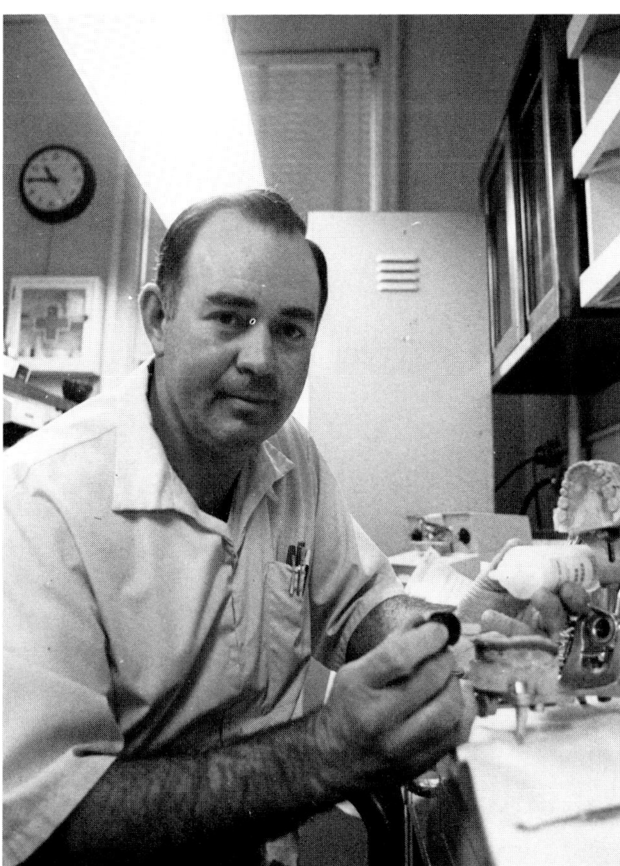

Lt. Col. Jack Rice working on a set of artificial dentures. Rice, as resources training officer, produced a successful Dental Therapy Assistant Program which began in 1972. Its purpose was to use a team approach in providing dental care for more servicemen through the use of dental therapy assistants. In a profession that prides itself on the independence of its practitioners, Rice and his colleagues demonstrated that teamwork could be a vital and essential part of dental practice. From Jack Rice.

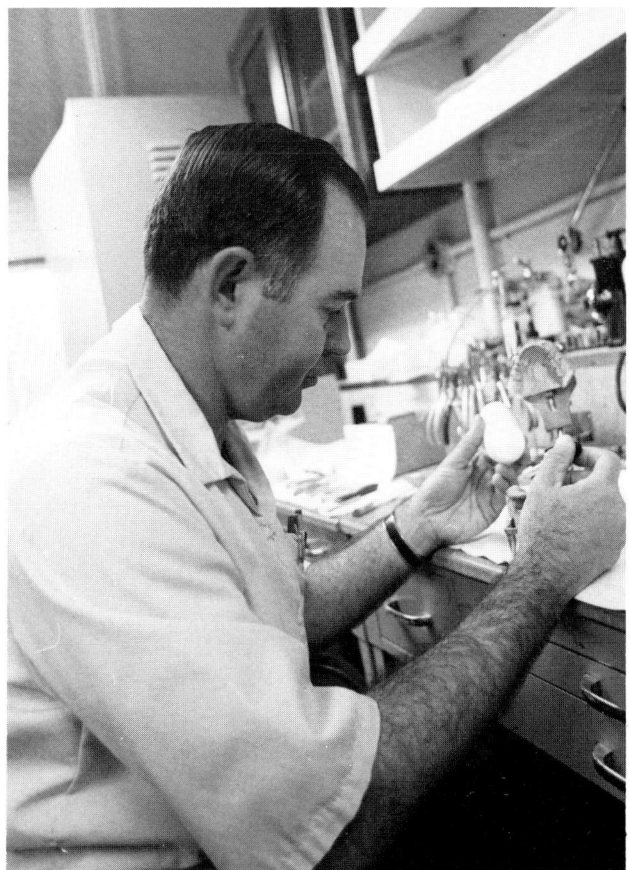

Dentistry in the Vietnam War. Dentists did not go into combat areas with the troops. The wounded and those in need of dental treatment were brought back from combat, for the most part in helicopters. The dental clinic in which Dr. Gary Lemen worked was a permanent structure, with corrugated metal on the exterior and half walled in brick to protect it from shells. The dental equipment was like that of a regular stateside office; it was not portable. In Vietnam, because troops could be easily transported by helicopters, they were brought back to permanent hospital and dental quarters. Therefore, the dental facilities were more like those in WWI where the front was more or less stationary, than WWII, in which troops moved a great deal and temporary dental units had to be moved with them.

Capt. Gary Lemen, who was promoted to major, served in the USAF from 1970-1974. He is shown with Capt. Steve Oldroyd and Capt. Donald "Diagus" McGhee, who served with him in Vietnam. From Gary Lemen, Sacramento, California.

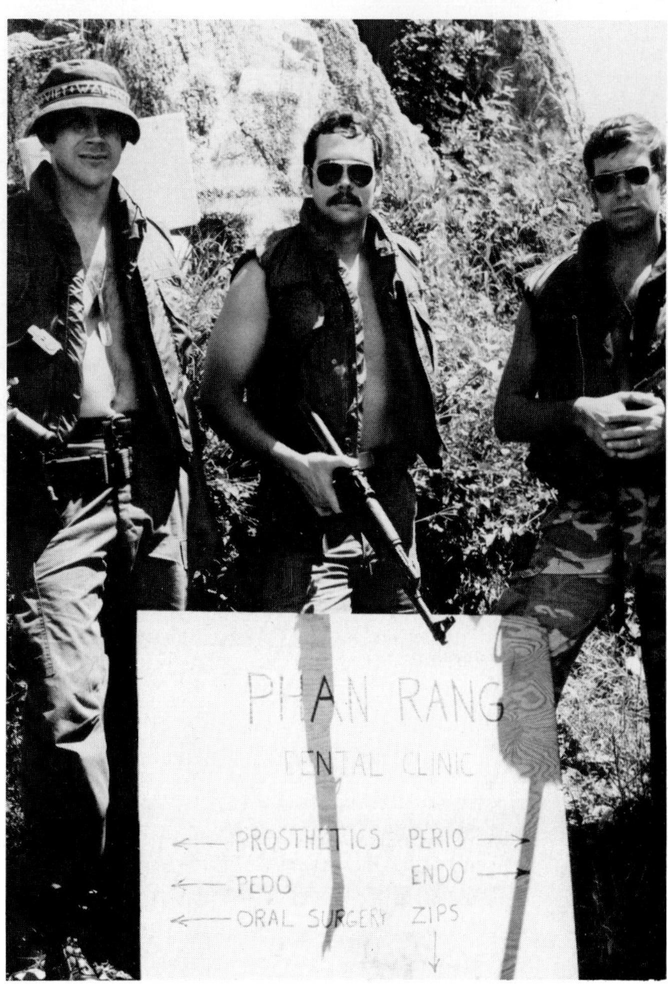

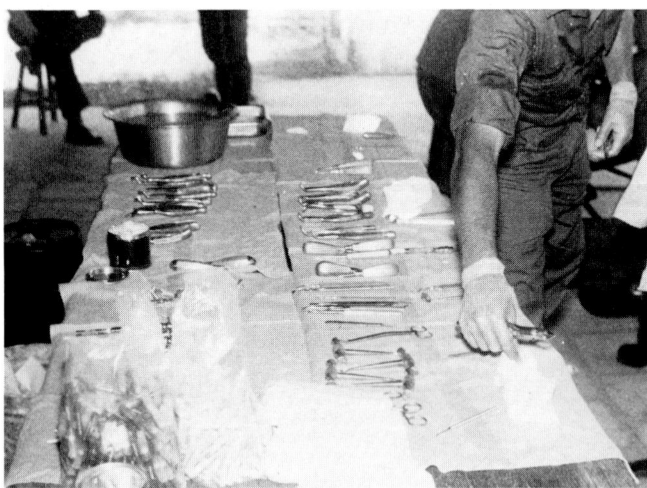

Table set with dental instruments under shade in Vietnam.

Dental Clinic sign, Vietnam.

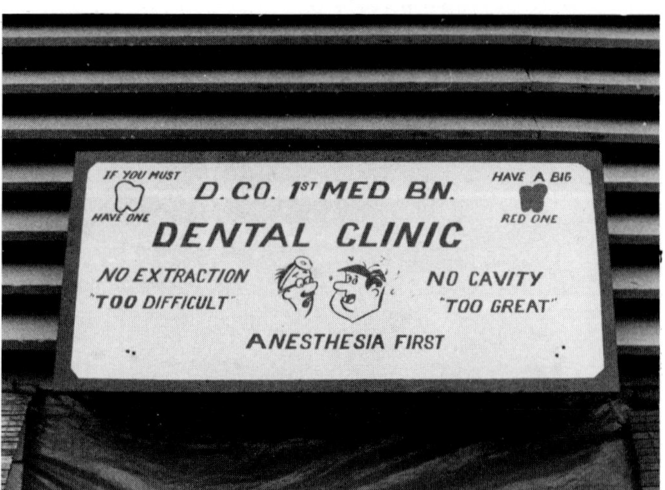

During the interim period of the 50s slower speed equipment was modified so that it would function at higher speeds. The optimal speed for the dental hand-piece was unknown and dentists were cautious about buying new and unproven equipment, therefore, manufacturers adapted existing hand-pieces to run at higher speeds. Modified equipment was more cumbersome and cluttered up the office, which interfered with the dentist's activies and displeased, if not alarmed, the patient. With modifications such as disconnecting the resistors, cleaning the engine armature, and cleaning and changing the slack in the belt the ordinary-speed hand-piece could be improved to run at speeds up to 12,000 rpm. In the late '50s dental units were produced with faster engines, resistor shunts, high-speed pulleys and coolants to control the heat resulting from higher speed hand-pieces. The water-turbine hand-piece required a separate unit placed next to the dental chair. Air-turbine hand-pieces employed a control box that was mounted on the bracket table arm of a dental unit.[246]

The high-speed hand-piece generated so much heat that water was required to cool the tooth and as a result high-speed suction units were necessary to remove the copious amount of fluid flowing out of the mouth. These portable suction units containing a collection bottle and motor were either attached to the dental units or placed in separate mobile units next to the chair. Even though constructed of soundproof materials all portable suction units were very noisy. The noise was eliminated only when the suction unit was replaced with a central suction unit, located in another area. Central units were also cleaner because collection bottles in the room did not have to be washed out and waste water went directly into the central plumbing.[247]

New equipment and gadgets did not insure that the dentist would improve his practice to the point of increasing his services to patients. The optimal arrangement of improved equipment was crucial to the dentist's ability to control the tone, temper and ease of operation of the office.

To determine how the dental office functioned and which changes might be appropriate, Marvin Mundel, a student of ergonomics in Milwaukee recommended that each dentist make a motion study of the daily activities in the office. Motion studies were originally developed for industrial activities, but were equally useful in non-routine, professional activities such as dentistry. The purpose of the studies was to find ways to save time, effort, and reduce tension.

The dentist was advised to keep a record of all the office activities on a minute-by-minute basis throughout the day. Records made on randomly selected days would reveal the amount of time spent on dental procedures, personal business, patient contact, etc. Based on actual data, the office could be rearranged to reduce some of the "wasted" time and excess effort. One example Mundel included showed how a dental office was improved after a motion study indicated changes should be made by rearranging the chair, cabinets, autoclave, X-ray unit, sterilizer and waste receptacle.[248]

Time and motion studies had their limitations too. One effect of the motion study, which was challenged as an unnecessary goal, a few years later, was the reduction in physical exercise of the staff as they went about their daily activities. The positions the dentist's body was placed in while working on teeth were also of concern. A study in 1963 of "Body Mechanics Applied to the Practice of Dentistry" revealed that the work habits and body motions dentists assumed to work on teeth were fatiguing, cramping, provided little exercise for muscles and the cardiovascular system, and generally, when practiced over a prolonged period, resulted in illness and a shorter career. The authors recommended changes in the shape and location of the chair the dentist sat upon while operating, with periodic rest and vigorous exercise throughout the day.[249] Thus the dentist had to select and arrange equipment to control the tone, temper and ease of operation of the office for the welfare of staff and patients.

A revival of interest in building new dental offices and installing radically different equipment led to another spate of articles on new and outstanding offices in the late '60s and early '70s in *Dental Survey*, *Dental Economics* and *J.A.D.A*. Dentists, who had practiced in the armed services under battlefield conditions and on foreign territory, were anxious to return home and build up successful practices in pleasant offices. Some of them bought new equipment and placed it in imaginative settings. The newly designed equipment incorporated military features such as the Sigma Instrument System and Orbiter Unit produced by the Ritter Company in 1972. Using computer-aided-design and advice from dentists, Ritter advertized the first organized dental environment. One of its features appealed to pilots for it was arranged like the cockpit of a jet with everything at the dentist's (pilot's) fingertips.[250]

Dr. Michael Uzelac's enthusiasm is typical of dentists returning from service overseas in Asia. In 1969, after serving for four years in the South Pacific, he looked forward to an attractive office with contemporary furnishings in the U.S.[251] Above all he wanted to project a feeling of warmth and comfort to reduce tensions and anxieties for the patient and dentist. His patients were seated in a contoured chair surrounded by customized cabinets with no dental unit or equipment in sight. Large windows overlooked a garden. Each of Uzelac's three patient rooms was equipped to support a specialized facet of dentistry including crown and bridge dentistry, prosthetics and surgery.

Daniel F. Specht of Columbus, Ohio, in the following year, went a little further in the direction of luxury and designed a spectacular entrance to his office. He also placed two aquaria, each 7 feet long and 3 feet high, holding 350 gallons of water, in view of the operatories, since he believed fish had a hypnotizing effect on the patient. Dr. Specht, like many of his contemporaries, objected to the arrangement of older offices. He complained: "Mazes of belts or gadgets are outmoded, old-fashioned dust collectors, always getting in the way of petite dental assistants, and looking like one-arm robots to frighten patients. Instead, I hang the high-speed handpiece under the arm of the chair and attach the water-air syringe on the back of the chair (along with a slow-speed turbine handpiece, where desired). This is simplicity with efficiency."[252]

Dentists joined an expanding list of individuals and businesses who engaged professional architects to build and design their offices. With the advice of psychologists and marketing consultants, the dentist and other professionals were urged to create a positive "image" to attract patients and clients. One feature of this plan was to create a warm and pleasant reception room that gave the effect of a private residence rather than a clinic.[253] The dental office no longer had to prove, by its appearance, that treatment was conducted under sterile conditions, which now were taken for granted. Richard V. Palmer who set up an office in Longview, Washington in 1972 wanted to avoid the look and odor of a typical dental office, but he had a limited budget to follow an architect's advice in selecting colors, carpets, furniture and drapes. He built a ramp leading to his front entrance rather than steps, and installed tinted windows and incandescent lights to provide a comfortable ambiance for his patients and his staff.[254]

Negative reaction to the common, small, compartmentalized office, divided by long hallways between the reception and other rooms, led N.J. Browne of Laguna Beach, California, in 1972, to set up an open-bay concept office with simplified traffic patterns, which he had observed in the offices of orthodontists and pedodontists. Radiating out from a central oblong area containing a local artist's sculptured fountain surrounded by planters, were two operatories, the X-ray, darkroom, laboratory, hygiene, lavatory, reception and business office spaces. A warm comfortable atmosphere, for those patients who noticed, was evoked by using rough-sawn wood, concrete tiles and many plants.[255]

In 1970, for the first time, a dental office won the American Institute of Interior Design Award. Anne McDonald designed the office for Thomas O. Ballard of San Francisco. The dental suite was filled with antiques except for the dental chair and contained such exquisite pieces as a brass lined porthole and hand rubbed walnut furniture.[256]

Coupled with the interest in opening up the rooms within an office in the late '50s was a change in office equipment—the contour, couch-like chair which reflected a major physical change in the dentist's method of working on a patient. He no longer stood up or leaned against the chair, but sat on a stool at the patient's side. Although not the first dentist to suggest a reclining dental chair for the benefit of the dentist, who could sit down beside the patient, a reclining chair was designed and manufactured by John L. Naughton of Des Moines, Iowa. His first chair, made in 1958, was operated by hand, using hydraulic cylinders and a brake to achieve the reclining position. The first model and the 100,000th manufactured chair were presented to the NMAH, Smithsonian Institution in 1982 by Dental Equipment Manufacturing Co. (Dental-Ez Co.).Studies of dentists demonstrated that years of standing beside the patient all day to operate on teeth resulted in rapid physical deterioration, especially of the legs. "Sit-down" dentistry was found to prolong the dentist's life by 17 percent.[257]

James E. Furr of Wilmington, North Carolina in 1971 engaged the architect, Charles H. Boney, to build an office in which the brick building was blended into the residential area it adjoined, and brought a feeling of the outdoors into the office. Generous glass windows allowed the ridged bark and gnarls of wild cherry trees to become a part of the office decor. An unusual collage placed on a wall consisting of dental "junk" such as rubber bands, burs, disks and orthodontic materials caught the patient's eye. Furr's collection of nautical items was displayed throughout the office.[258]

In other offices, like the one of Owen (Rich) Herold of Whittier, California, the noisy and cumbersome items including a compressor, water heater, suction pump, vacuum cleaning system and telephone relay were placed in a mechanical room outside the building for easy access and service.[259]

The transition from older techniques and equipment could be seen in practices shared by a father and son. Ollie J. Weigel of Des Moines, Iowa, graduate of the class of 1951 of the University of Iowa Dental School, used the conventional equipment for standing up to work on a patient, while his son John (1969) employed the new "lie-down" equipment.[260]

Among the criteria dentists used to select a location for their offices was proximity to other medical offices, hospitals, clinics, etc., as well as, the more usual access to downtown shopping areas and public transportation. By placing the dental office near other medical facilities, the dentist could employ an anesthetist more readily, on a part-time basis, and have adequate medical resources to draw upon in an emergency.[261]

Larger offices in which two or more dentists joined their practices and engaged a secretary, hygienists, laboratory technicians and other chair-side assistants became more fashionable as dentists decided they no longer wanted to work 50, 60 or 70 hours a week. Group practice offered dentists a means to increase their range and effectiveness, while easing the burdens upon the individual practitioner.[262] One group practice was oriented toward preventive dentistry and introduced such novelties as showing films to instruct patients about dental care. Laren W. Teutsch of Omaha, Nebraska reported in 1970 that he also sent a bimonthly newsletter, *The Dental Educator*, to all his patients.[263] He further indulged his patients and staff by installing an exer-cycle and treadmill, as well as a staff lounge. Thus the dental office of the 70s became similar to the large business office or factory in which space was allotted for the staff to rest and rejuvenate their energies.

One group practice gradually evolved from the practice of one dentist, who over 25 years, built up his staff to include six full-time dentists, six part-time dentists and four hygienists, five people in the business office, 14 dental assistants and two dental educators. In a two-floor office, previously occupied by two stores in Mattapan Square, Boston, were placed a lobby, business office, reception area, private office, nine operatories, two lavatories, supply room, darkroom, panorex room and small laboratory. One of the advantages of this unusually large practice was the employment of young graduate dentists who brought new techniques and ideas with them. Dentists worked four days a week. Local dentists benefited by having their patients attended to, while they were away, by dentists in the group practice.

Another group practice which led to the opening of offices in eight other locations began as a single office in West Haverstraw, New York in 1967. Dentists realized that to meet the demands for increased dental care growing out of private insurance plans, increased Medicaid and federal-state dental insurance plans that were in the offing, increased productivity and efficiency would be needed on the part of all dentists. Offices were opened by the group at the rate of one per year, and by 1971, nine dentists and 22 nurses practiced as a cluster of three groups. The financial and legal relationships became increasingly complex as third-party plans to pay for dental care evolved, population increased, and specialties advanced.[264]

Precision was added to comfort in another large office located in Baltimore, Maryland in 1971. I. Norton Brotman and Howard L. Rothschild, graduates of the University of Maryland School of Dentistry practiced with six auxilliary staff and five laboratory technicians. They engaged an office manager to schedule each day's appointments on a precise regimen. Every day all staff met for 20 minutes to review the day's plans and a schedule was posted in each of the five treatment rooms. As dentists to the Baltimore Colts football team, they adopted sit down dentistry, working on patients lying in chairs suspended by an air-foil mobile base, which allowed the patient to be placed anywhere in the room. Brotman and Rothschild believed "By catching the eye, stimulating the imagination and occupying the mind, the visual characteristics of the office plays an important role in keeping the patient calm and cooperative."[265]

Avoiding what were believed to be excess income taxes motivated the first dental group to incorporate in 1965 within the guidelines of the U.S. Internal Revenue Service. The structure of this practice resembled a corporation with each dentist acting as a department head in charge of one facet of the office. The group of six dentists, who operated in Independence, Missouri, owned 25 shares of stock in the corporation valued at $250 per share in 1972. In a 7,500 square foot space they worked out of 18 operatories, along with four hygienists, a dental educator, X-ray technician, credit manager and four people in the business office. The laboratory technician worked to suit his own needs and extra laboratory work was sent out as needed. An executive director with a degree in accounting handled all employee problems, purchasing, payouts, hiring and firing. The advantages of this incorporated office extended beyond paying lower taxes. Additional advantages included friendship among the dentists, higher incomes, more time off than if each worked alone, built-in peer review and a competitive atmosphere which stimulated all to produce to the maximum of their potential.[266]

By 1987, architects experienced in designing dental offices, counseled dentists on a common pitfall of modern offices. John Crane, architect, who had assisted on 750 projects over 19 years in Seattle and San Fancisco, reported that 90 percent of dentists do not like their air-handling systems. Crane recommended a zone air-conditioning plan to meet several requirements, one of which was stipulated by law, that an office must function with a limited amount of energy. All systems such as purchasing, scheduling, air handling and others could be controlled by a computer for optimal efficiency and energy consumption. To obtain this ultra-modern office the dentist had to invest 6-1/2 to 8-1/2 percent of the construction costs for architectural services and could expect to pay between $55 and $85 per square foot to build an office in 1987 compared to approximately $35 for the same space, two decades earlier.[267]

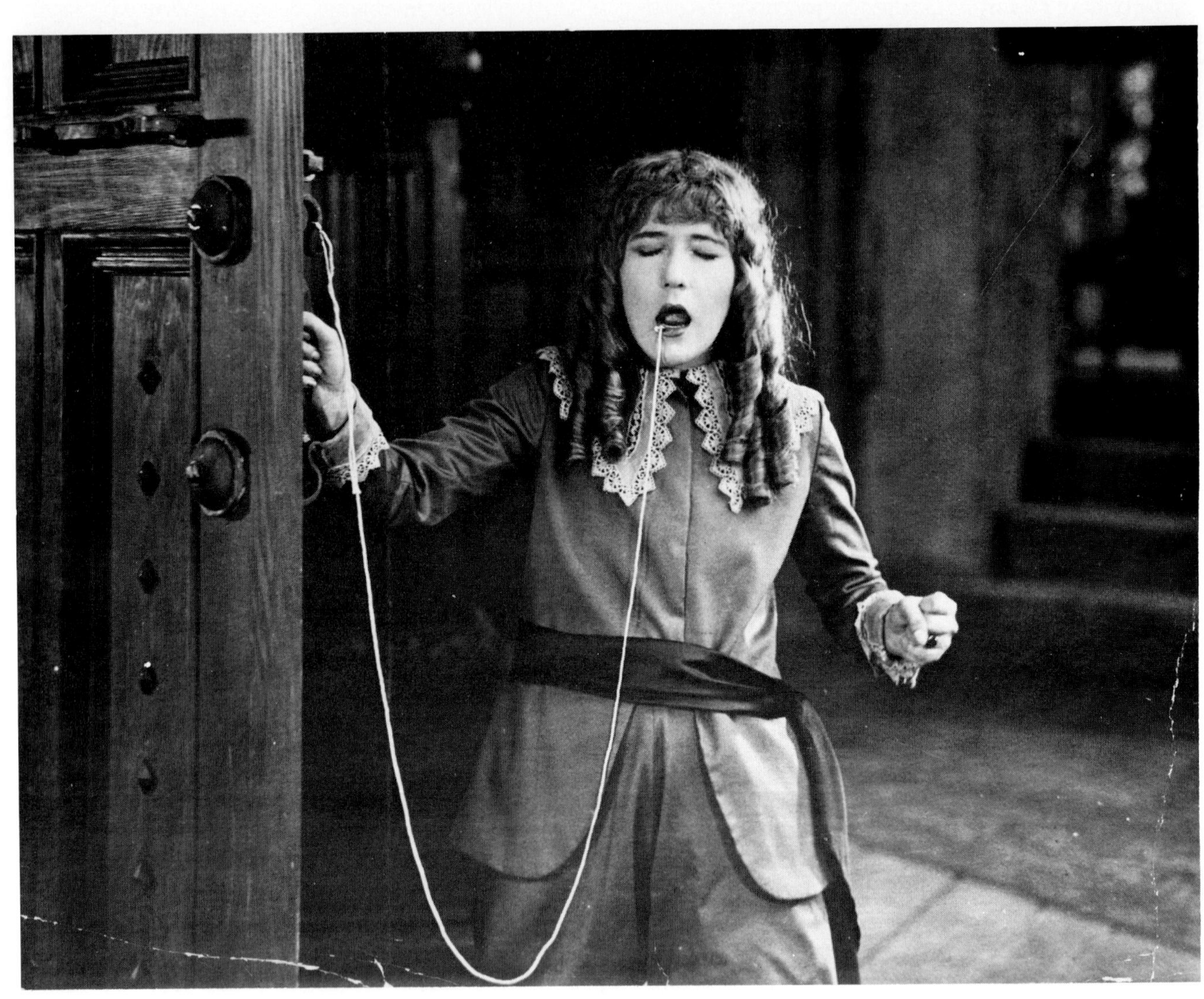

Mary Pickford extracting her own tooth by a "homemade method" in "Little Lord Fauntleroy," produced in 1921.

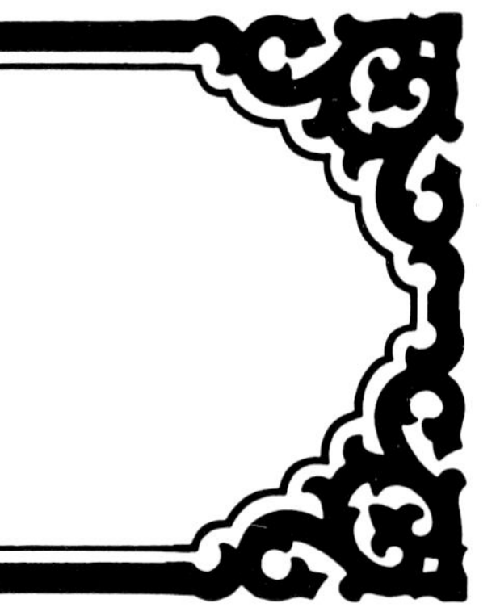

CHAPTER TWENTY

The Dentist in Films

Before we discuss the dentist in films, a brief investigation is in order into how the dentist perceived his role in society and the impact of his profession on his patients and himself. A Baltimore dentist, B. Holly Smith, after a quarter century of experience, described dentists in 1907 as "the hardest-worked professional men . . . that . . . work under more trying circumstances and for longer hours."[268] Smith reviewed and contrasted other medical specialities with dentistry. He singled out the oculist who sits in a chair from 9 a.m. to 1 or 2 p.m. examining and applying a spray, curette or knife. Then, after lunch, the oculist may spend an hour or two at the hospital or infirmary. He never spends more than a few minutes with a patient and receives a good fee of between $2 to $5 for each treatment. The gynecologist and surgeon operate for a few hours each day with the assistance of nurses, technicians and attendants who take charge of the patient after the operation is completed. The general medical practitioner may work as many hours as the dentist but he is not confined to one room and he is respected and praised by patients who make him feel that he and God are "the great dispensers of healing and comfort."

In contrast the dentist works from 8 or 9 a.m. to 5 or 6 p.m., seven days a week. He is under constant tension primarily induced by the patient's dread of dentistry—an impression left from the period when "painless dentistry" was not possible. In addition to absorbing the patient's discomfort, the dentist must inhale bad breath and the unpleasant odors of chemicals and disinfectants required to practice. He stands throughout the day on one foot, pedaling the dental engine with the other, while twisting his head, neck and arms to treat teeth within the enclosure of the mouth.

When the effect of all these unnatural and physically exhausting exertions has produced poor health, the dentist is unable to continue his profession, unlike the physician, who even in advanced age, is accepted by his patients as a wise advisor. The dentist devoted to his art demands precise instruments and machinery, but often overlooks his body's need to keep fit and well. Smith recommended that dentists shorten their office hours, perform the most difficult procedures in the morning, and charge, at least, minimal fees for all the advice and minor treatments their patients receive. The time saved by shortening their hours in the office after it became more efficient could be spent out-of-doors, communing with nature or pursuing a hobby that refreshes the mind and body.

R.O. Williams of Council Bluffs, Iowa provided another vantage point for the dentist to reduce the toll of practicing dentistry on his health. In an article entitled "Little Things" he urged the dentist to proceed in small stages to change his practice and help his patients. He, too, realized that the dentist who is intensely engrossed in treating a patient, overlooks obvious small changes that would enable him to perform the operation more comfortably. For instance, during a long procedure, the dentist twists and bends to accommodate himself to the tooth, rather than lowering or raising the chair a trifle or tilting the headrest, which would save him from contorting his body.[269]

Williams urged that the dentist add "little by little, as you can" useful and labor-saving devices and do his best "no matter how trifling the operation" in order to improve his reputation among patients and the ease with which he provides his services.

If the dentist chose to watch movies in his spare time he was in for a shock when he observed those films in which dentists appeared. Several dozen films, some of them classics, depict the dentist in very unflattering roles. A review of the major films reveals some of the common characteristics attributed to the dentist.

At the end of the 19th century in the period when motion pictures were introduced, the physician was respected for relieving pain, while the dentist inflicted more pain to treat the patient. For the most part people were terrified of a dental office. The image of the compassionate physician sitting by the bedside of a desperately ill child was contrasted with the aggressive dentist torturing his patient sitting helplessly and frightened in the fearsome dental chair.

To deal with these negative feelings patients found relief in making fun of the dentist, rather than facing up to the realities of their treatment and care. The resulting caricatures and comical images of the dentist are seen in a few motion pictures dating back to the inception of the commercial film. The first film shown in the U.S. appeared in New York City on April 23, 1896.[270]

The earliest film with a dental scene was made in England by George Albert Smith in 1902 and called "At Last! That Awful Tooth." Smith, formerly a portrait photographer, who was among the first to edit a film, varied the camera's views from long-range to close-up. In his first film, "My Grandma's Reading Glass," which he made in 1900, a boy with a magnifying glass focuses on a newspaper, a watch and a canary. In his next film made in 1902, one of the objects scrutinized is a tooth. Among the first American films with a dental scene was "The Fair Dentist," made in 1911. It starred Mary Pickford at the age of 18. Unfortunately, other than a still photograph of Pickford extracting a tooth nothing else is known about this picture. Noted for her roles as a child in this period, it is unusual to see her acting an adult part. She became not only a famous actress but a successful career woman.[271]

Films in this period derived some of their characters and scenes from vaudeville acts. Dentists were commonly mimicked in vaudeville skits. One of these vaudevillian derived films dealing with the subject of going to the dentist was "Laughing Gas," written, directed and acted-in by Charlie Chaplin. This Keystone Comedy was released in 1914. The short film explores the comic possibilities of the subject. Chaplin plays the role of an assistant to the dentist, Dr. Pain. While the dentist is distracted from his patients, Chaplin takes charge. One patient, who is a pretty girl, has her nose held by a forceps while Chaplin kisses her.[272]

The one-reel comedy, "The Dippy Dentist," starring Harry "Snub" Pollard, released in 1919 by Hal Roach, is one of the most humorous films ever produced based on going to the dentist. Harry, as a small man with a drooping moustache, who in some ways acted like Charlie Chaplin in "Laughing Gas," treated his patients in various unprofessional ways. A final scene shows Pollard giving gas to a beautiful woman patient, and then, kissing her after she is asleep.[273]

From a technical point of view this is an important film, since it shows an early urban office in a multi-story building. The film may have been shot in an actual office. The office contains commercially made equipment including a dental unit with plumbing and an electric dental engine.

"Greed" was the first non-comical, full-length silent film to center on the life of a dentist and his wife. This film, considered one of a dozen best films produced in the U.S., was adapted from the novel, *McTeague*, written by Frank Norris and published in 1899. It depicts the disintegration of a man's life, marriage, and subsequent death stemming from his increasing and unremitting greed.[274] The fact that a dentist was selected to portray the impact of greed on a person's life, affirms in a popular medium that at the end of the 19th century when dentistry was entering its modern renaissance, its cost in the patient's eyes, was centered on the unreasonable quest for money by the dentist. Physicians and surgeons are also financially successful, even more so than many dentists, however, their ministrations were acceptable with less acerbic criticism of their fees, at least until later.

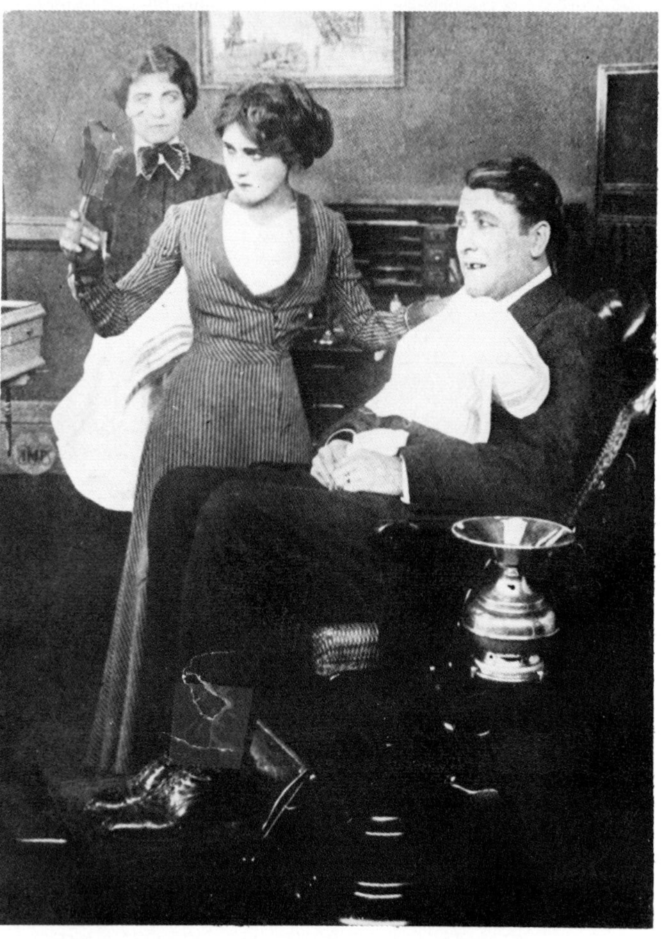

"The Fair Dentist," 1911. This picture of Mary Pickford when she was 18, in the role of the dentist, is the earliest showing a movie actress as a dentist. This scene is not listed among Mary Pickford's films and may have been incorporated into, or cut from, another film. From Independent Moving Pictures Co., New York.

The novel and the picture tells the story of McTeague who married and lost his license to practice dentistry after it was revealed that he was unqualified. After seeking and not finding another job he became brutish and ill-tempered. He began to drink, lost his possessions, and murdered his wife for her money. While running away from his crimes he died of thirst in the desert, handcuffed to the corpse of a man whom he had killed.[275]

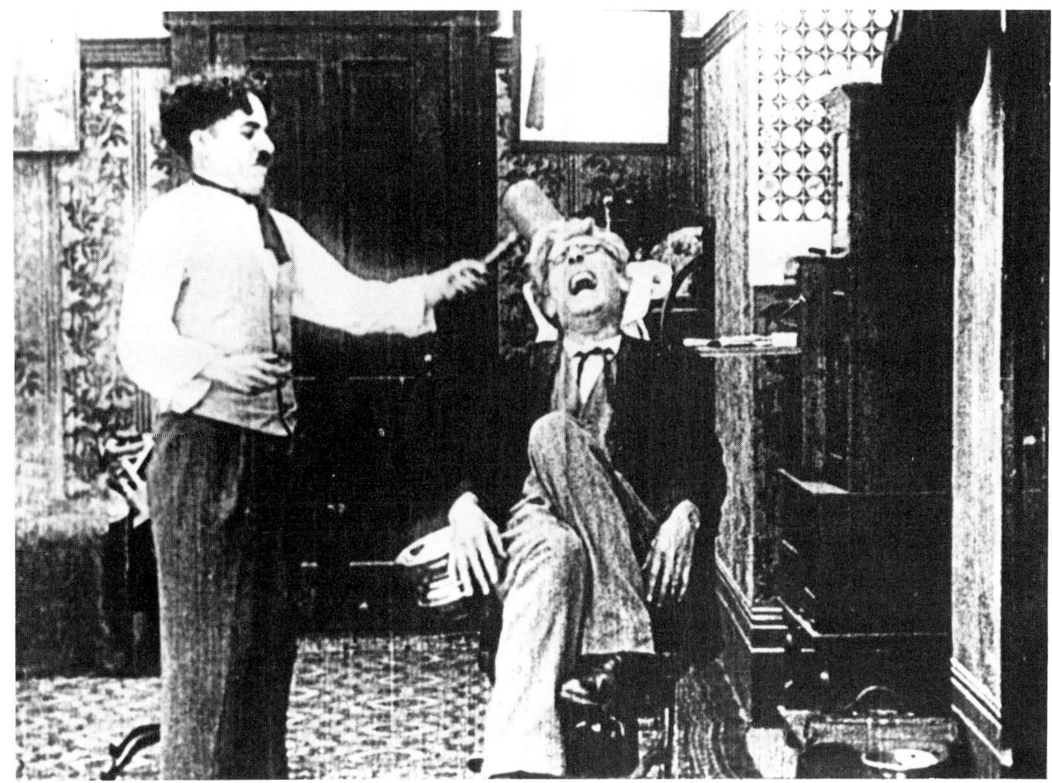

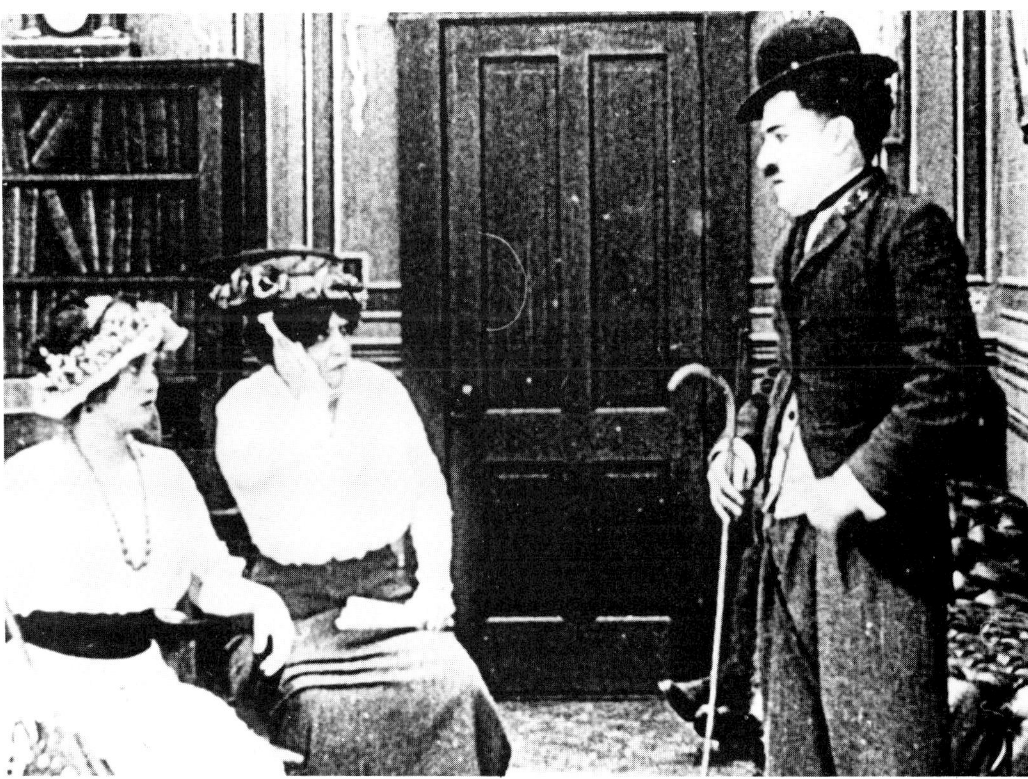

TOP: "Laughing Gas," 1914. Written, directed and acted in by Charlie Chaplin. This short comedy appears to be the first commercial movie to deal with the subject of going to the dentist. The office and equipment are typical of those found in this country from the 1880s to World War I. This office had no plumbing or electricity, therefore a foot-powered dental drill was installed and a spittoon was attached to the chair. In this scene, the patient woke up after being given laughing gas, so Chaplin, the dentist's assistant, found a more efficient method to knock him out by striking the patient on the head with a mallet. Mallets were also a part of dental office equipment in the 19th and early 20th centuries. The mallet wielded by Chaplin may have been used to beat gold into thin layers for use in filling teeth. From Museum of Modern Art/Film Stills Archives, New York City. BOTTOM: "Laughing Gas," 1914. Waiting room outside dental office. Chaplin, the dentist's assistant, confronts a patient with a toothache. From Museum of Modern Art/Film Stills Archives, New York City.

Erich von Stroheim directed the film for Metro-Goldwyn which became Metro-Goldwyn-Mayer at the time the film was released.[276] Von Stroheim's idiosyncratic genius resulted in a film that went through successive cuttings from its original eight hours on 42 reels, until it was edited down to two hours on two reels for commercial distribution. "Greed" was von Stroheim's great achievement. His discovery of *McTeague* when he arrived in the U.S., poor and uncertain of his future, inspired von Stroheim to become a film maker.[277] Norris' novel, set at the time he wrote it, was advanced to 1908 when it was filmed under the title "Greed" in 1923. In the picture the actors dress in turn-of-the-century costumes, while people in the background wear clothes of the style of 1923. Von Stroheim respected Norris' book and was exhaustive in adapting it to film to the extent of embellishing its characters beyond their lives in the book. As he did in other films, von Stroheim presented all the facts in developing his characters with the effect of "breaking through social hypocrisy and reasserting the corporality of experience."[278] In going beyond the book, the director made a film that had no precedent and has never been surpassed in depth of character development.[279]

The realism of the film fooled even friends of Norris. Several decades after the book appeared Norris' contemporaries believed that McTeague's office was modeled after an actual dental office on the street in San Francisco where the story evolves. Norris' brother published pictures to prove that the fictional dental parlor was located over the branch post office. However, this is an instance of life imitating fiction, for the street directory shows that it was not until some years after Norris had written his book that a dentist moved into this location. Norris managed to deceive so many because the rest of the street is reliably depicted in the book. Norris introduced one fictional element, the dentist's office, while meticulously drawing the rest of the street's profile from reality, observing the most trivial details from the actual locations of shops to the correct names of their owners. The film used the actual site for its setting, one of the first films to use real interiors as a movie set.[280]

The fictional dentist, McTeague, is accurately described. Norris, attended Harvard as a special student in 1894, while he wrote the story. To prepare himself for the development of McTeague's career he familiarized himself with the technical details of dentistry. To do this, Norris read Thomas Fillebrown's *A Text-book of Operative Dentistry* published in 1889. Norris leaned heavily on Fillebrown by incorporating the technical details almost verbatim from the text book.

The office Norris chose and von Stroheim filmed is authentic for the period and suits the type of dentist McTeague became. The office lacked plumbing, therefore, a spittoon was attached to the dental chair. Although there were electric lights, including one placed over the chair, the main source of light was the large bay window to which the chair faced. The drill was foot-powered. To have made the office more advanced would have belied McTeague's inadequate dental training and lack of ability to advance his skills.

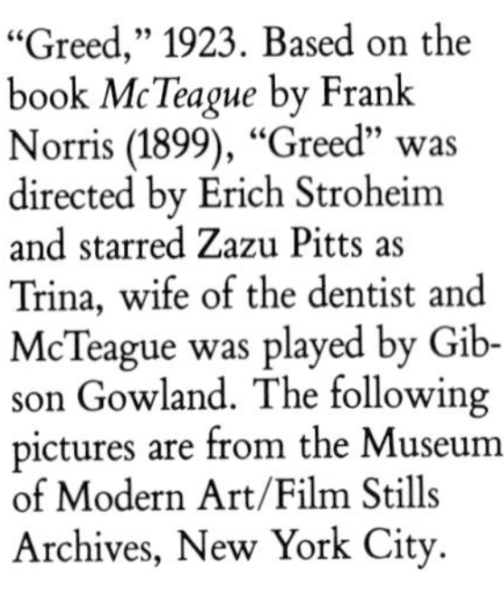

"Greed," 1923. Based on the book *McTeague* by Frank Norris (1899), "Greed" was directed by Erich Stroheim and starred Zazu Pitts as Trina, wife of the dentist and McTeague was played by Gibson Gowland. The following pictures are from the Museum of Modern Art/Film Stills Archives, New York City.

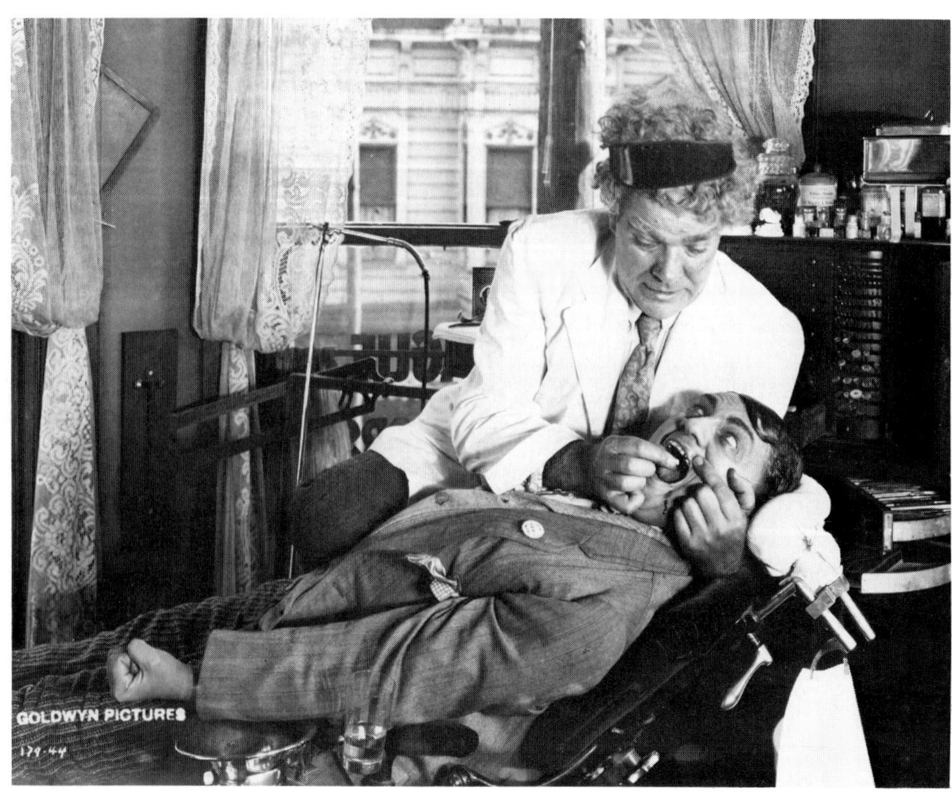

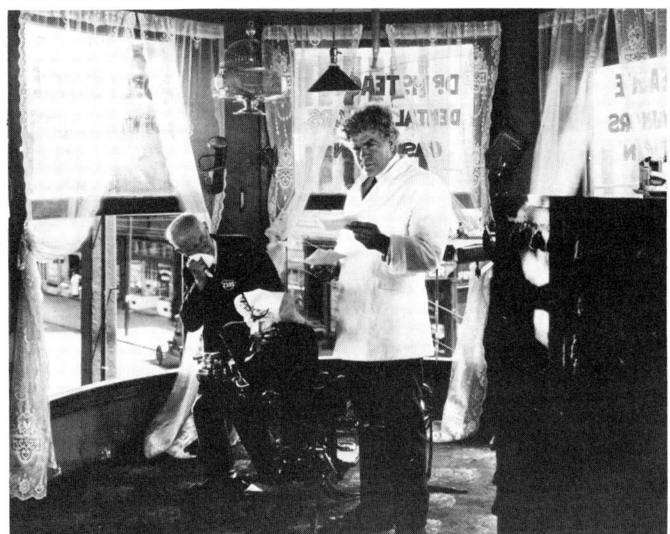

"Doc McTeague's Dental Parlors." A patient, a car-conductor, holds his face as he gets up from the chair. The bay windows face Polk Street in San Francisco.

Erich Stroheim directing a scene from "Greed." The ether can (Squibb) stands on the bracket table to the left just under the dental drill. The patient, Trina, was put to sleep before an extraction.

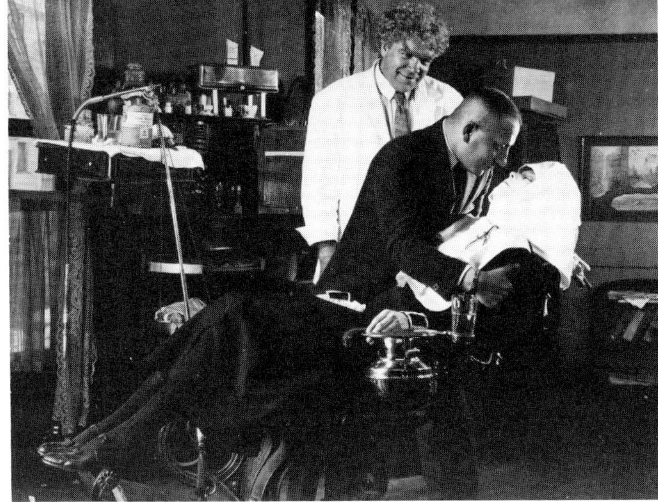

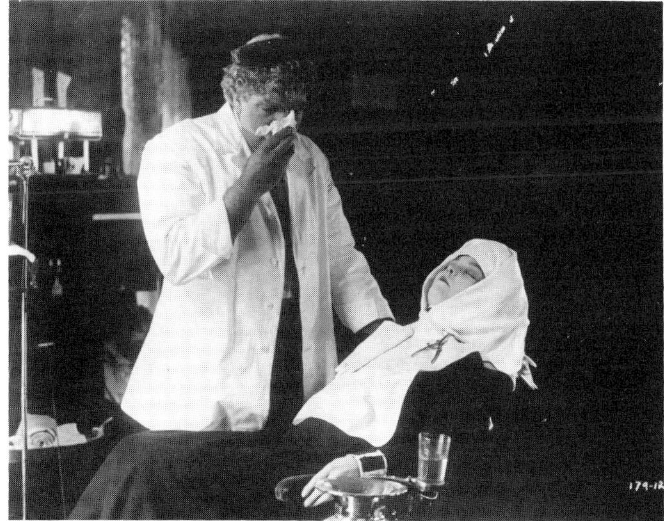

This is the first scene in a motion picture in which a dentist is shown acting in a lecherous manner. The caption for this scene states:
". . . and she was absolutely without defense. Suddenly the animal in the man stirred and woke. . . . It was a crisis . . . for which he was totally unprepared. Blindly . . . McTeague fought against it. . . . He turned to his work, as if seeking a refuge in it. But as he drew near to her again, the charm of her innocence and helplessness came over him afresh. It was a final protest against his resolution."

McTeague unpacks a huge, gold-gilded tooth which symbolizes his dream of perfect contentment as a dentist. Gold is used throughout the movie to epitomize the continuing greed which the characters display. In the original copy of the film each image of a gold piece, including the gold in tooth fillings, was tinted by hand in gold to emphasize the obsession of the characters.

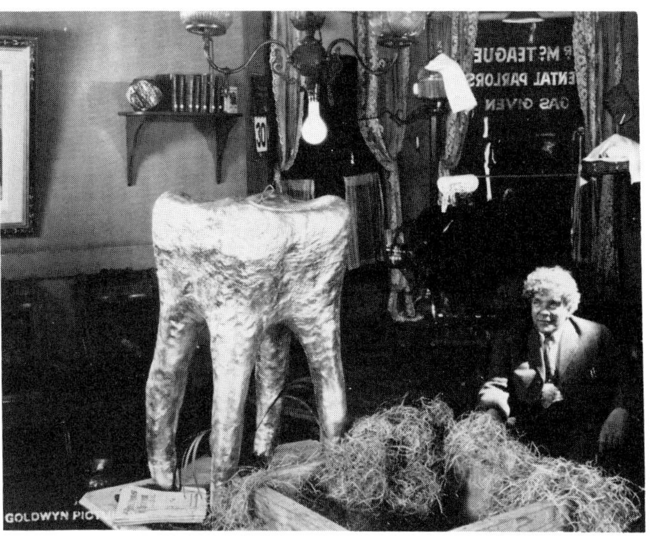

Five years after the film "Greed" appeared, Hal Roach wrote and produced a short two-reel silent movie called "Leave 'Em Laughing" (working title: "A Little Laughing Gas"). Released in January 1928, one of 23 films they made in 1928-29, the film starred Stan Laurel and Oliver Hardy.[281] This comedy poked fun at the dental profession and is an excellent example of how Laurel and Hardy could turn a little material into a well-focused and warm comedy. Stan Laurel immigrated from England with Charlie Chaplin and became Chaplin's understudy in vaudeville. Oliver Hardy, who was born in Harlem, Georgia, began to study law, but turned to the theater in 1910 and operated a movie house for three years.[282] Laurel and Hardy acted in vaudeville scenes ridiculing the dentist and carried some of these acts into silent films. One classic pie throwing scene in one of their first films as a comedy team appears in the film "The Battle of the Century," (1927). In the film a pie lands in the face of a man in a dentist's chair.[283]

In the film "Leave 'Em Laughing" Stan Laurel wakes up at 3 a.m. with a toothache. He ties a bandage around his head in the classical manner, and later in the morning his friend, Oliver Hardy, takes him to the dentist. The caption under this scene states "Stan is finally coerced into the chair of pain . . ." An attempt is made to give him laughing gas (nitrous oxide), but when this is unsuccessful Hardy sits in the chair to show him how easy it can be. After a series of comical events Hardy's tooth is extracted instead of Laurel's. The film ends with both of them on the street staggering around from the effects of the gas.[284]

The film was made in a typical dental office of the 1920s that was supplied with plumbing and electricity. The age of sterility also had arrived as witnessed by the white metal dental cabinet, polished linoleum floor and the white uniforms worn by the dentist and nurses or dental hygienists.

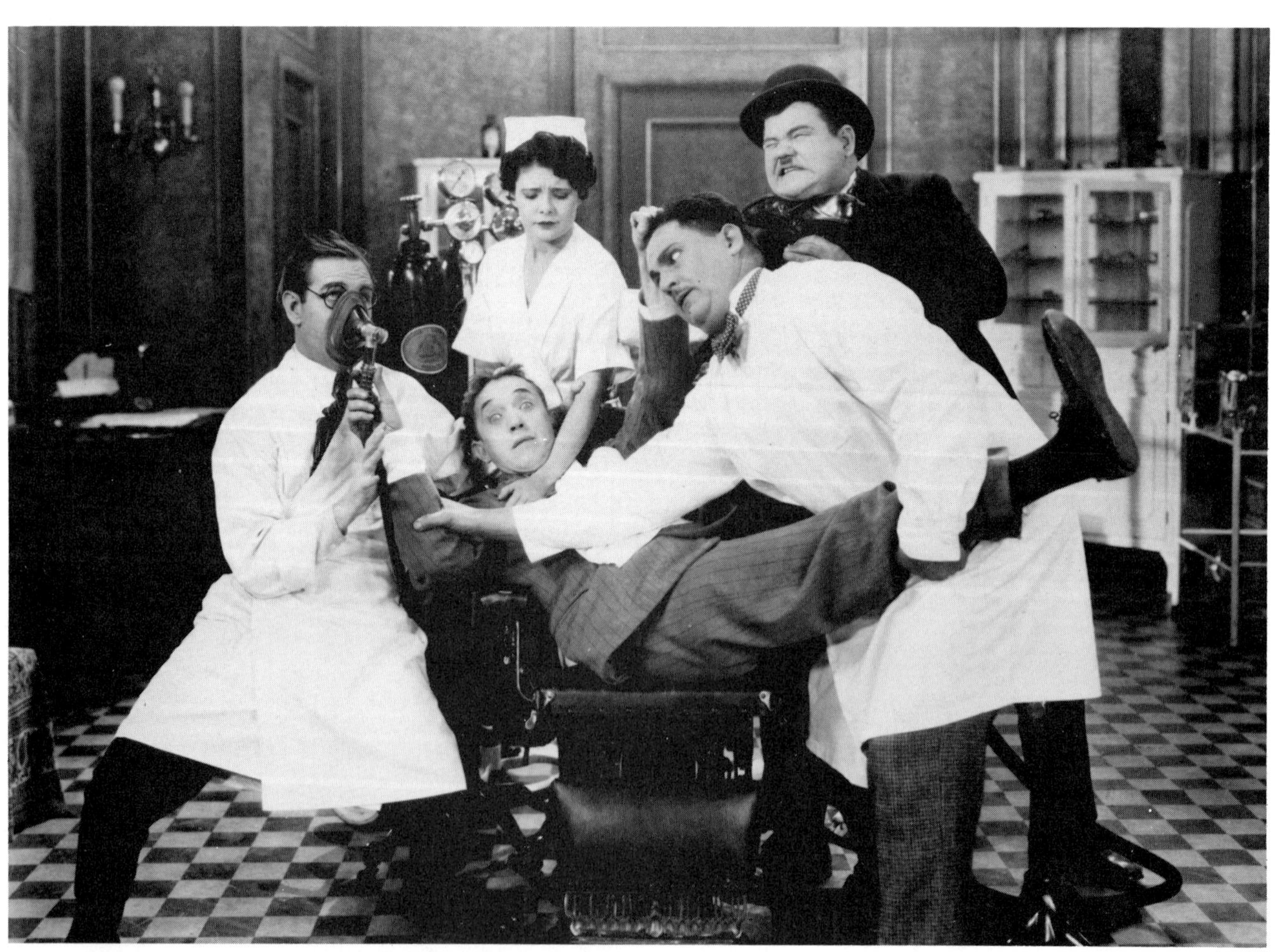

Here Stan struggles to avoid the mask which is used to apply nitrous oxide (laughing gas). The office is typical of the 1920s with both plumbing and electricity. The white coats, white metal cabinet, and linoleum floor which could be easily cleaned, were the mainstays of a sterile office in this period.

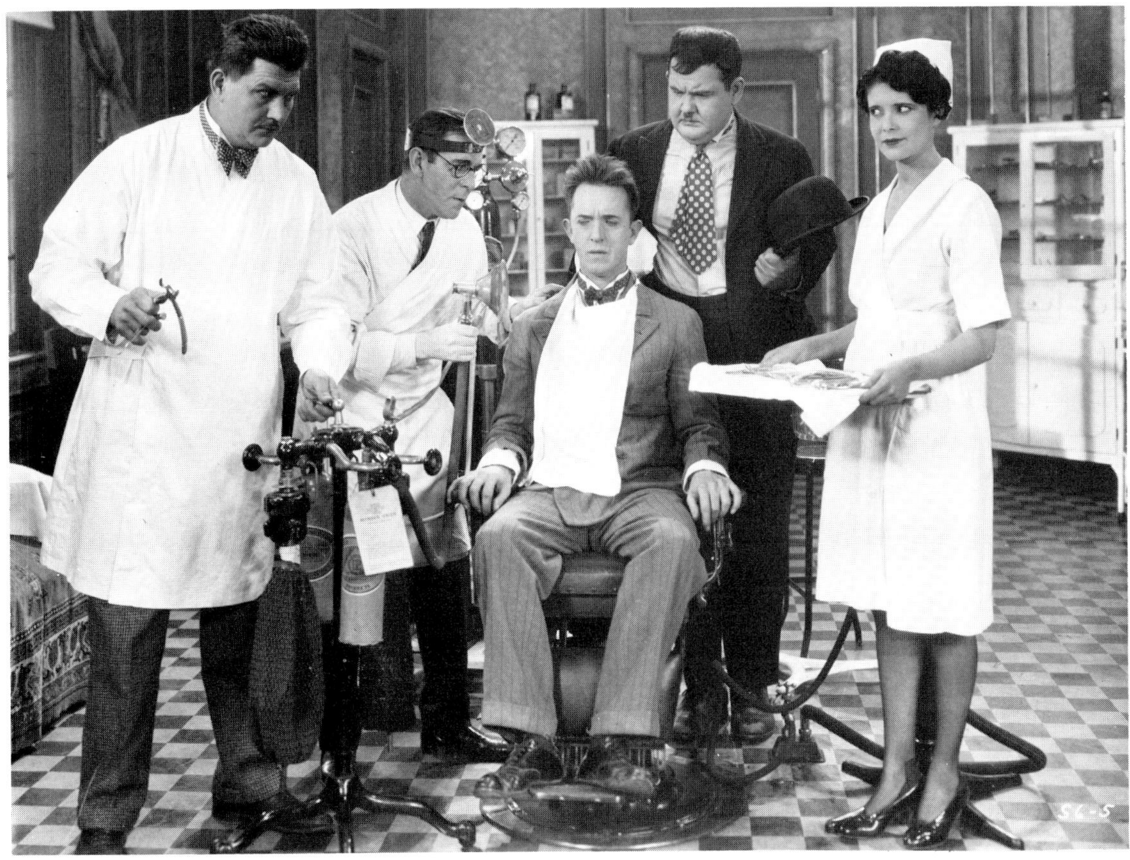

"Stan is finally coerced into the chair of pain..."

The tables are turned. Oliver Hardy ends up in the chair and is about to have one of his teeth extracted.

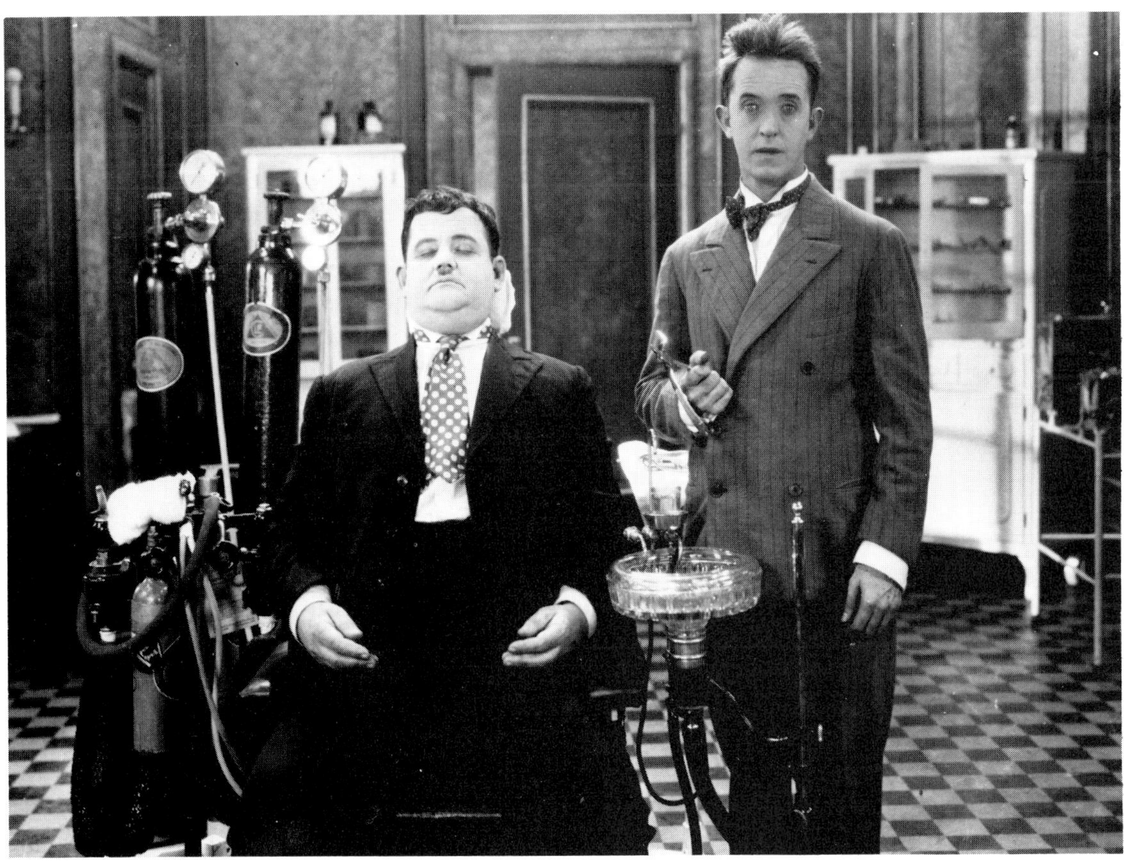

"Pardon Us," another Hal Roach comedy, stars Laurel and Hardy in their first all-talking feature film (1931). They did a scene at the dentist which was similar to their 1928 silent short comedy, "Laughing Gas." The film displayed a series of skits, much in the manner of music hall acts, of which the dental scene was one.

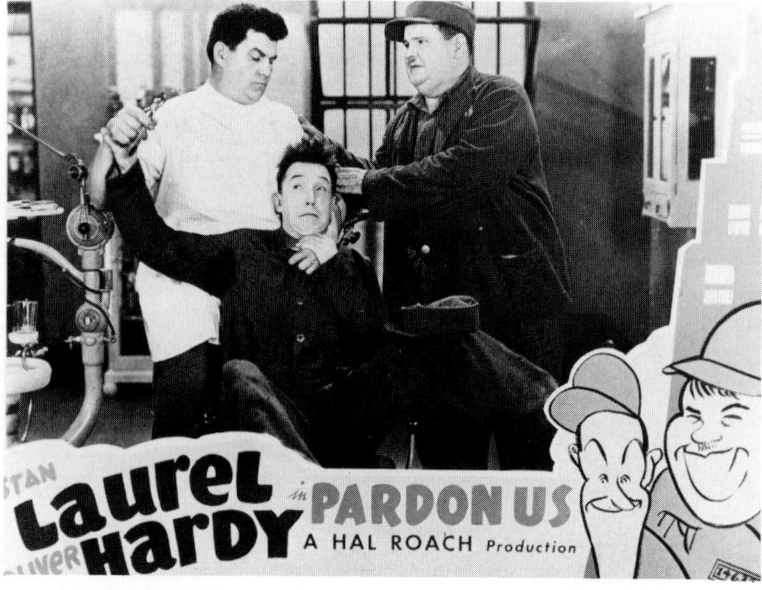

Stan Laurel is escorted to the dental chair by his friend Oliver Hardy and a dental assistant.

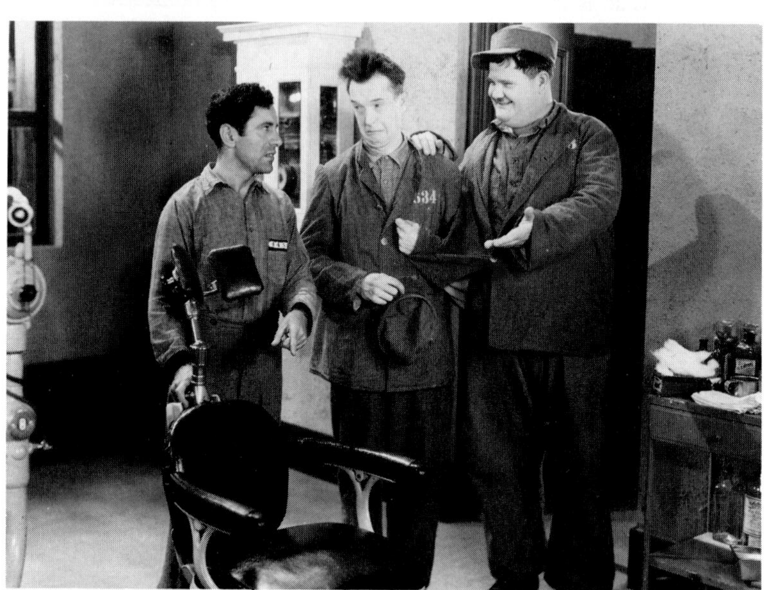

Patients sit in the waiting room as Stan Laurel is wheeled into the office. Note the man on the left with his swollen jaw bandaged, a typical response to an infected tooth in the period before sulfur drugs and antibiotics.

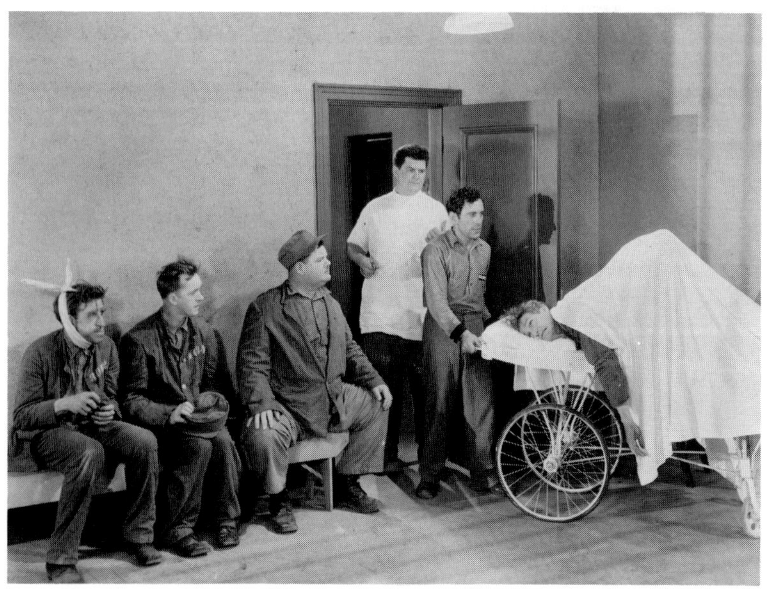

Another popular comedy team specializing in violent, vulgar slapstick was the Three Stooges. They began their acting careers in vaudeville in 1923 and remained a team for almost 50 years.[285] The original team consisted of Moe and Skemp Howard and Ted Healy. Jerome (Curly) replaced Skemp in 1930 and Larry Fine replaced Ted Healy. The Three Stooges appeared in feature films in 1934 and began the longest-running series of two-reel comedies in the history of sound films. They acted in over 200 shorts which were produced by Columbia Pictures between 1934 and 1958. Skemp returned to the act in 1946 after Curly left the team in 1946 and was succeeded in 1955 by Joe Besser.[286]

The Stooges achieved their humor by exaggerating life in their films. Comedy revolved around the team in the act of brutally bopping each other on the head with mallets, tweaking one another's noses, gouging their eyes and kicking each other in the shins. They turned stereotypical situations into comedy through slapstick. For instance, they acted out going to the dentist, perceived as painful by the public, and made it into an even more painful procedure to make people laugh.

The Stooges made two films which cast aspersions on medicine including "From Nurse to Worse" and "Dizzy Doctors."[287] and three films containing material about going to the dentist. They were "All the World's A Stooge," released in 1941, "I Can Hardly Wait" (1943) and "The Tooth Will Out" (1951). In the film "I Can Hardly Wait" they used material from the Laurel and Hardy film "Leave 'Em Laughing," but made it more physical. The Three Stooges wanted instant laughter, whereas Laurel and Hardy were more subtle and took more time to develop a visual joke. The Stooges' films were difficult to produce and sometimes resulted in accidents. In one scene, in which they were portraying dentists, plaster was thrown around. The property men became too enthusiastic and hit Larry Fine in the eye. In another short, he lost a tooth, and once was stabbed in the forehead with a quill pen.[288]

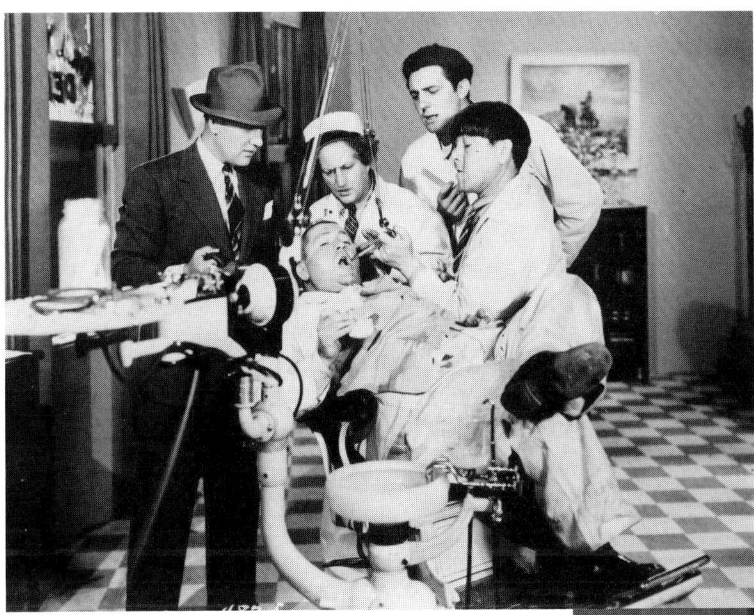

"All the World's A Stooge," produced in 1941 as a short comedy. The Three Stooges are window washers-turned-dentists. The 1930s-40s dental equipment faces away from the window, rather than toward the window, as would be expected in a dental office.

In another Stooge film, "I Can Hardly Wait," produced in 1943, Curly develops a terrible toothache, while eating a ham bone. Because of the pain he falls asleep with difficulty and dreams that Moe and Larry rush him to the dentist. To prove that there is nothing to be frightened of in the dentist's chair, Moe sits in the chair, and before he can prevent it, has one of his teeth extracted. The two dentists in the film are Dr. Yank (acted by Bud Jamison) and Dr. Tug (acted by Dick Curtis). Laurel and Hardy used the same "extracting tooth gag" in their film "Leave 'Em Laughing" in 1928. The intense fear of the pain the dentist would inflict extended up to the period of the 1950s when the high-speed drill was introduced and made removing decay from a tooth much less irritating and painful.

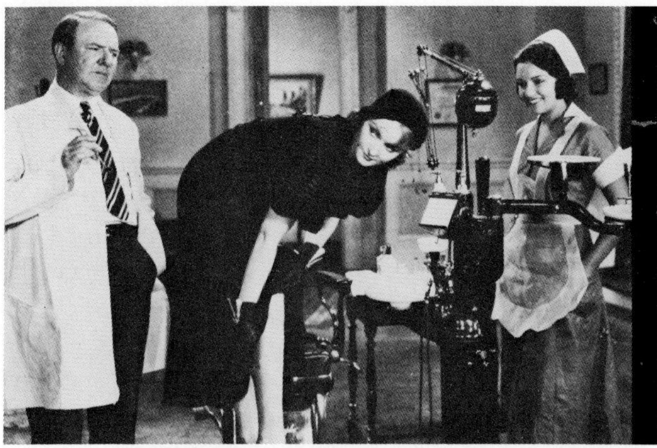

Before seating his attractive patient in the chair, Fields looks at her legs when she shows him where she was bitten by a dog. This photograph provides a good example of the lecherous dentist.

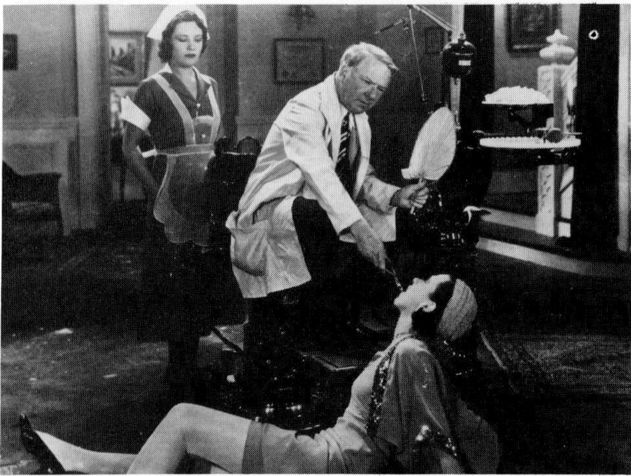

After extracting actress Elsie Cananna's tooth, Fields remarks tongue-in-cheek, "There you are; it din't hurt a bit, did it?" Before taking out the tooth, he attempted to save it. He ordered his nurse "Just hand me that 404 circular buzz saw." He then hummed a tuneless song as he drilled while repeating the word "grubbing."

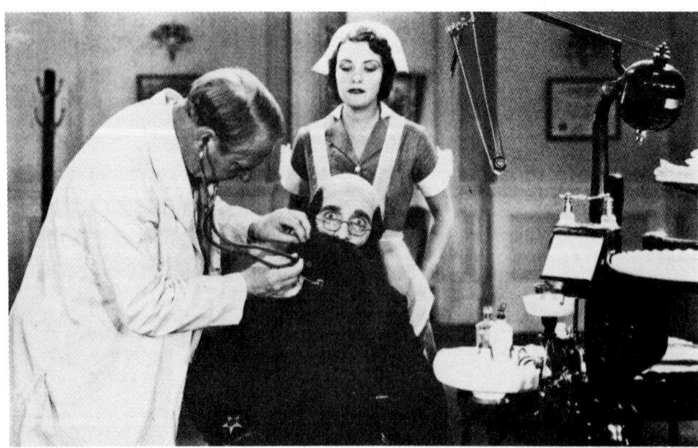

Fields conducts a search for this patient's mouth. He tells him to say "Ah," and then, using a stethoscope, traces the source of the sound. Without asking the patient which tooth is bothering him, he begins drilling. The patient spits out a few teeth. After this, a bird flies by and Fields grabs his rifle to shoot it.

"The Dentist," a Mack Sennett comedy, produced in 1932 starred W.C. Fields. Fields enjoyed making fun of the hardships and troubles of others for he believed that "comedy was tragedy happening to someone else." Fields' dental office is in his home, not atypical for dental offices up to this time.

In the 30s films continued to be made which poked fun at the dentist. The classical film of this decade was a 20 minute short comedy with sound made in 1932. Called "The Dentist" it was written by and starred W.C. Fields. The film was produced by Mack Sennett, directed by Leslie Pearce, and distributed by Paramount Pictures.

"The Dentist" was the only Fields' film to show him entirely unsympathetic. He displayed a complete lack of consideration and outright cruelty to others. As a dentist he treated various patients, always in a comical way, including a scene where he becomes lecherous and verges on becoming a sadist. Without even a token attempt to justify his behavior, Fields must have known that this film presented a serious flaw for a comedic image that he intended to continue in other films. In succeeding films he displays a warmer personality.[289]

The office is in the dentist's home and contains a hydraulic dental chair, dental cabinet and dental unit with electric hand-piece attached.

One of the early sound films to feature a dentist was the film "The Strawberry Blonde." It was produced three times beginning in 1933 when it was called "One Sunday Afternoon" and starred Gary Cooper, Frances Fuller and Fay Wray who were employed by Paramount Pictures. In 1941 with its title changed to "The Strawberry Blonde" and starring James Cagney, Olivia De Havilland, Rita Hayworth, Alan Hale, George Tobias, Jack Carson and George Reeves, it was produced by Warner Brothers, which made a third version of it as a musical in 1948 with Dennis Morgan, Janis Paige and Dorothy Malone.[290]

This film is a sentimental turn-of-the-century movie in which the comedy is pleasant. The second version takes place in Brooklyn, New York rather than the small town of the original version. The atmosphere of the period is well presented. In the second version James Cagney portrays the dentist, who graduated from a correspondence school. He loses Rita Hayworth, the neighborhood strawberry blonde, to a crooked contractor, Jack Carson. Then he marries her girlfriend, Olivia De Havilland. After working for Carson he is sent to jail and upon his release joins his wife and sets up a dental practice in his home. When Carson arrives for emergency dental care, Cagney plans to kill him with laughing gas, but at the last minute he decides that he is the happier man and has married the right woman. Cagney softens his anger and merely extracts Carson's tooth without giving him an anesthetic.

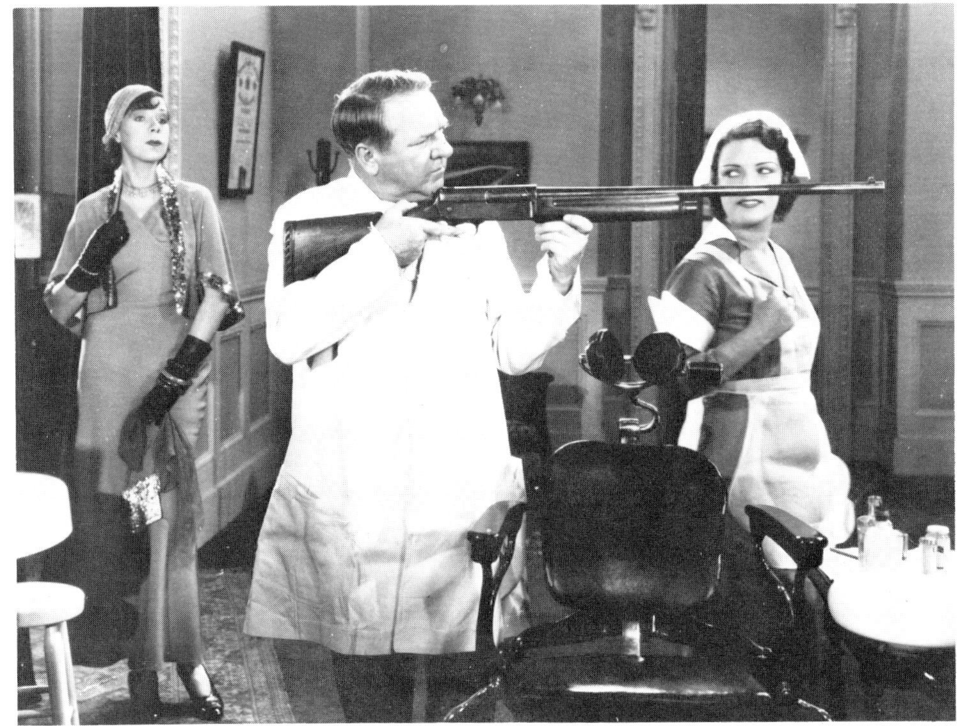

In between patients Fields takes aim with his hunting rifle, emphasizing the fact that he is at home and has access to all his personal items.

"Strawberry Blonde," produced in 1941 by Warner Brothers, provides some excellent scenes of the dentist working out of his home around the turn of the century. James Cagney plays the dentist, who learned his trade from a correspondence school course.

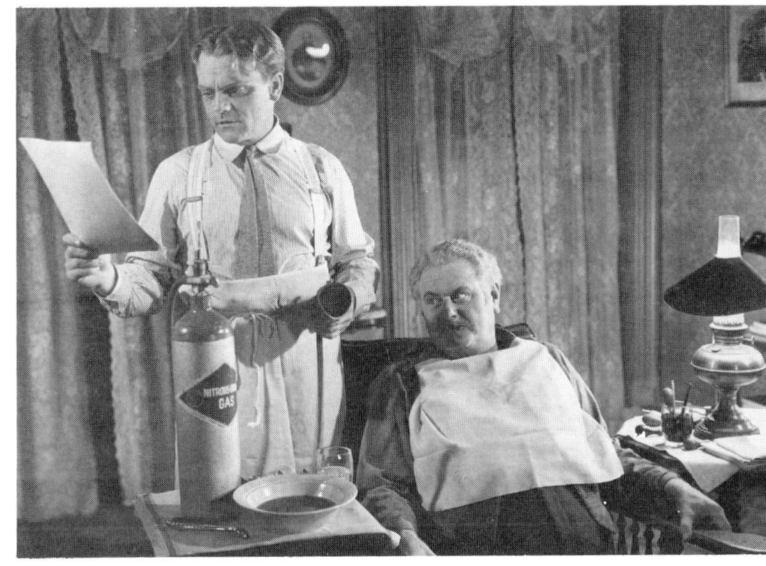

Alan Hale sits in a household chair, which serves as a dental chair, while James Cagney, the dentist, studies his correspondence school material on how to use laughing gas (nitrous oxide), so that he can put Hale to sleep before extracting a tooth.

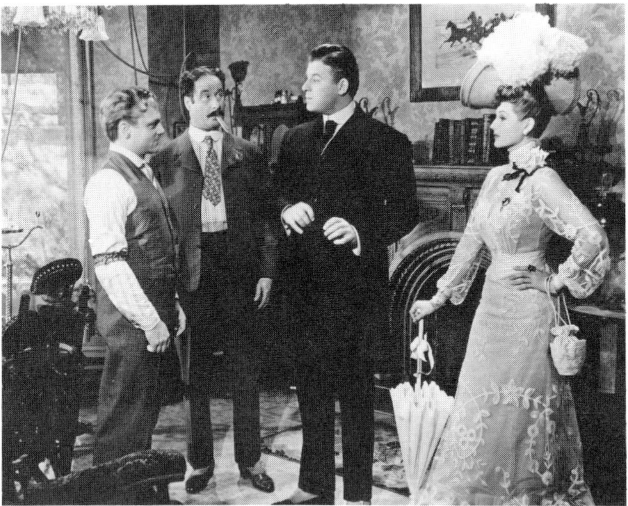

Jack Carson, Cagney's rival for Rita Hayworth, now Carson's wife, comes to the dentist to cure his aching tooth. Now more successful, Cagney owns a commercially manufactured chair which faces the window for light and is also provided with artificial light.

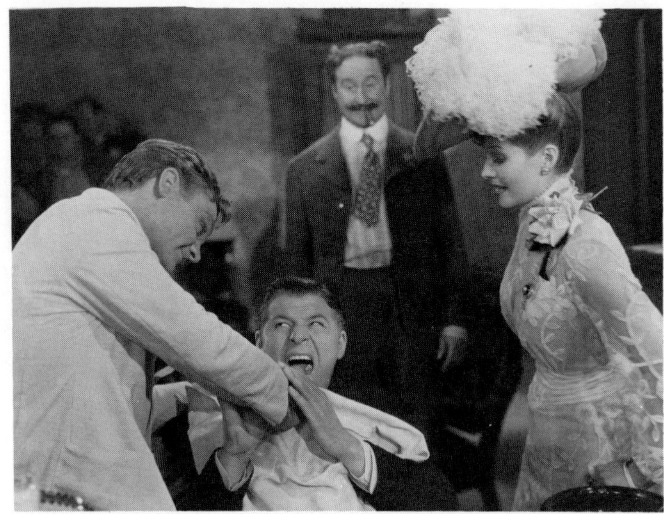

James Cagney, dentist, extracts Jack Carson's tooth without anesthesia to get even with him for marrying the woman he courted, Rita Hayworth.

"Texas," produced by Columbia Pictures in 1941, is a full length drama about two veterans of the Confederate Army, who go to Texas to set up a cattle business. Set in 1866, the film starred William Holden, Glenn Ford, Claire Trevor, George Bancroft, Edgar Buchanan and others, who carry on in true Hollywood western fashion by rough riding, stagecoach holdups and much shooting.

Columbia produced another film in 1941 called "Texas" which is the story of two veterans of the Confederate Army who go to Texas after the Civil War to set up a cattle business. The film was set in 1866 and starred William Holden, Glenn Ford, Claire Trevor, George Bancroft, Edgar Buchanan, Don Beddoe and others. Edgar Buchanan portrays the dentist and a bandit, who is always prepared to check a tooth for a cavity, even in the midst of a shoot-out.[291] The dental office in a home is authentic in having the proper furnishings, however, the dental engine is anachronistic since it was introduced in 1872, six years after the time frame of the film.

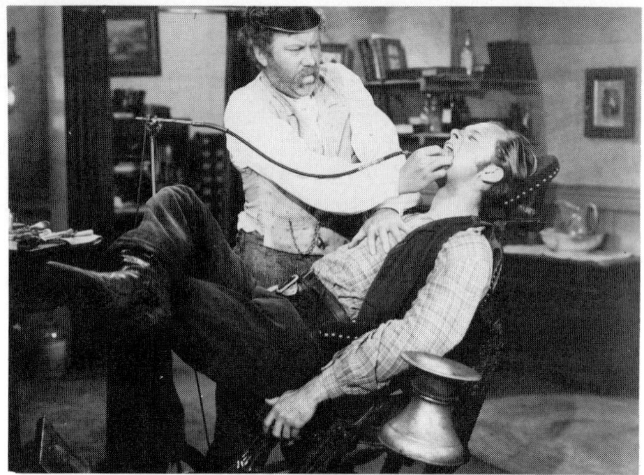

Edgar Buchanan studied dentistry and graduated from the University of Oregon, before he decided to become an actor. Here he treats a cowboy with a foot-pedal drill, which is an anachronism, since this drill was only introduced in 1872, six years after the time frame of the film. The eye-shade indicates this dentist had other professional functions, perhaps including banker, physician, etc.

Edgar Buchanan (1903-1979) who played the dentist, was originally a dentist who graduated from the University of Oregon. Unhappy with his profession, he drifted into making films beginning in 1940. He soon became a favorite western character playing roles such as a corrupt sheriff or judge or a rugged old-timer. In spite of the shady characters Buchanan played, he remained a friendly personality to American audiences. He appeared in almost 100 films and co-starred in the TV series "Petticoat Junction."[292]

The specialist dentist or oral surgeon was given a more sinister role in the film "Footsteps in the Dark" produced by Warner Brothers in 1941. In this light comedy patterned after the *Thin Man* films, Ralph Bellamy plays the part of the oral surgeon who is a murderer.[293]

Another film set in the West was made in 1948 by Paramount Pictures. The film "The Paleface" stars Bob Hope and Jane Russell. The film was remade under the title, "The Shakiest Gun in the West" in 1967. The second version is a dreary farce, which is much less subtle in depicting a cowardly dentist becoming a western hero.[294] The story takes place in the 1870s. Painless Peter Potter (Bob Hope), an itinerant dentist, who earned his dental credentials through a correspondence school, is chased out of town after extracting the wrong tooth of a patient. Calamity Jane (Jane Russell), working as an undercover

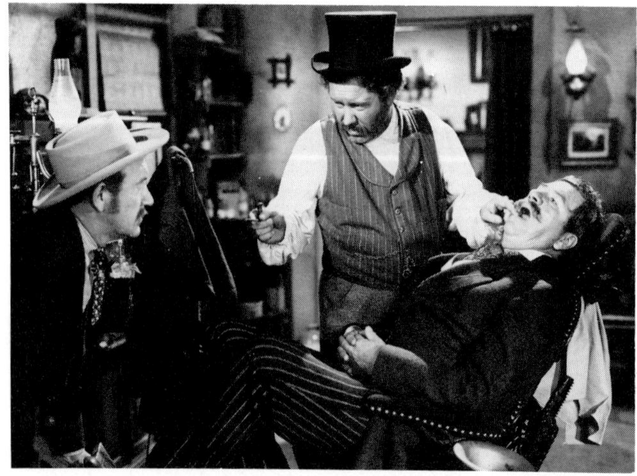

Edgar Buchanan talks to George Bancroft as he holds Addison Richards' jaw open with his fingers. The dentist's jacket draped over the drill provides a touch of humor, but also indicates the informality of the 19th century dental office. From M.B. Paul, photographer, Columbia Studios.

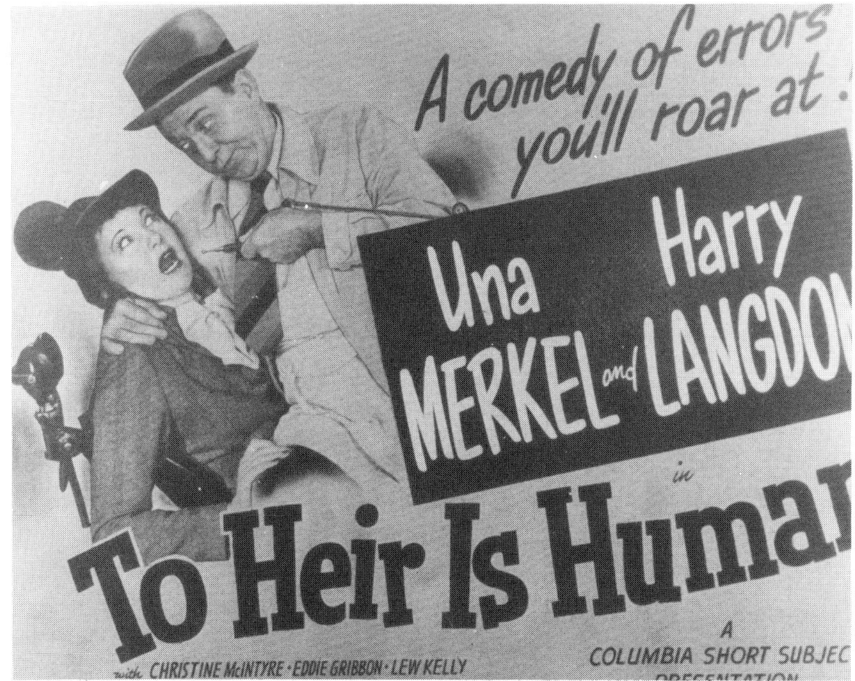

"To Heir is Human," released by Columbia Pictures in 1944, starred Una Merkel and Harry Langdon, here seen pointing a drill at Merkel's mouth while he sits on her lap in the dental chair. His attire, which includes an apron, conveys the message that he is not an expert, and may even be a butcher. From Columbia Pictures No. D-572-5.

Advertising poster for the film "To Heir is Human."

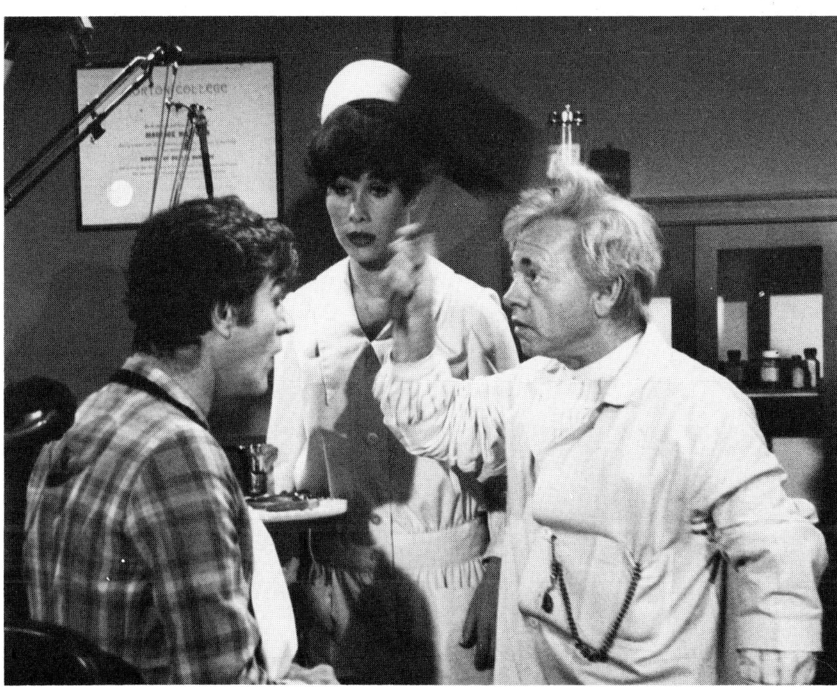

Mickey Rooney is the dentist in this scene of an unknown film. The office equipment is of the 1930s-40s type.

agent for the government, marries the timid dentist and proceeds to get him into all kinds of jams and lets him and everyone else believe that he shoots his way out of them, when, in fact, she does the shooting. Painless is convinced that he is a hero and the villains are convinced that he is the government agent. Painless and his wife are captured by Indians. He escapes and frees his wife, after which they fall in love.

In this period it was common for the dentist to travel to patients among a circle of towns and set up his equipment in a hotel or inn. Dentists more often learned their profession by apprenticeship to another dentist, who they observed and assisted with his patients. It was less likely for a dentist to obtain an education through a correspondence school. This detail in the film seems more likely to be based on the belief of the period in which the film was made, that this was a good way to convince contemporary audiences that the dentist was incompetent, rather than being historically accurate to the story.

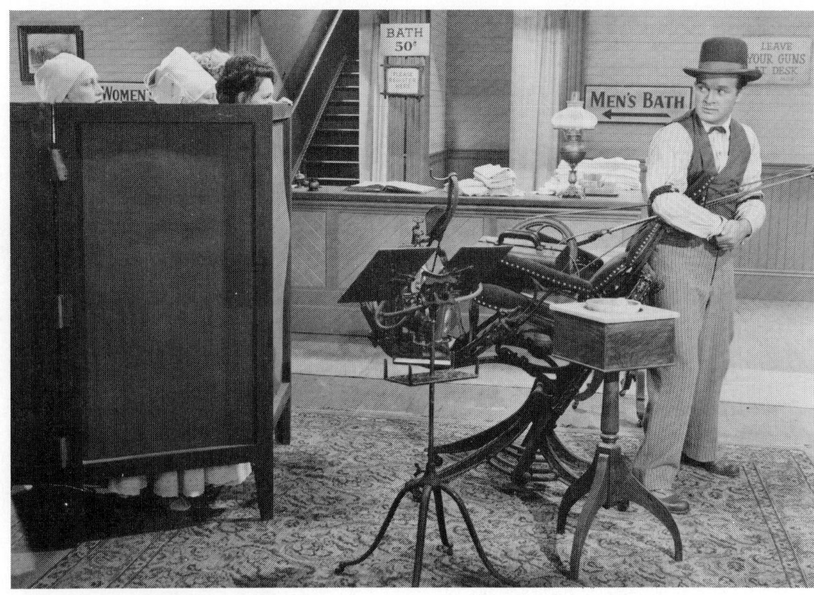

"Paleface," produced by Paramount Pictures in 1948, starred Bob Hope as an itinerant dentist, Painless Peter Potter. The film is a loose take-off on the practice of Painless Parker. In this picture he is shown arriving with his dental equipment at a hotel in a small western town in the 1870s. He is carting a dental chair (not the usual small, portable-type carried by itinerants), a foot engine, spittoon, nitrous oxide apparatus and a small case of instruments placed on the seat of the chair. From National Screen Service Corporation.

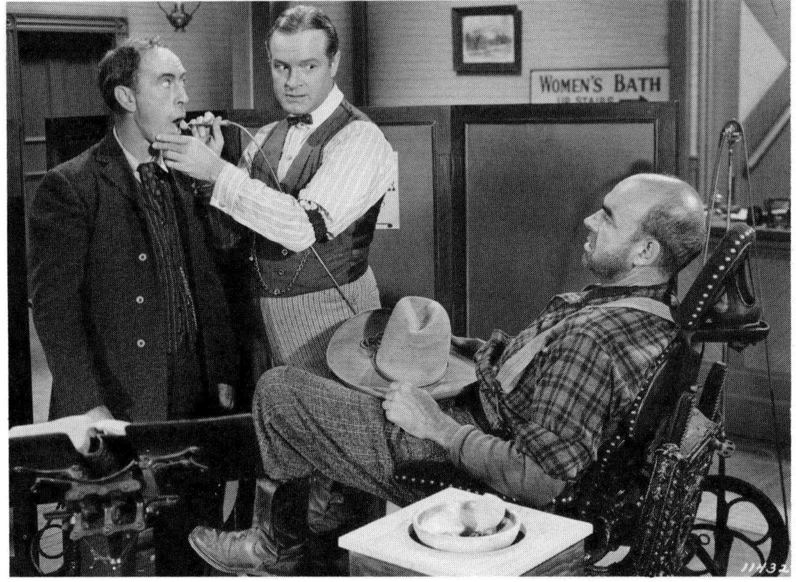

Painless Potter, in "Paleface," demonstrates to a patient that "it doesn't hurt." Note marble-top cuspidor in lower center of the picture. From National Screen Service Corporation.

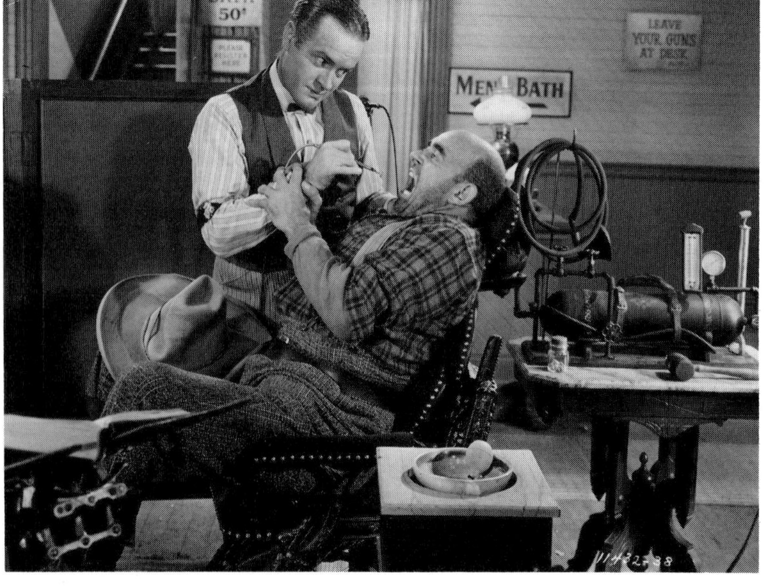

Bob Hope is about to start drilling on a very reluctant patient. While pumping the foot-pedal drill with his foot he applies the drill to the patient's teeth. Part of the comedy was created by Painless Peter Potter's reversing the action of his hands and feet. Note the signs in the background which add humor to the scene, but also reflect the reality of the settings in which itinerant dentists worked in the last quarter of the 19th century.

HOPE'S ALWAYS PULLIN' 'EM IN "THE PALEFACE"

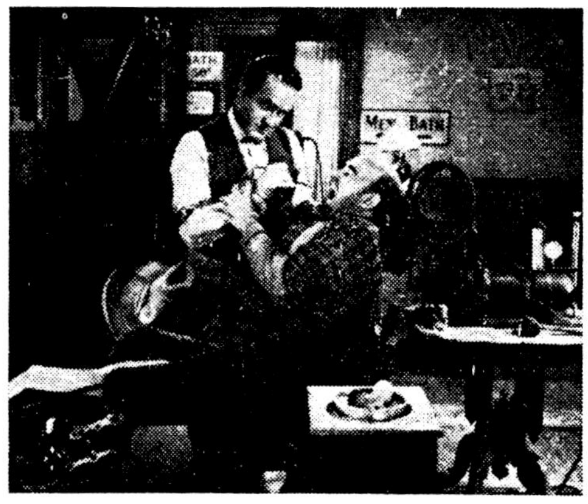

See your dentist twice a year for healthy teeth.

See Bob Hope as Doc "Painless Potter" in

"THE PALEFACE"

for the healthiest laffs you ever had!

SCREENING FOR DENTISTS

Since Bob Hope plays a traveling dentist in "The Paleface" you have a peg on which to hang a promotion with dentists. You might invite a group of them to a screening, and use their comments in newspaper ads and lobby display.

Ethics of the profession prohibit use of dentists' names, but testimonial gag could be worked out this way:

Dr. X, one of Blanktown's leading dentists, says of Bob Hope in "The Paleface":

"That Hope and his gags! . . . Always pulling them!"

OPEN WIDE, PLEASE! . . . and let all those laughs come out . . . Dr. Bob Hope is extracting laughs in "The Paleface".

A recent film casts the dentist as an extremely evil person. The film "Marathon Man" produced in 1976 by Paramount Pictures provides the ultimate example of a dentist acting as a torturer. In this complex thriller Laurence Olivier plays a cold-blooded Nazi dentist who tortures the character acted by Dustin Hoffman, by removing the nerve of a tooth without an anesthetic.[295]

With these films and others including "Why Worry?" with Harold Lloyd (1923), "Pardon Us" with Laurel and Hardy (1931), "The Awful Tooth" featuring Our Gang (1937), "A Southern Yankee" with Red Skelton (1948), originally "The General" with Buster Keaton (1926), "The Noose Hangs High" with Abbott and Costello (1948), "Don't Raise the Bridge" with Jerry Lewis (1968), "Cactus Flower" featuring Goldie Hawn and Walter Matthau (1969), "Little Shop of Horrors," which introduced Jack Nicholson in its first version filmed in 1961, "The In-laws" with Alan Arkin (1979), "10" with Bo Derek and Dudley Moore (1979), "Reuben, Reuben" (1983) with Tom Conte, who was nominated for an Academy Award, and "Compromising Positions" (1985), the patient may assuage his fears and turn them into laughter before or after visiting the American dentist.[296] By making the dentist, who is considered the "enemy," a clown, the patient uses the film as a vehicle for turning his anxiety into laughter. The dentist, who can bear to watch these films at all, must learn to accept them as an occupational hazard that reduces his feeling of self-worth.

Although dentists were more commonly represented in comedies and made the brunt of derision, physicians have more often been portrayed in stag films. There are at least four times as many stag films (17) in which the physician appears as those in which the dentist is depicted. The physician, who has been the pre-eminent subject of public trust and reverence also becomes the object of erotic tension when this trust is broken. To intrude upon a patient's sexual persona while he/she is vulnerable as a patient produces the epitome of erotic pleasure, especially when viewed by others.[297]

In the film "Greed" one scene captures the complexity of the sexual aspect of the dentist-patient relationship. The dentist, McTeague, gazes at the helpless and innocent-looking patient, Trina, who is asleep under an anesthetic. He satisfies his desire for her by kissing her tenderly before inflicting pain on her in caring for her teeth.[298] This episode could have ended more violently. There have been instances in which women have accused their dentists and physicians of overstepping their professional duties while treating them.

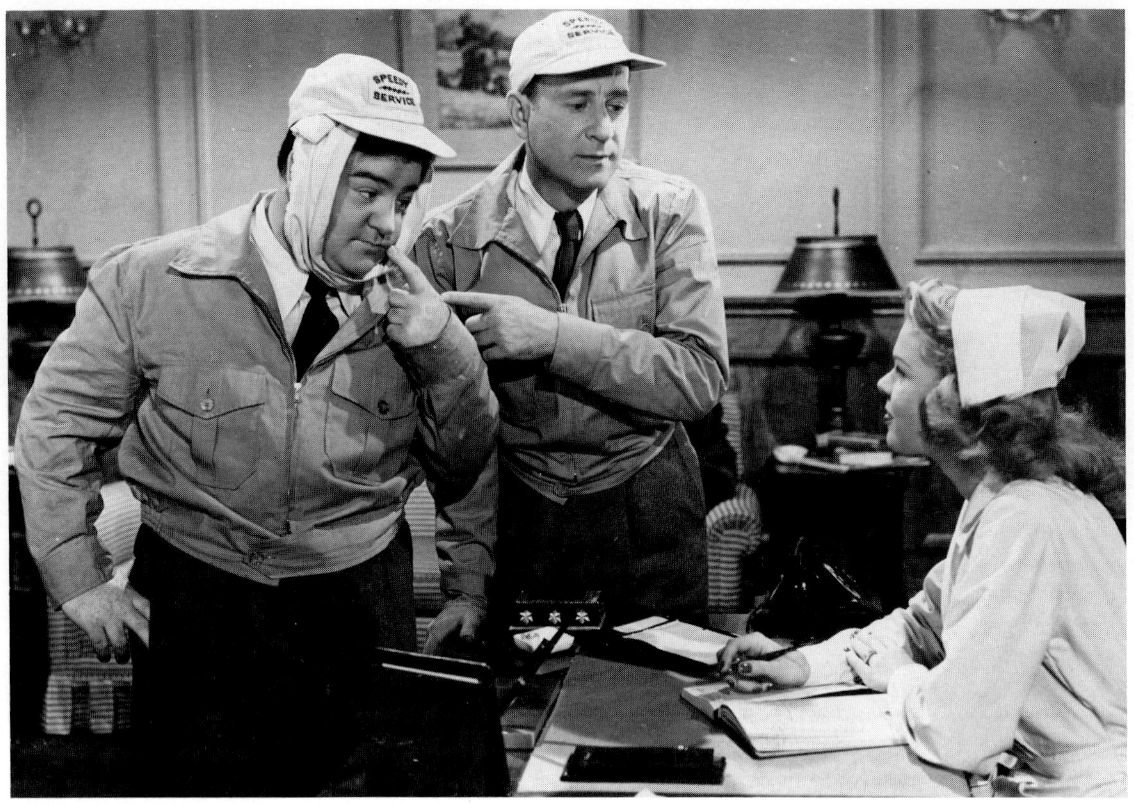

"The Noose Hangs High," with Bud Abbott and Lou Costello, produced by Eagle Lion Films in 1948, shows Costello approaching the dental nurse-receptionist with a toothache. This film was made when Abbott and Costello were at the height of their popularity.

"The Great Impostor," starring Tony Curtis, was produced in 1961 by Universal-International. The film told the story of Ferdinand Waldo Demara who impersonated a marine, Trappist monk, Harvard research fellow, prison warden and school teacher. In this photograph Curtis shows him as a naval doctor about to extract the tooth of co-star, Edmund O'Brien.

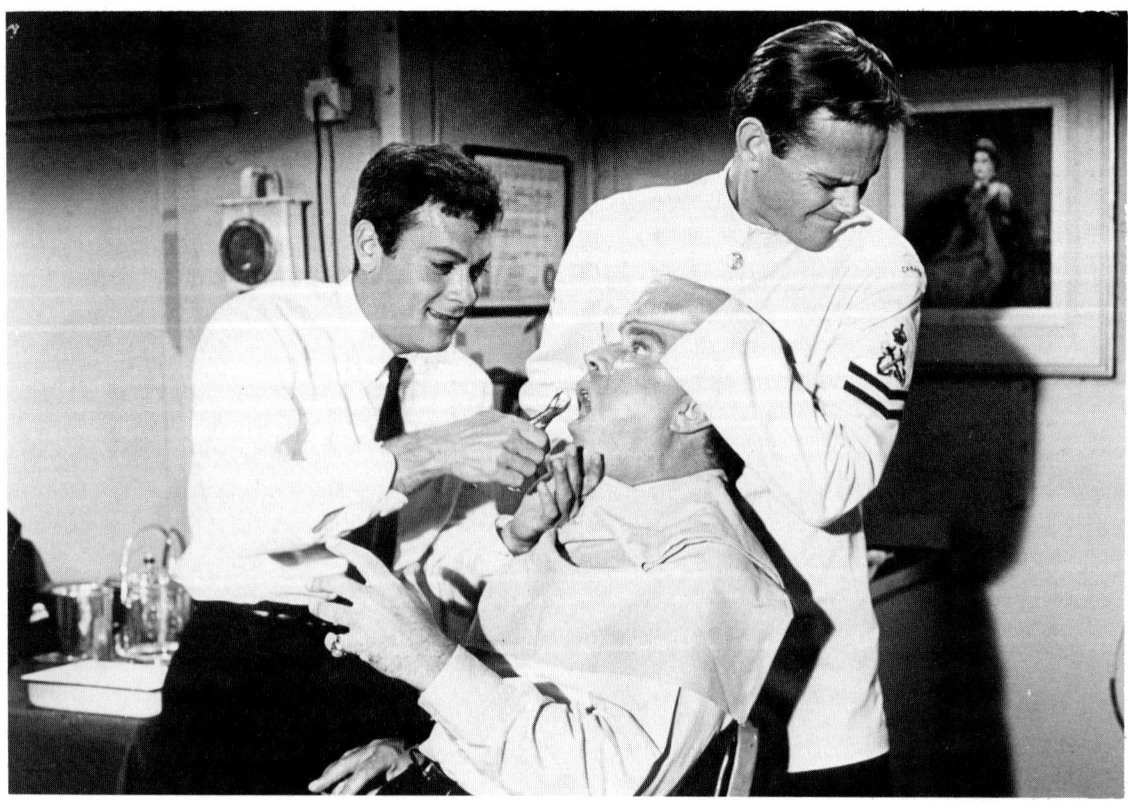

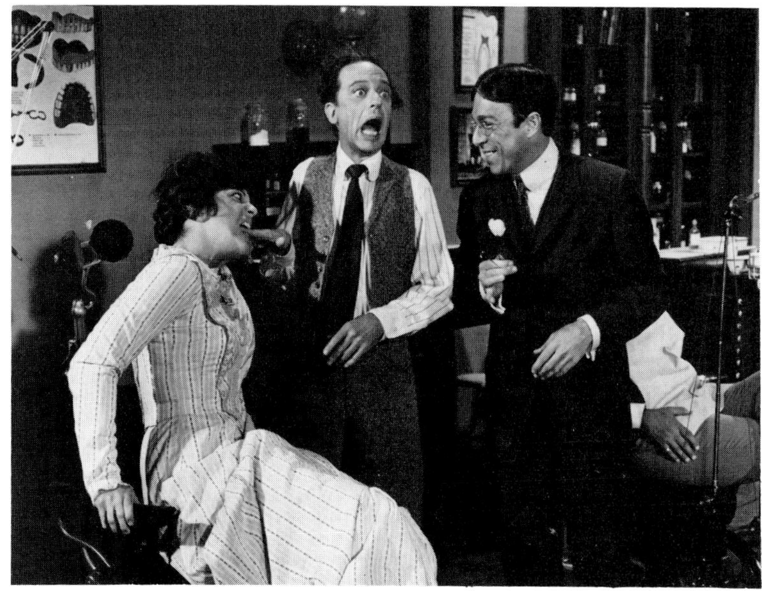

"The Shakiest Gun in the West," made by Universal in technicolor in 1967, is a less sophisticated remake of "Paleface." Here Don Knotts, as a dental student in the school clinic, gets his patient, Barbara Luddy, to open her mouth but then she quickly closes her mouth and bites his finger.

"Don't Raise the Bridge, Lower the River," produced by Columbia Pictures in 1968, starred Jerry Lewis. The office equipment is standard for the period for stand-up dentistry. The contour chair could be lowered for use by the dentist sitting down next to the patient. In this scene the dental assistant is particularly cozy with the patient.

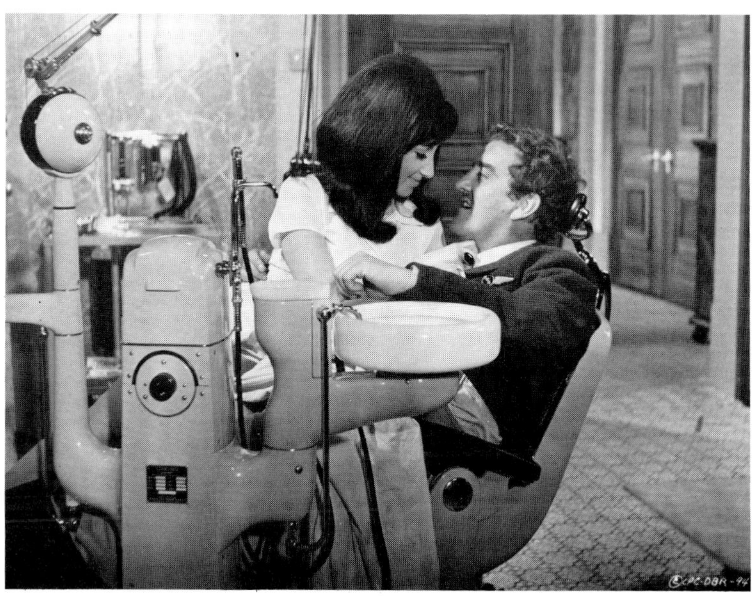

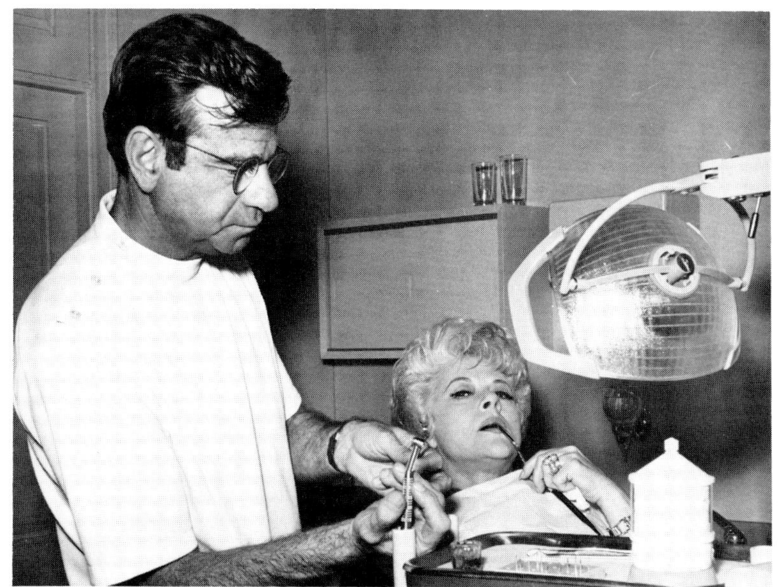

"Cactus Flower," produced by Columbia Pictures in 1969, starred Walter Matthau as the dentist and Ingrid Bergman as his assistant. Matthau is preparing his high-speed drill for use on his patient.

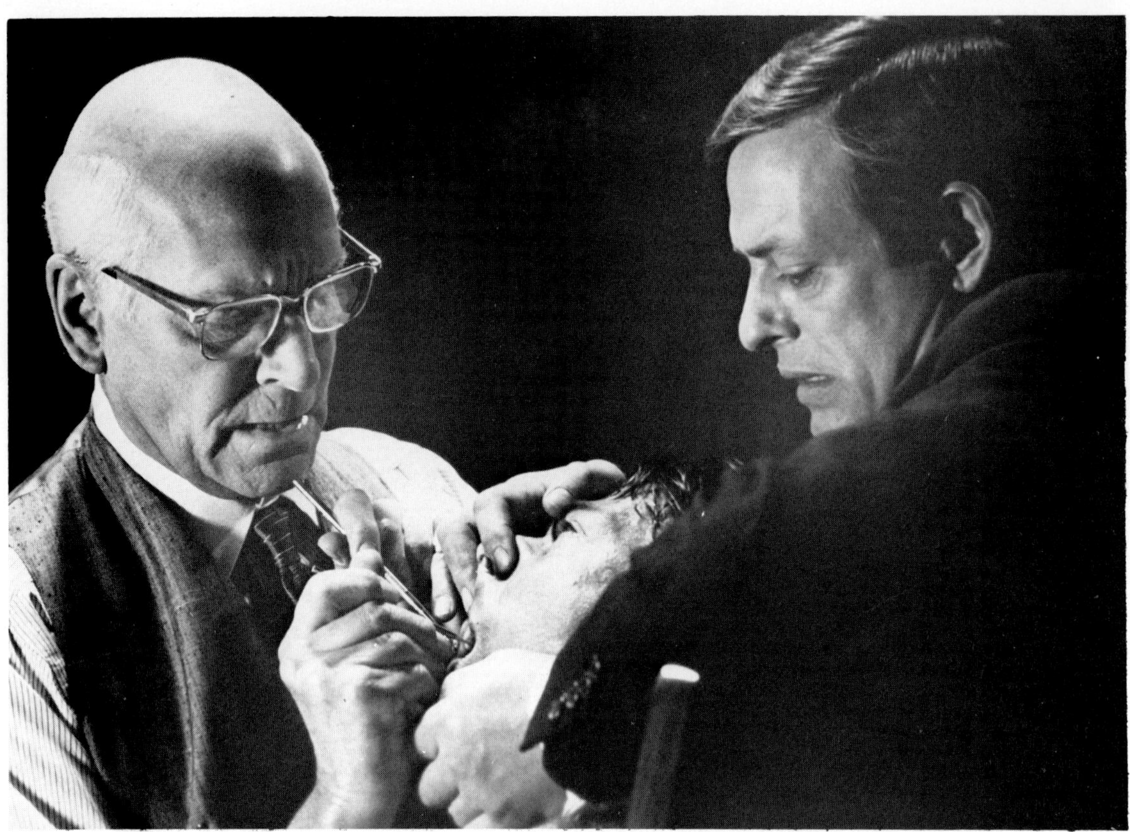

"Marathon Man," produced in 1976 by Paramount Pictures, is a complex mystery story. It contains the ultimate example of dental torture. Lawrence Olivier, a cold-blooded Nazi dentist is about to remove the nerve of a tooth without an anesthetic from his victim, Dustin Hoffman.

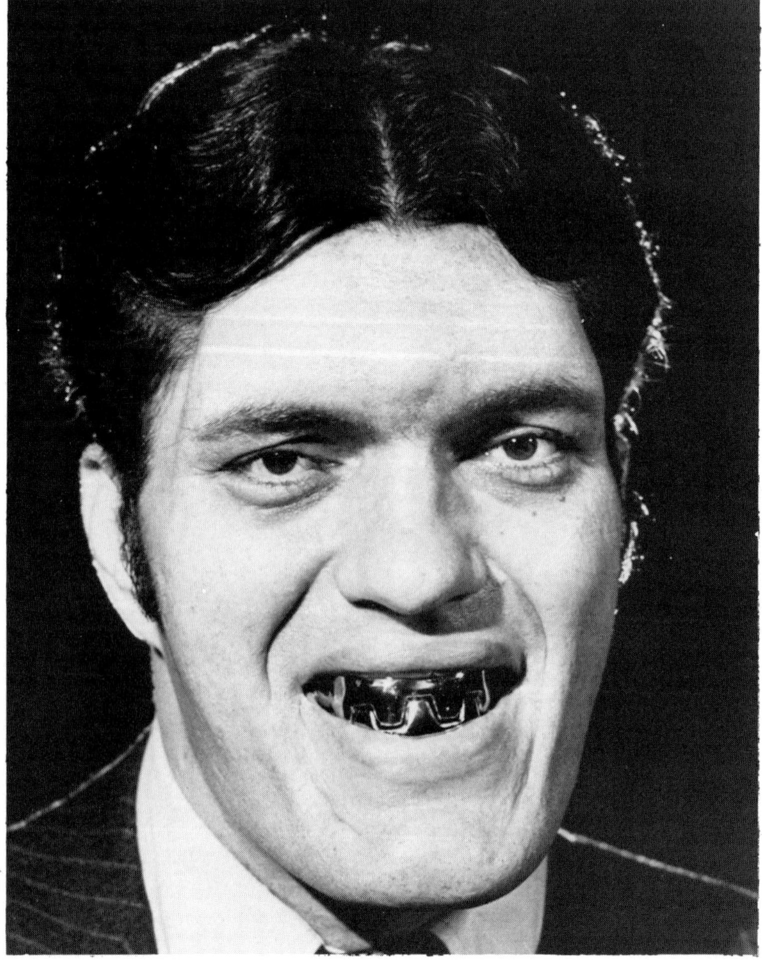

"The Spy Who Loved Me," produced by United Artists in 1977, shows Richard Kiel as a murderous giant with a mouthful of steel teeth. The possibilities for using dentistry to make characters more realistic continues as new materials and techniques are developed.

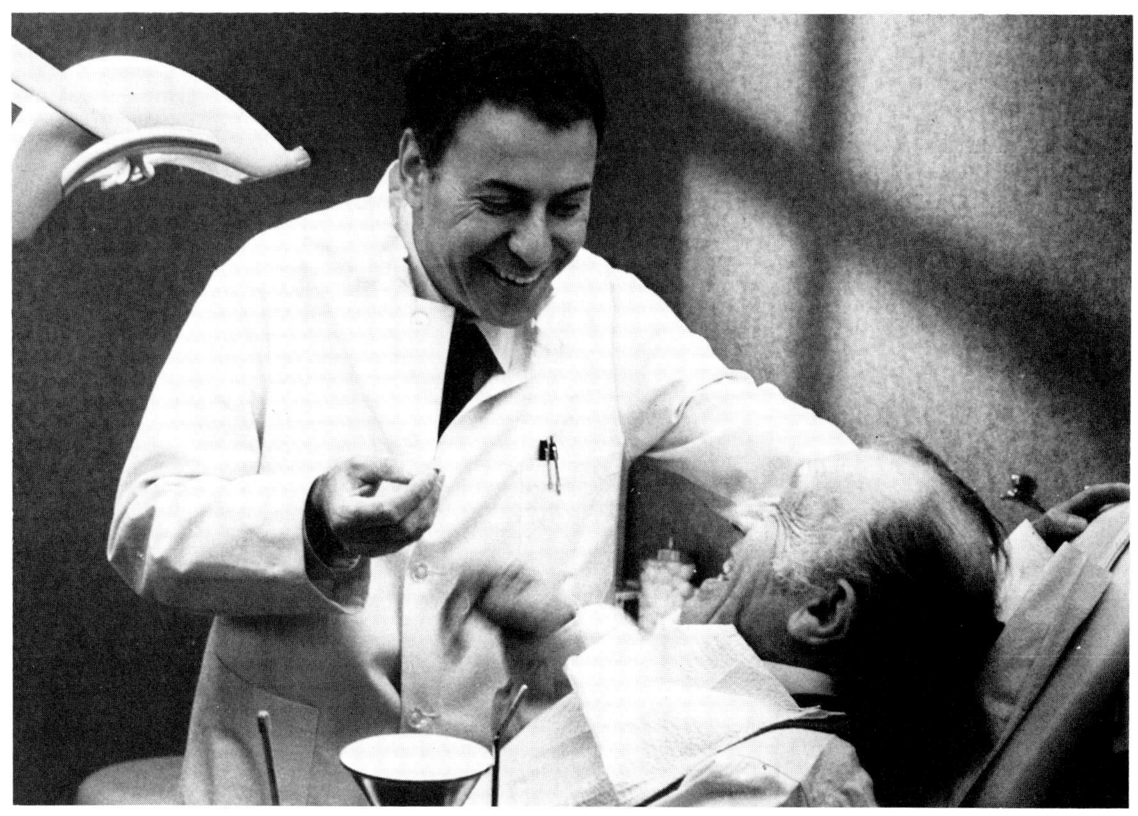

Allan Arkin, in "The In-Laws," as a dentist.

"Compromising Positions," produced by Paramount Pictures in 1985, shows another dental specialist played by Joe Mantegna, who makes advances to his patient Susan Sarandon, shortly before he is murdered. The theme of lechery in dentistry continues up to the present, having also appeared in the 1914 film "Laughing Gas" and in 1919 in the "Dippy Dentist" to name a few.

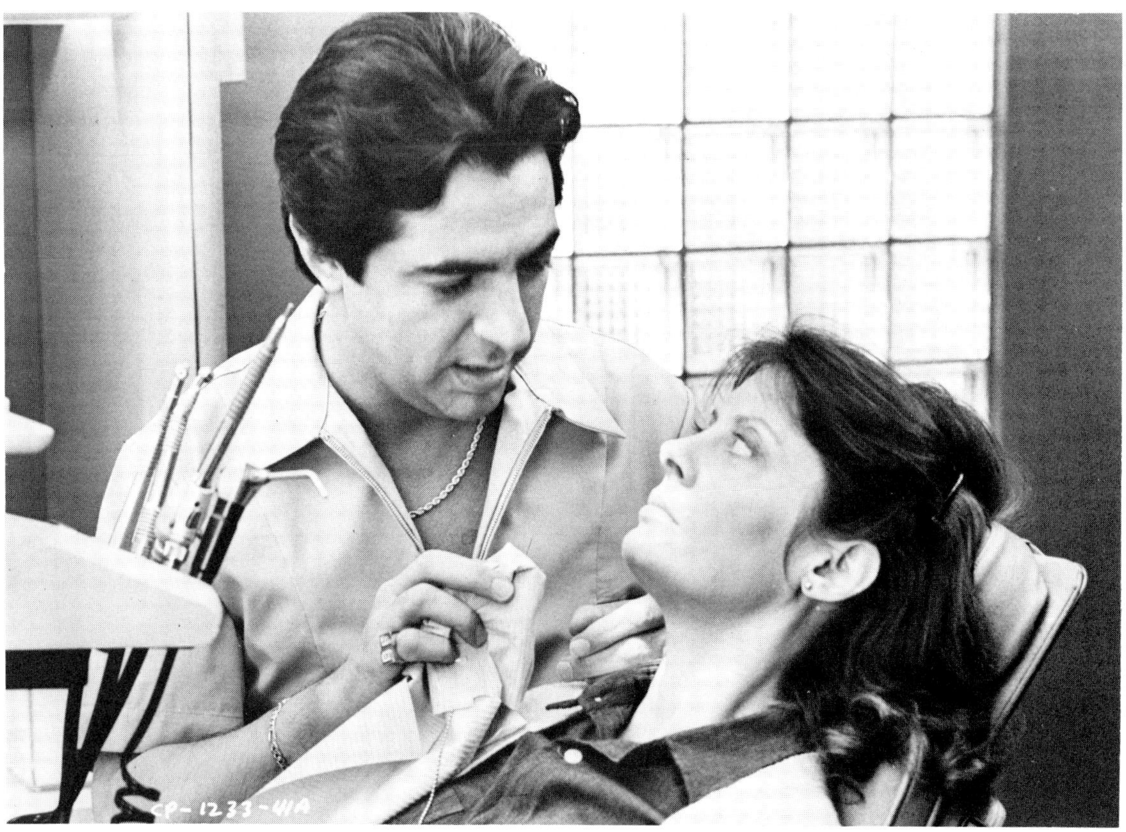

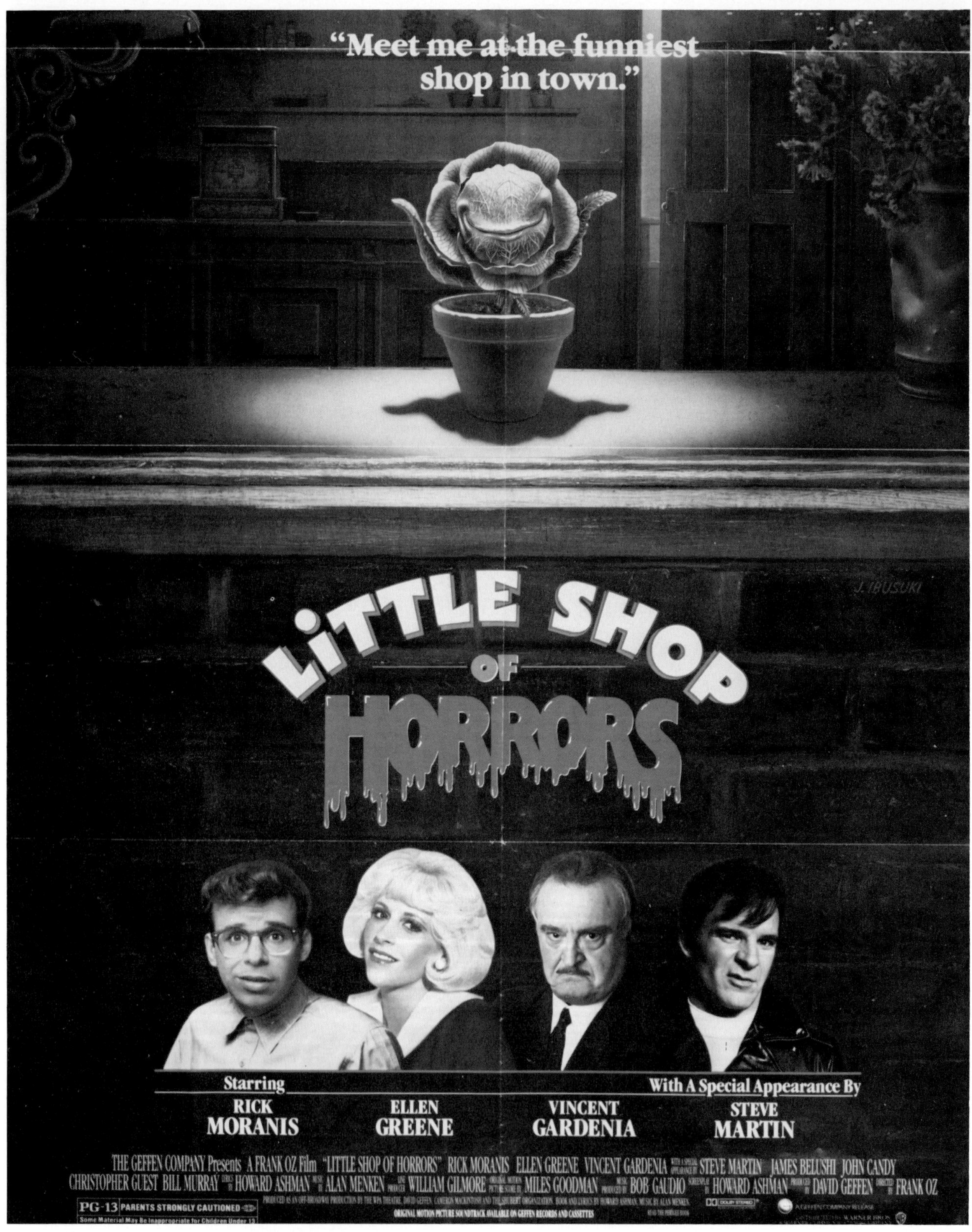

"Little Shop of Horrors," re-filmed in 1986, was first produced in 1961 with Jack Nicholson playing the patient in his first motion picture. In this film the dentist is portrayed as a sadistic person, who is murdered by a patient and his body is fed to a blood-eating plant. This song about the dentist sums up the sadism: "When I was young, my mom noticed funny things I did. Like shooting puppies with a B-B gun. He poisoned guppies and bashed in the head of a pussy cat. His mother said you'll be a dentist. Your temperament is wrong for the priesthood. He's like the Marquis de Sade. I'm your dentist I get high on the pain I inflict, I thrill when I drill a bicuspid, although it may cause my patients distress. Here he is folks Leader of the plaque, 'Wait I'm not numb,' 'That's ok,' 'that hurts', 'oh shut up and open wide,' You have a talent for causing great pain. Somewhere up there I know my mother's proud of me, I'm a dentist and a success, Say ah, say ah, say aah, say aaah..."

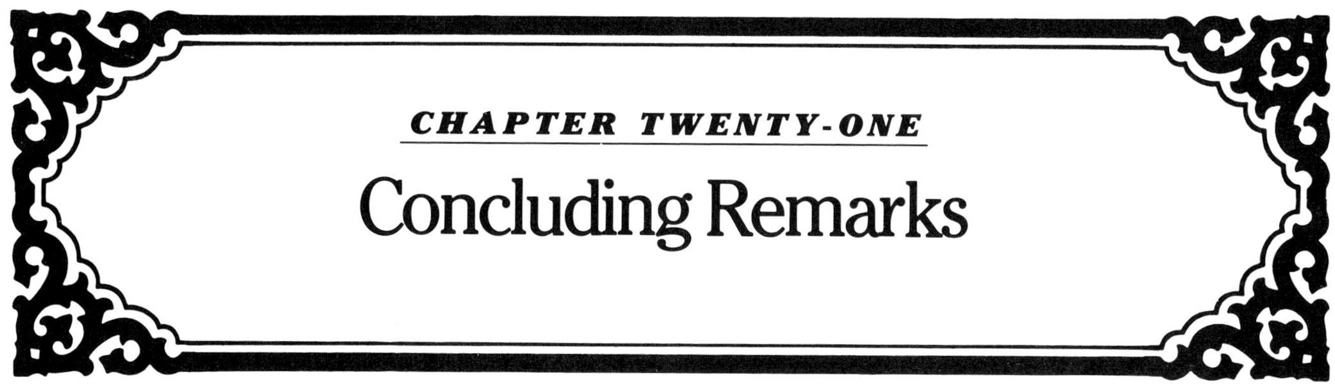

CHAPTER TWENTY-ONE

Concluding Remarks

The American dentist's operating theater developed from a small, simply furnished room with multiple uses centered around the dental chair, into a complex of several operating and specialized rooms between the early 19th century and the present. In the early part of the last century the patient sat in a low rocking chair, and the dentist, without a dental mouth mirror, in a poorly gaslit room stooped over his patient to get a view of a cavity in the upper jaw. Later, to drill a patient's tooth, the dentist balanced himself on one foot in order to pedal his foot engine with the other foot. Without plumbing until the end of the 19th century, he had to empty and clean his spittoon after each patient. In dramatic contrast is the modern dentist who works on his patient sitting down in a well-lit and air-conditioned office with vastly refined instruments including a high-speed drill and a quiet and effective evacuation system.

As the technology required to preserve, repair and replace teeth evolved into a big business, the dentist changed his skills to master the equipment sold to him and broadened his approach to include prevention and treatment of a greater range of dental diseases. The dentist's widening horizons were reflected in the location of his office and the furnishings he chose to install. Decor and equipment were selected to please the patient, especially the female patient, who was revolted by a homely, unkempt office containing disquieting exhibits such as skulls, artificial teeth, strange and mysterious dental instruments, etc. In his effort to calm the patient, the dentist modified the appearance of his operating room, cleaned his equipment after each use, and employed assistants to cope with the increasing demands of his patients, as well as to reduce the time that he spent working on a patient.

A major reason, attributed by successful dentists, for the transformation in dental offices at the turn of the century, was the desire to attract and please female patients. Female patients and assistants were the driving force in encouraging the American dentist to change his office from a factory for the extraction and reconstruction of teeth into a unique space with amenities to comfort the patient and provide convenience for the dentist. Cleanliness was the first order of business. One editorialist equated the "Dentists on Pleasant Street with someone who could be as sweet and clean in body and mind as a woman."[299]

The simple, specific tasks necessary in keeping a dental office clean appeared less significant to many dentists who were absorbed in the mechanics of saving teeth and curing dental diseases. However, a few American dentists could step aside from their daily practices long enough to observe the impact on the patient of their methods, habits, attitudes and physical arrangements. Others lectured and published on the importance of the overall appearance and cleanliness of the dental office. Rodrigues Ottolengui, a new editor in 1896, introduced a series of illustrated articles to describe the variety of dental offices in the U.S. and foreign cities in the journal, *Dental Items of Interest*. This series reveals the common and controversial issues of the period and provided benchmarks for each dentist to measure his own practice against.

Not all dentists had become convinced of the need for cleanliness. J.M. Weems of Sherman, Texas reported in 1910 that one dentist who practiced in a soiled office explained to him: "I know my office is not as clean as it should be, but leaving these soiled napkins, strips and pellets around makes the new patients believe that I have been very busy."[300] Weems advised all dentists to employ an assistant to make sure that each day the office was dusted, instruments were sterilized and all linen changed. In many offices a carbolic-creosote-oil-of-cloves-dirty-spittoon smell permeated the operatory, which was ignored by the dentist, who by constant exposure, became insensitive to this disagreeable olfactory assault.[301]

Waiting rooms were decorated to "court forgetfulness" of the dental procedure or to provide scenic views that would instill calmness and a sense of grandeur. The elaborately furnished offices of M.L. Rhein of New York, Frank Faber of Constantinople, Turkey, the dental boat of F.H. Houghton piloted along the Florida coast, and C.E. Kells' office facing the Mississippi River and Lake Pontchartrain are examples of dentists, who offered an unusual setting to please their patients and relieve the stress of going to the dentist. Patients, when suffering from the pain of dental disease, preferred dentists who pacified them and provided a calm, efficient service.

Dental offices changed not only because of technological advancements in dental equipment and patient expectations, but also as a result of new concepts in dental treatment. Such was the case of the arrival of the "Age of Sterility" in the early 1900s. Oriental rugs gave way to linoleum or tile floors, occasionally designed to look like a rug, for those dentists who wanted to preserve the appearance of a residential dwelling considered more inviting to patients. Sterilization was translated into changes in equipment such as chairs made only of metal and with rounded corners so they could be readily cleaned. Patients accepted their responsibility to seek professional dental care when the enormous consequences of neglect were brought home to everyone under the focal infection theory. Promulgated after WWI as a major cause of difficult to cure diseases, the focal infection idea provided a new group of patients for the newly sanitized dental office. The dentist obtained a new and vigorous sense of his services which had important consequences not only for the teeth but for the overall health of the body. Primarily middle- and upper-class Americans could afford the more extensive dental treatment recommended.

The surgical operating room in the hospital provided another incentive for the dentist to make the office look spick-and-span. O.W. Randall of Port Huron, Michigan argued in 1902 for the installation in the dental office of porcelain floor tiles of the type that were used in hospital operating rooms, because they could be easily sterilized. To mitigate the tiring effect of the tiles on the leg muscles and feet, Randall recommended that a wool or rubber rug be placed on the floor or rubber-soled shoes be worn by the dentist.[302] By 1920 sterility was a major concern. Metal cabinets had replaced wooden ones. Everything, including chairs and cabinets, had to be white in color to underscore the impression of cleanliness in the operatory. By the 1930s, dental offices looked immaculate, but the white, sterile look was too harsh for the patient and too tiring on the eyes of the dentist. Therefore, white-painted equipment and furniture was replaced with easily sterilized and cleaned equipment and cabinetry manufactured in pastel and dark colors. Appearance continues to be a major objective in successful offices which help patients to feel comfortable. Whether the professional office be that of the dentist, physician, lawyer, etc., soft colors, good lighting, music and other amenities contribute to the visitor's sense of welcome and security.[303]

Duties within the dental office illustrate and mirror the male-female dichotomy in the work place expected of each gender throughout this period. The male dentist (we found only a few descriptions of female-run dental offices and none of them employed assistants) worked with his instruments in the operating room and laboratory, creating disarray, soiling clothes and leaving debris, which the female assistant cleaned up, goaded by the complaints and criticisms of patients. Dentists were repeatedly reminded of their responsibilities to maintain a clean office in addition to sterilization of their instruments and other apparatus used on the patient.

Alfred Fones, who emphasized preventive dentistry, and C.N. Johnson, recognized the importance for the dentist of working with educated nurse assistants or dental hygienists. Fones opened a school for dental hygienists in 1913, in his own office building devoted entirely to dentistry and closed it in 1916, when several dental schools began to teach dental hygiene courses. The inauguration of the female dental hygienist came about to keep women subservient to the male dentist and to restrict her role to that of performing only those procedures which could be reversed, as well as assisting the busy dentist.

Once accepted by the community as a well-trained, effective professional, the dentist attracted patients and kept their good will as long as he/she operated an organized, clean and economical office. His assistant had a major role to play in running the office by "standing between [the dentist] and many of the petty annoyances which would otherwise fall to his lot." She was expected to take care of patient and billing records, send notices to patients, make appointments, calm nervous patients, clean the office, and assist with dental procedures. To complete her "girl Friday" duties she was also expected to accept the blame when the dentist was at fault, to remember things he forgot, and to write his letters and memoranda.[304]

The dental hygienist, whose services are increasing, aided the dentist and took over some of the chores associated with cleaning the teeth and teaching the patient to practice dental hygiene at home through daily cleansing rituals. After the first trained dental hygienists graduated in 1914, their role in the dental office increased. They followed the pattern of other professional groups in organizing and developing standards and goals of their own.

Beginning in 1958 the dental assistant served the dentist more directly as she sat on one side of the patient while the dentist sat on the other, to work on the patient reclining in the new, contoured dental chair. "Four-handed" dentistry remains in vogue. In the last few years there has been a renewed impetus to control infection, highlighted by the public fear of contracting AIDS. Procedures, recommended by the Center for Disease Control in Atlanta and the American Dental Association, are designed to assure the patient and consist of wearing uniforms composed of long gowns with long sleeves, rubber gloves and eye protection, and increased precautions of disinfection and sterilization after each patient. Office debris is discarded with precautions for safety.

The sensitive dentist became attuned to the temperament, whims, prejudices, fancies and peculiarities of patients in the management of his practice. General belief was that if he was "a steady, sturdy plodder," he would, "win in the end" and become a successful dentist. However, dentists who lacked acumen into human nature could be fooled by superficial observation of their patients and lose those they would have preferred to serve. For instance, one successful dentist had hoped to treat the governor of his state. One day when an individual appeared for treatment, who seemed unprepossessing, the dentist turned him over to a colleague, only to discover later that the man was the governor.[305]

Mastering the technical side of dentistry provided one path to an effective practice. Insight into personality, patient adaptability, and patient and staff psychology were equally crucial to the dentist's management of the office. Dentists "needed to study people" in addition to books to establish a dental practice.[306] The patient has been rising in the dentist's esteem over the past century from one of the "little things" to understand and treat on an individual basis, to a major determinant of methods of dental treatment. Dentists, as a result are more accepted by patients. In a recent poll of 1,000 adults published in *USA Today*, dentists ranked number one in consumer satisfaction, receiving approval from 68 percent of those asked if they were satisfied with the service they received from their dentist. Only 61 percent of those polled were satisfied with their physicians.[307]

Films, jokes, paintings, photographs and popular discussions throughout the centuries have placed the dentist in humorous, terrifying and other ignominious roles. Some of the most extreme and memorable characterizations grew out of the fears and experiences of patients in the dental office at the time the motion picture industry began in the early 20th century and extends back to the poignant paintings of tooth-drawers in earlier periods. One value of these films lies in their cathartic function for the patient. Since the dentist has often denied the pain ("this won't hurt much") he has had to inflict in order to save teeth, the patient's denial and mocking of the dentist's behavior, was an obvious and natural response. The American patient is relieved of personal trauma by exposure to skits, plays, movies, cartoons, jokes, etc., in which the unpleasant aspects of dentistry have been exaggerated and lampooned. The trip to the dentist is shared, disguised and forgotten in laughter. The commercial films and photographic stills deliver these messages graphically.

Dentistry was incorporated into the military bureaucracy in this century. The Army through its dental corps, legislated into existence in 1901, became the first U.S. military branch to provide regular dental care, followed in 1912 by the Naval Dental Corps. Confronted with logistical problems in their first overseas operation in the Philippines, Army dentists learned the importance of specially designed equipment that could be transported and the hazards of climatic extremes on dental instruments. The first World War presented unusual opportunities for Army and Navy dentists to keep soldiers ready for combat. The greatest challenge for the military dental corps came in World War II when physical standards for inductees were lower than during World War I. One-fourth of all soldiers required dental treatment before they became physically fit to carry out their military assignments. A proportion of the dental care was elaborate, expensive and time-consuming since over three-fourths of a million soldiers required artificial dentures; many to replace missing and broken dentures.

The military draft in the 1940s demonstrated a serious weakness in the American dental care system, in that, young and otherwise healthy men, had not or could not afford, proper care of their teeth. The American Dental Association had recognized that a larger number of dentists than were trained were needed to provide dental care for Americans even before the war. An Oklahoma dentist witnessed the results of lack of dental care and commented on its impact on the dental profession after the war. L.L. Willis wrote in 1943 that his experience for 18 months, on shipboard, taking care of military personnel led him to believe "that something must and will be done after the war to improve the present debilitated oral condition of the average American. Figures don't lie. Of the first 2,000,000 of the country's best, examined for service, about 1,000,000 were rejected because of their oral condition."[308]

While American dental care achieves unusual results today, the education necessary to alert Americans to the personal and professional aspects of dental hygiene falls short of its goal in reaching everyone and preventing loss of teeth. The dentist's image has an impact on how readily patients consult the dentist. Exposure to dentistry in films, the military services, schools, hospitals, etc., offers opportunities for dentists to reinforce their methods, goals and services.

Of great significance, although only touched on briefly in this essay, in improving American dental health, are public health programs such as fluoridated water and an improved diet, which prevents or reduces cavities in children's teeth. Screening programs for school-age children provide an additional incentive to improve dental hygiene. Many of these nationwide programs were supported and grew out of research conducted by the National Institute of Dental Research which celebrated its 40th anniversary in 1988.[309]

Series of three photos showing how the history of dentistry was displayed at the Smithsonian Institution until 1964. A pegboard was placed along the rear of a glass case with brackets suspended from it to hold shelves and instruments.

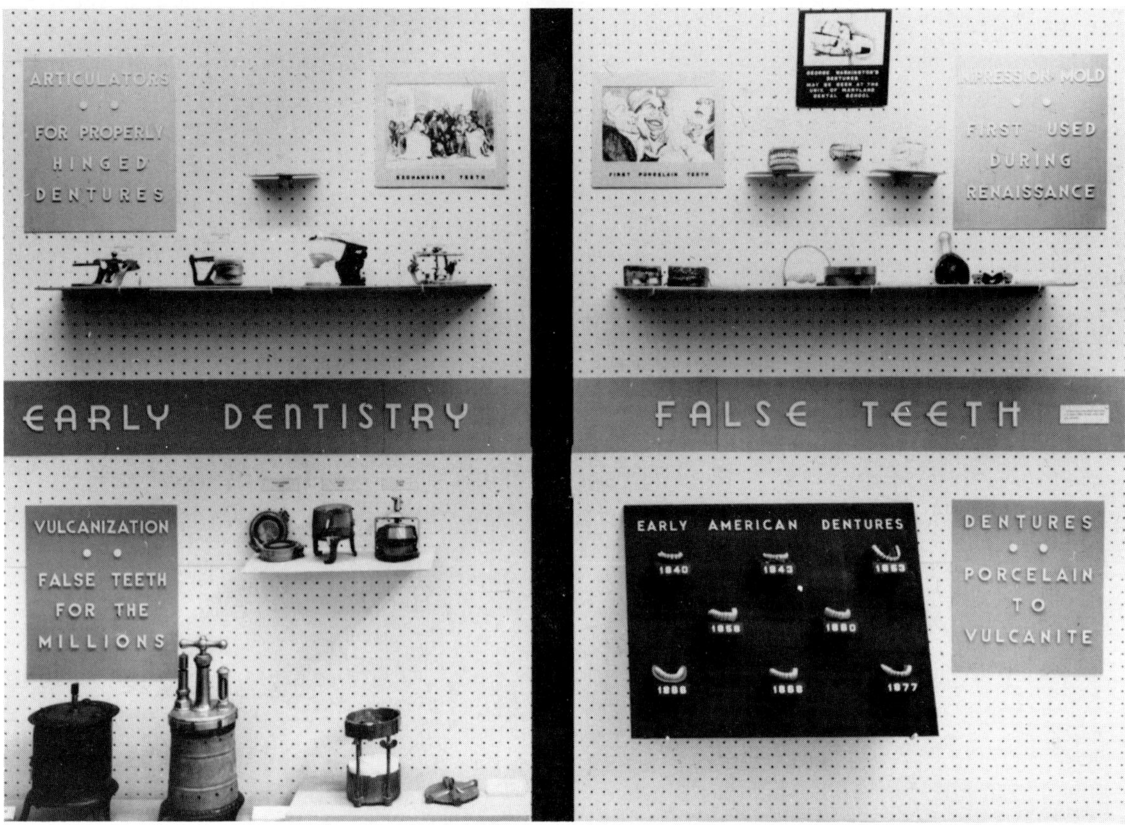

Panel divided into four sections. Upper left quadrant: extraction implements; upper right quadrant: hand-propelled drills; lower left: instruments used in filling teeth with gold; lower right: pluggers for packing fillings into the teeth.

Panel divided into four sections. Upper left quadrant: dental articulators used in making artificial teeth; upper right quadrant: molds for making artificial teeth; lower left: vulcanizers for making artificial teeth out of hardened rubber; lower right: varieties of artificial teeth.

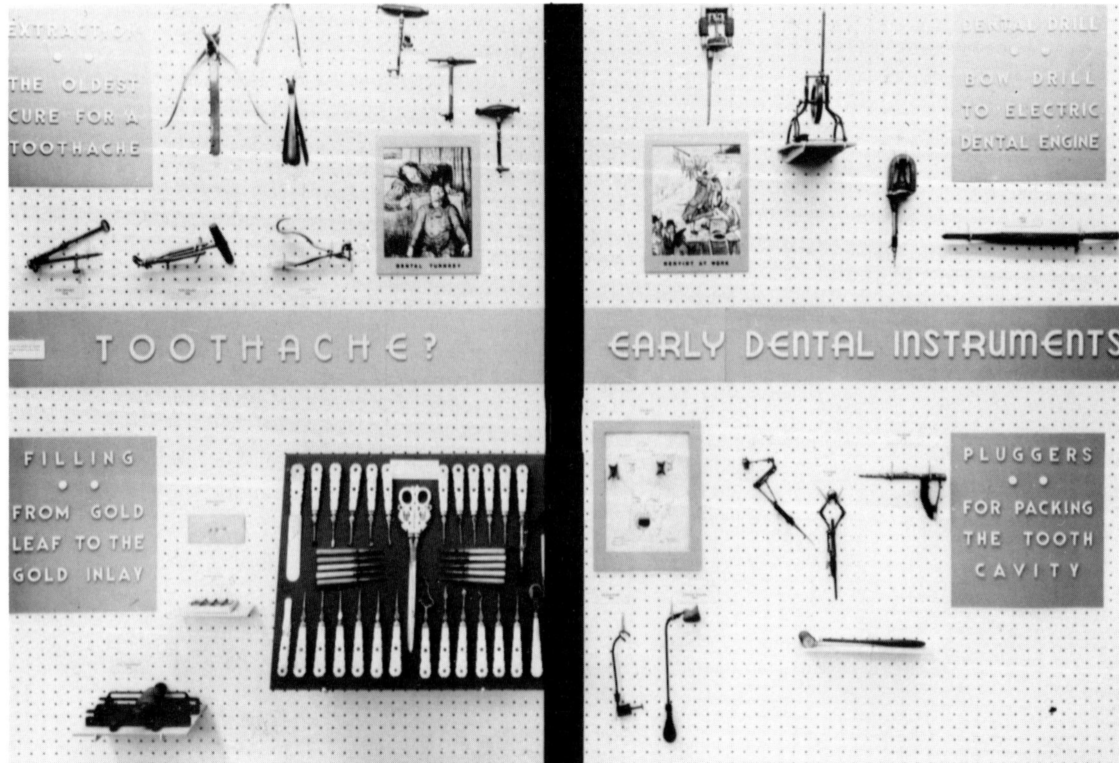

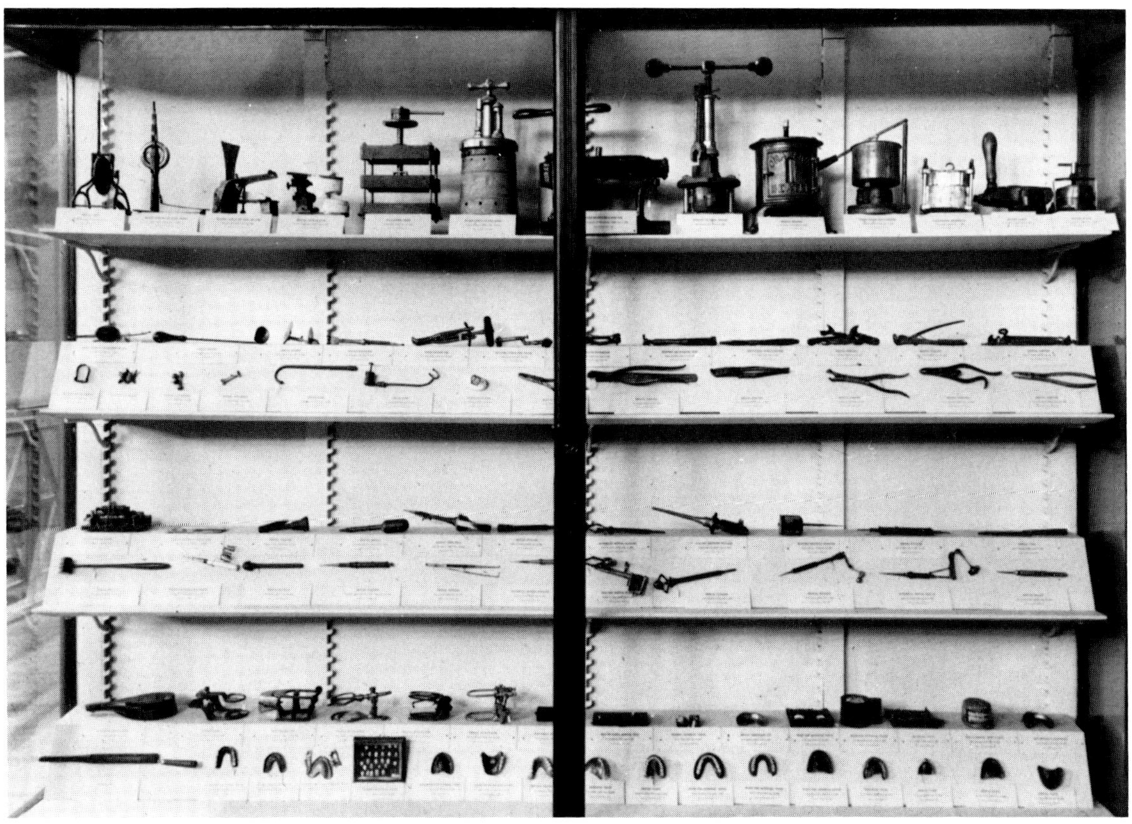

Original patent models, part of the almost 400 patent models of dental items in the National Museum of American History, Smithsonian Institution collection. On the top shelf are vulcanizers, the next shelf contains forceps, on the third shelf are displayed pluggers which were designed to force gold into teeth and on the bottom shelf are arranged articulators and examples of artificial teeth made from different materials.

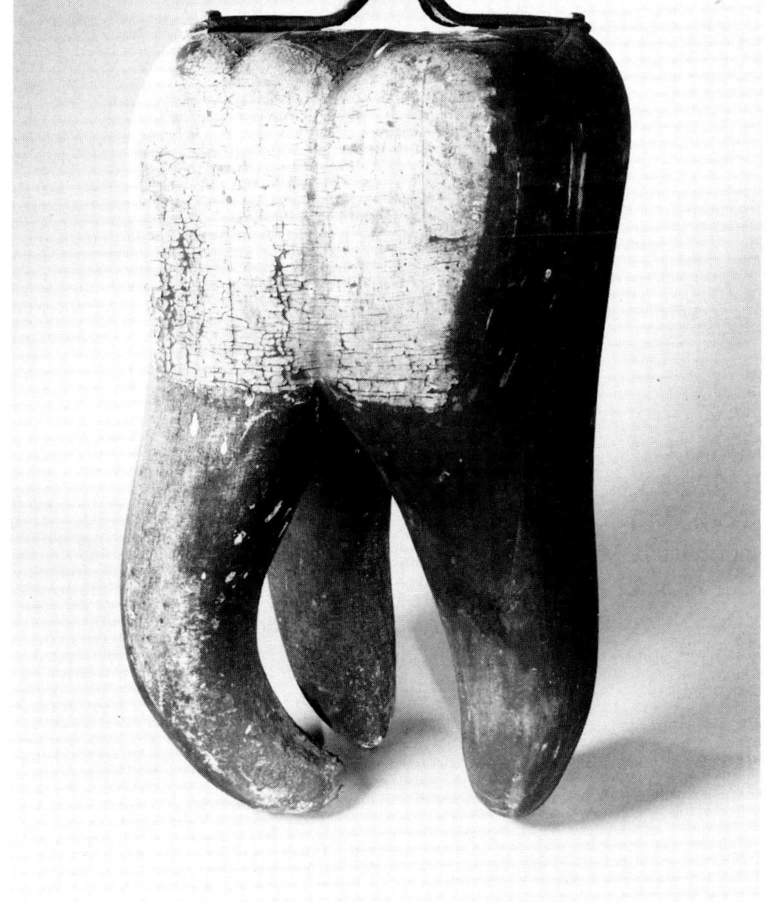

Wood model of tooth used as sign for dental office in the 19th century. It is currently on display outside G.V. Black's office in the National Museum of American History. Neg. No. 79,10203.

DENTAL OFFICE
EQUIPMENT OF
DR. G. V. BLACK,
PIONEER
DENTIST
INVENTED
DENTAL
NORTHWESTERN

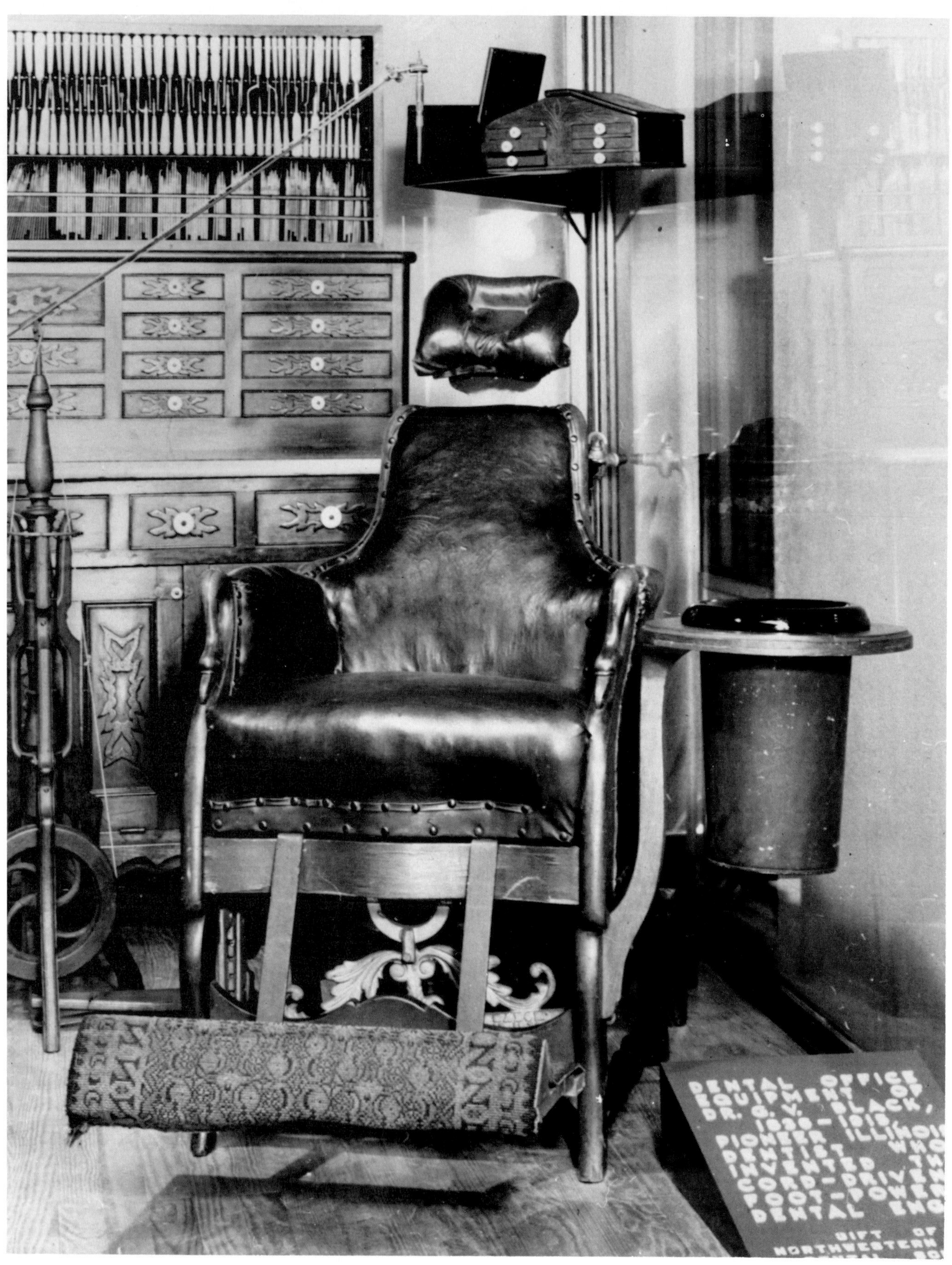

Archer's Chair (introduced in the 1860s) and foot-pedal drill, designed by Black in 1871, as they appeared on display at the Smithsonian Institution from 1955 until 1964. The items were donated by the Northwestern University Dental School. Note the array of ivory-handled implements arranged in a cabinet along the back wall.

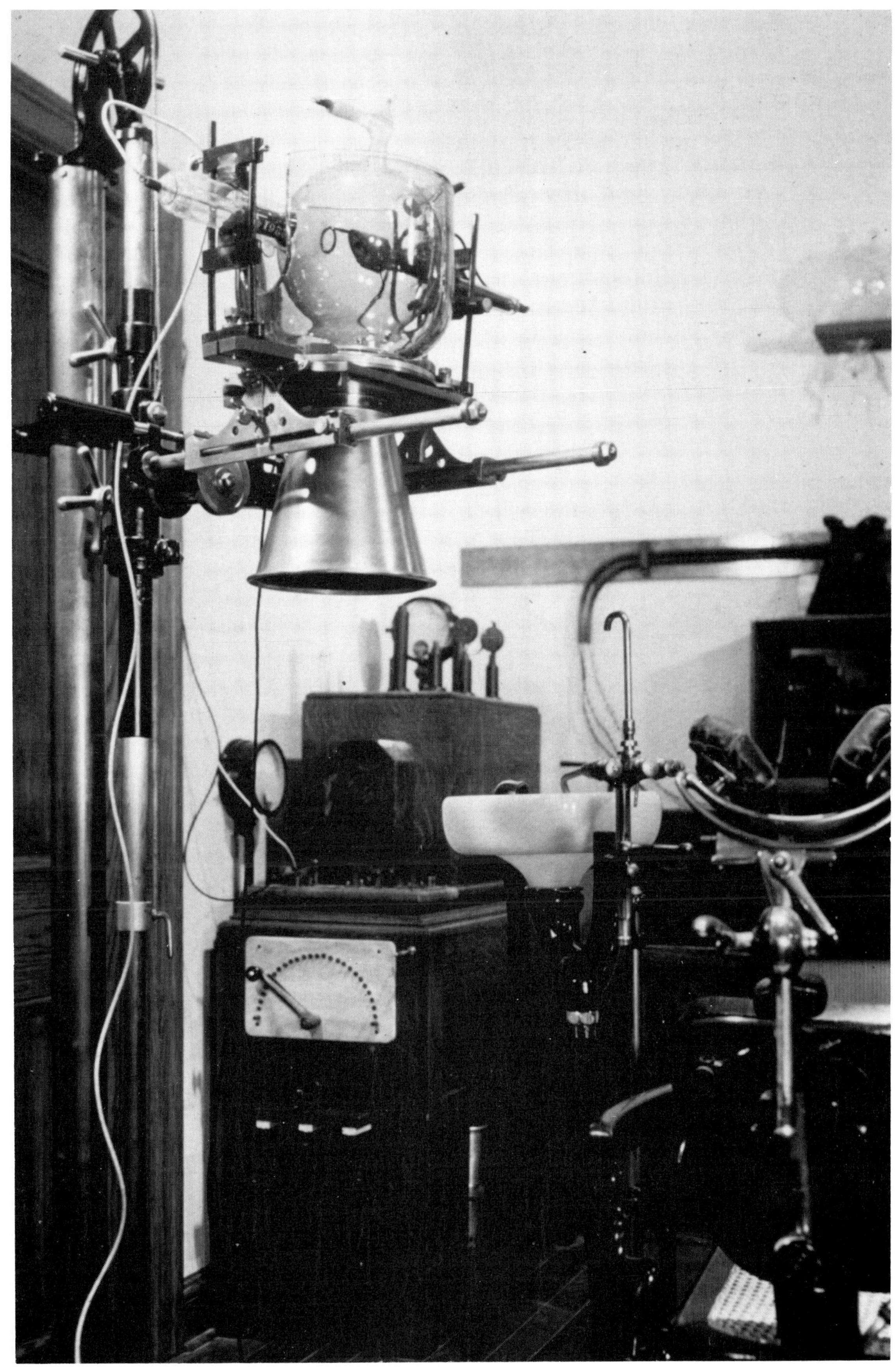

C. Edmond Kells' office with early x-ray device in its present location on exhibit in The National Museum of American History, Smithsonian Institution.

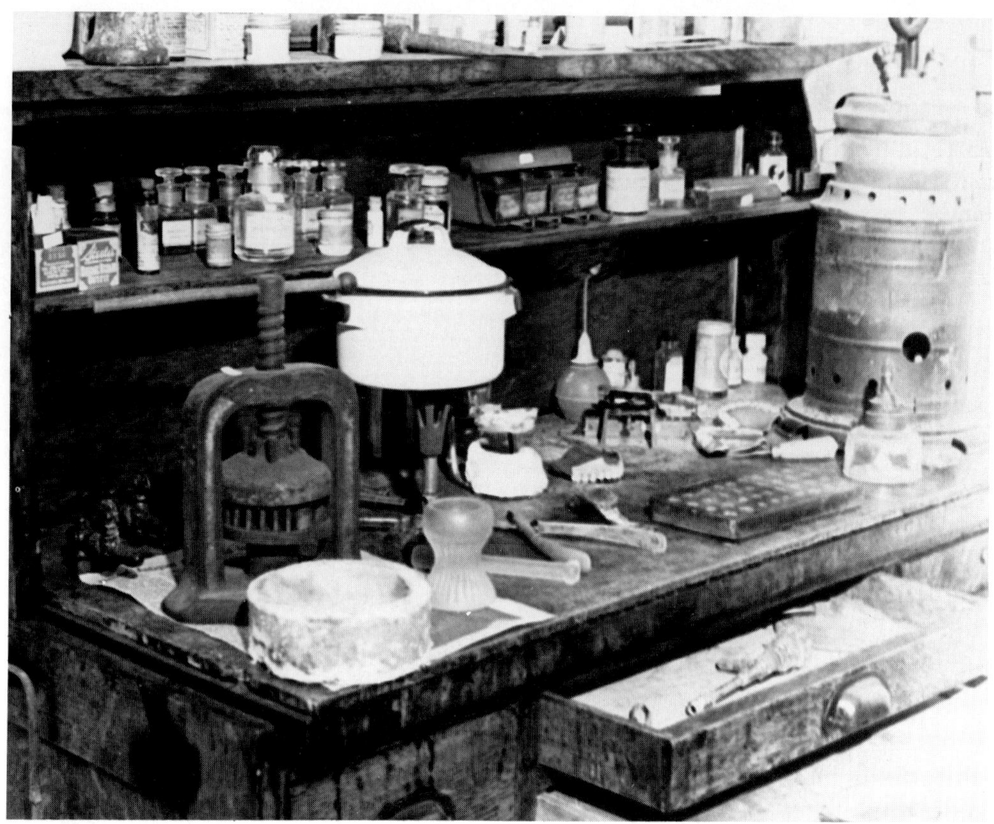

A dentist's workbench circa 1900 on display at the Orange County Dental Society Museum, Orange, California in 1980s. The vulcanizer stands on the extreme right and the flask on the left. Various solutions and chemicals used in making teeth are displayed on the top two shelves.

Display at the Kansas State Historical Society Museum mounted with a $350 grant from the Kansas State Dental Association, circa 1960.

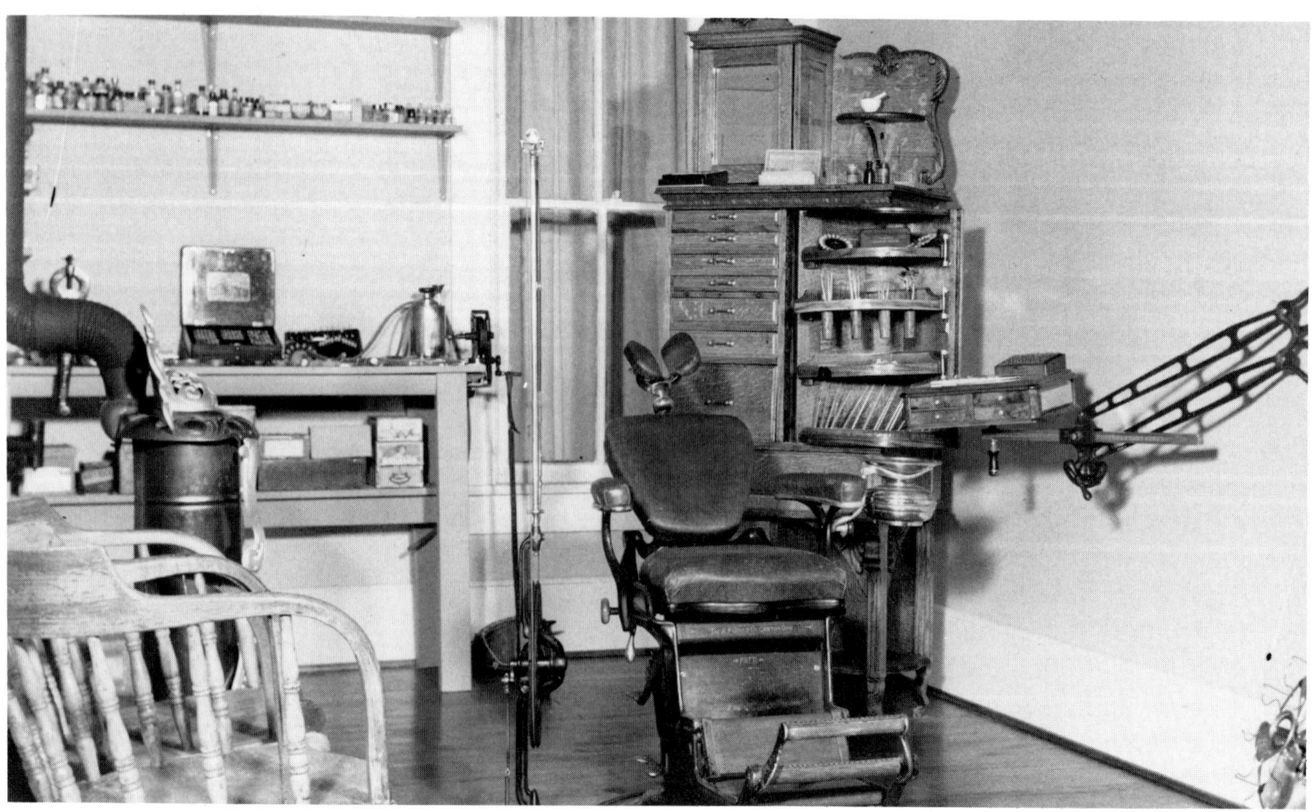

Notes

Introduction

1. Milton S. Asbell, *A Century of Dentistry: A History of the School of Dental Medicine, University of Pennsylvania.* (Philadelphia: Univ. of Pennsylvania Press), 1977, pgs. 2, 117.

2. Richard Rudisill, *Mirror Image: The Influence of the Daguerreotype on American Society.* (Albuquerque: Univ. of New Mexico Press), 1971, pg. 52.

3. Stanley B. Burns, *Early Medical Photography in America (1839-1883).* (New York: The Burns Archive), 1983, pg. 1259.

4. Examination of published photography texts and sales catalogs reveals no European occupational images of dentists. European archives also are devoid of dental occupational images.

5. C.W. Ceram, *Archeology of the Cinema.* (New York: Harcourt, Brace and World, Inc.), 1965, pgs. 78-9.

6. Margaret Supplee Smith, "The Agnew Clinic: 'Not Cheerful for the Ladies to Look At,' " *Prospects*, II, 1987, pgs. 161-183.

7. Diana Long, "The Medical World of 'The Agnew Clinic:' A World We have Lost?" *Prospects*, II, 1987, pgs. 185-198.

8. Floyd and Marion Rinhardt, *The American Daguerreotype.* (Athens, Georgia: Press), 1981, pg. 416.

9. Ibid., pg. 40. Robert Taft, *Photography and the American Scene: A Social History 1839-1889.* (New York: Dover Publ., Inc.), 1964, reprint of 1938 ed., pg. 459.

10. William Welling, *Photography in America: The Formative Years 1839-1900.* (New York: Thomas Y. Crowell Co.), pg. 10.

11. Floyd and Marion Rinhardt, "Wollcott and Johnson: their Camera and their Photography," *History of Photography*, April 1977, pg. 129.

12. Welling, *op. cit.*, pg. 9.

13. Rudisill, *op. cit.*, pgs. 69-70.

14. Welling, *op. cit.*, pg. 17.

15. Ibid., pg. 16.

16. Rinhardts, *The American Daguerreotype*, pg. 412.

17. Ibid., pgs. 400-1.

18. Welling, *op. cit.*, pg. 276.

19. Personal communication with Irish photohistorian and researcher Roberta McGrath.

20. Rudisill, *op. cit.*, pg. 83.

21. Joel-Peter Witkin, ed., and Stanley B. Burns, *Masterpieces of Medical Photography: Selections from the Burns Archive.* (Pasadena, California, Twelve Trees Press), 1987, photos #33, 40.

22. R. Rudisill, *op. cit.*, pg. 155.

23. Burns, *Early Medical Photography*, pg. 1938.

24. W. Ayer, "Account of an eye-witness," in *The Semi-Centennial of Anesthesia.* (Boston: Massachusetts General Hospital), 1897.

25. Ibid.

26. Burns, *op. cit.*, pg. 1260.

27. Ibid., pg. 1938.

28. Asbell, *op. cit.*, pg. 48.

29. Alison Gernshein, "Medical Photography in the Nineteenth Century," *Medical and Biological Illustration, 2*, 1961, pgs. 85-86.

30. pg 286.

31. Asbell, *op. cit.*, pg. 48.

32. James Robinson, "An Address to the Society of the Alumni of the Baltimore College of Dental Surgery," *American Journal of Dental Surgery*, July 1850, Vol. 10, pgs. 225-256.

33. C. Edmund Kells, *The Dentist's Own Book*, (St. Louis: The C.V. Mosby Co.), pgs. 203-205.

34. Burns, *op. cit.*, pg. 1253.

35. Daniel M. Fox and James Terry, "Photography and the Self Image of American Physicians, 1880-1920," *Bulletin of the History of Medicine, 52*, 1978, pgs. 435-457. Fox and Terry show that a culture of medicine distinct from normal life becomes visible in photographs made in the closing decades of the 19th and early 20th centuries. See also Daniel M. Fox and Christopher Lawrence, *Photographing Medicine: Images and Power in Britain and America since 1840*, (Westport, Connecticut, Greenwood Press), 1988.

36. Estimate from books and pioneer collectors.

37. Christraud Geary, lecture, "Reality Recorded? German Photographs in Bamum (Cameroon)," June 28, 1988, The National Museum of African Art.

38. Eric Margolis, "Mining Photographs: Unearthing the Meanings of Historical Photographs," *Radical History Review, 40*, 1988, pg. 47.

39. Fox and Lawrence, *op. cit.*

Chapters 1-21

1. Robert M. Warner, *Profile of a Profession: A History of the Michigan State Dental Association.* (Detroit: Wayne State Univ. Press, 1964), pg. 1.

2. Pierre Fauchard, *The Surgeon Dentist or a Treatise on the Teeth.* (Birmingham, Alabama: Classics of Dentistry Library, 1980), Introductions by Lilian Lindsay and J. Menzies Campbell.

3. C.H. Cramer, *The Story of Dentistry and the School in University Circle.* (Cleveland: The School of Dentistry Case Western Reserve Univ., 1982), pg. 21

4. Fauchard, *The Surgeon Dentist*, pg. 163.

5. Warner, *Profile of a Profession:*, pg. 1.

6. Curt Proskauer, *Iconographia Odeontologica.* (Hildesheim: Georg Olm, 1967) Curt Proskauer and Franz H. Witt, *A Pictorial History of Dentistry.* (Cologne: M. DuMont Schaubert, 1962).

7. For those unfamiliar with dental history we wish to call attention to the first important history of colonial American dentistry by Bernhard Weinberger. The volume was first published in 1948 and reprinted by the Classics of Dentistry Library in 1981. The book is the most thoroughly documented account of American dentistry culminating with the dental treatment of George Washington. Weinberger preceded this volume with an equally impressive text on the evolution of dentistry from antiquity to the 18th century. Bernhard Weinberger, *An Introduction to the History of Dentistry.* (St. Louis: C.V. Mosby Co., 1948), Vols. I and II, reprint Birmingham, Alabama, 1981.

8. J. Ben Robinson, compiler, "Eighteenth Century Dentistry in America." (Photocopy of newspaper extracts bound in Division of Medical Sciences, NMAH, Smithsonian Institution, 1940, Vol. 1. History Committee of the State Dental Association. For another account of colonial dentistry see Milton B. Asbell, "The Dental Art and its Practitioners in Colonial Philadelphia," *The Bulletin of the Philadelphia County Dental Society*, 46, March 1981, pgs. 6-13.

9. *The History of Dentistry in Missouri*. (Fulton, Missouri: The Ovid Bell Press, 1938), pg. 19.

10. Ibid., pg. 20.

11. Cramer, *The Story of Dentistry*, pg. 49.

12. Warner, *Profile of a Profession*, pg. 4.

13. Claudius Ash, *A Century of the Dental Art: A Centenary Memoir 1820-1821*. (London: C. Ash, 1921), pg. 36.

14. Curt Proskauer and Franz H. Witt, *A Pictorial History of Dentistry*.

15. Randy L. Burningham, "The Evolution of the Dental Office," *Bulletin of the History of Dentistry*, 28, 1980, pg. 23.

16. Milton S. Asbell, *A Century of Dentistry: A History of the University of Pennsylvania School of Dental Medicine*. (Philadelphia: Univ. of Pennsylvania, 1977), pgs. 3-5. Asbell's book is a model history of a dental school minus its typographical errors.

16. Warner, *Profile of a Profession*, pg. 7. City directories should be mined for the names of dentists, who may be investigated through historical society records, archives, libraries and other sources. Knowledge of their lives and careers is required to reveal more about the reality of American dentistry, which at present, relies heavily on the biographies of its leaders.

17. Foster Kidd, ed., *Profile of the Negro in American Dentistry*. (Washington, D.C.: Howard Univ. Press, 1979), pg. 1.

18. M.L. Rhein, "Office and Laboratory of M.L. Rhein," *Items of Interest*, Vol. 19, 1897, pg. 515.

19. Kidd, *Profile of the Negro in American Dentistry*, pg. 1.

20. Robinson, advertizement February 16, 1786, *North Carolina Gazette*, Le Mayeur

21. Clifton O. Dummett and Lois Doyle Dummett, *Afro-Americans in Dentistry: Sequence and Consequence of Events*. (Los Angeles: Dental Society, 1978), pg. 3.

22. Ibid.

23. James Morse Dunning, *The Harvard School of Dental Medicine: Phase Two in the Development of a University Dental School*. (Cambridge, Massachusetts: Harvard School of Dental Medicine, 1981), pg. 3.

24. C. Willard Camiliar Sr., *One Hundred Years of Dental Progress in the Nation's Capitol*. (Washington, D.C.: District of Columbia Dental Society Centenary), 1966, pgs. 236, 246. Malvin E. Ring, *Dentistry An Illustrated History*. (New York: Harry N. Abrams, Inc.) 1985, pg. 287. Joseph L. Henry, "History of Howard University College of Dentistry," *Bulletin of the History of Dentistry*, 23, 1975, pgs. 5-9.

25. Cramer, *The Story of Dentistry*, pg. 19.

26. Warner, *Profile of a Profession*, pg. 4.

27. Cramer, *The Story of Dentistry*, pg. 24.

28. Warner, *Profile of a Profession*, pg. 5.

29. *The History of Dentistry in Missouri*, pg. 13.

30. Warner, *Profile of a Profession*, pg. 4.

31. Ibid., pg. 5.

32. Burningham, "Evolution of the Dental Office," pg. 23

33. Richard Glenner, *The Dental Office A Pictorial History*. (Missoula, Montana: Pictorial Histories Publ. Co., 1984), pg. 23.

34. Malvin E. Ring, "Oddments in Dental History," *Bulletin of the History of Dentistry*, 17, 1964, pg. 26.

35. James Snell, *A Practical Guide to Operations on the Teeth*. (Philadelphia: Carey and Lea, 1832), pg. 61.

36. Ibid., pgs. 65, 66.

37. J.L. Asay, "A Retrospect of a Half Century," *Transactions of the California State Dental Association*, 26, 1896, pg. 22.

38. Ibid., pgs. 59-60, 65.

39. Ibid., pgs. 68-69.

40. Richard Glenner, *The Dental Office*, pgs. 23, 25-26.

41. George H. Monks, "The Museum of the Harvard Dental School," *Harvard Alumni Bulletin*, 37, 1925, pg. 905.

42. J.L. Asay, pgs. 22-23.

43. Editor, "Dentistry in America of the 1850s as seen by a Foreign Visitor," *Bulletin of the History of Dentistry*, 28, 1980, pg. 96.

44. Ibid., pg. 97.

45. Dummett, *Afro-Americans in Dentistry*, pg. 4.

46. D. Henderson, "Greene Vardiman Black (1836-1915), The Grand Old Man of Dentistry," Medical History, 5, 1961, pgs. 132-143. Aletha A. Kowitz, H.J. Loevy, "American Dentistry of the Past: G.V. Black," *Dental Historian* No. 13, October 1987, pgs. 1-6.; Aletha Kowitz, Hannelore Loevy, "On the Occasion of the 150th Anniversary of the Birth of G.V. Black," *Bulletin of the History of Dentistry*, 35, 1987, pgs. 129-136. Bessie M. Black, "Greene Vardiman Black, 1836-1915," *Illinois Dental Journal*, September-October, 1986, pgs. 501-506.; Carl E. Black and Bessie M. Black, *From Pioneer to Scientist*. (St. Paul, Minnesota, 1940); Charles N. Pappas, *The Life and Times of G.V. Black*. (Chicago: Quintessence Publ. Co., 1983)

47. *History of Dentistry in Missouri*, pg. 424

48. Ibid., pg. 422. Walter Hoffmann Arthelm, *History of Dentistry*. Trans, H.M. Koehler, (Chicago: Quintessence Publ. Co.) 1981, pgs. 302, 305.

49. Monks, "The Museum of the Harvard Dental School," pg. 906.

50. Glenner, *The Dental Office*, pg. 25.

51. Ritter Dental Manufacturing Company, *Practice Building Suggestions*. (Rochester: Ritter Manufacturing Co., 1924), pg. 23.

52. Glenner, *The Dental Office*, pg. 24.

53. Kowitz, Loevy, "American Dentistry of the Past," pg. 4.

54. Rodriguez Ottolengui, "Office of Dr. C.J.B. Stephens," *Items of Interest*, Vol. 19, 1897, pg. 600.

55.Francis A. Walker, ed., *International Exhibition Reports and Awards*. (Washington, D.C.: Government Printing Office, 1880), 8, pg. 314. Malvin E. Ring, "Oddments in Dental History: The Dental Exhibit at the Centennial, 1876," *Bulletin of the History of Dentistry*, 24, 1976, pg. 97.

56. "Cleanliness in Dental Offices," *Items of Interest*, Vol. 9, 1887, pg. 90.

57. D.W. Barber, "Neatness in the Dental Office," *Items of Interest*, Vol. 15, 1893, pg. 718.

58. "For Our Patients: A Lady's Suggestions to Dentists," *Items of Interest*, Vol. 8, 1886, pg. 129.

59. Glenner, *The Dental Office*, pgs. 47-48.

60. Thomas L. Gilmer, "Proceedings," *Dental Review*, 7,

1893, pgs. 489, 493.

61. Chapin Harris, *The Principles and Practice of Dental Surgery*. (Philadelphia: Lindsay and Blakiston, 1845), pg. 28.

62. Jacob Sharp, *A History of the Connecticut State Dental Association 1864-1956*, (New Haven), 1956, pg. 40.

63. William Gies, *Dental Education in the United States and Canada*. (New York: The Carnegie Foundation for the Advancement of Teaching), 1926, Bulletin #19, pgs. 45-46.

64. Rodriguez Ottolengui, "The Office of Fielden Briggs," *Items of Interest*, Vol. 20, 1898, pgs. 296-303.

65. Robert J. Bruckner, J. Henry Clarke, Janice S. Bruckner, "Dental Preceptorships of the 19th Century: What Were They Like?," *Bulletin of the History of Dentistry*, 36, 1988, pg. 12.

66. Ibid., pgs. 14-15.

67. A. Hibbard, "Our Old Wheel Horses," *Dental Items of Interest*, Vol. 12, 1890, pg. 78.

68. Ibid.

69. C. Edward Mills, "Bainbridge, Ross County, Ohio, the Cradle of Dental Education," *Journal of the American Dental Association*, 19, 1932, pgs. 361-389.; J. Ben Robinson, "The Claims of Bainbridge, Ohio, to Priority in Dental Education," *Dental Items of Interest*, Vol. 63, 1941, pgs. 3-27.; C.E. Mills, "The Claim for Bainbridge, Ohio, to Priority in Dental Education," *Dental Items of Interest*, Vol. 63, 1941, pgs. 517-536. H. Burton Macauley, "The Mythical Dental School Of Bainbridge, Ohio," *Oral Hygiene*, 56, 1966, pgs. 60-66.

70. Charles R. Turner, "Seventy-Five Years of Dental Education and Legislation in the U. S.," *Dental Cosmos*, 62, 1920, pg. 56.

71. Charles Kelsey, "An Early View of a Dental Clinic at the University of Michigan School of Dentistry," *Journal of the Michigan Dental Association*, 53, 1971, pg. 152.

72. Ibid. pg. 62.

73. Ibid., pg. 57.

74. Charles C. Kelsey, ed., "An Interview with Roy G. Hayward, Class of 1911," *Alumni Bulletin School of Dentistry*, (Univ. of Michigan) 1973, pg. 42.

75. Anonymous, *A History of the University of Missouri-Kansas City, School of Dentistry*. Centennial Publication, 1982, pgs. xvii, xix.

76. G.V. Black, "Management of the Infirmary Clinic in Dental Schools," *Dental Cosmos*, 1902, pg. 309.

77. Ibid., pgs. 310, 312-313.

78. Marcus L. Ward, "Landmarks in Dental Education," *Dental Cosmos*, 76, 1934, pg. 22

79. *Quarterly Bulletin of the Dental School*, 2, January 1906, pg. 27. Taught by Charles R.E. Koch one lecture per week in second semester.

80. Anonymous, "Tufts Centennial Issue," *Bulletin of the History of Dentistry*, 18, 1970, pg. 26.

81. Wilma E. Motley, *History of the American Dental Hygienists' Association 1923-1982*. (Chicago: Association of Dental Hygienists, 1986), pg. 6.

82. William G. Adair, "Sketch of Lucy Hobbs Taylor, D.D.S.," *Journal of the Ohio State Dental Association*, May 1949, pgs. 89-91.

83. Kidd, *Profile of the Negro in American Dentistry*, pg. 46. Anonymous, *The Baltimore College of Dental Surgery: Heritage and History*. (Baltimore: University of Maryland School of Dentistry), 1975, pg. 12.

84. J.A. Chapple, "Coeducation in Dental Colleges, and Is Dentistry a Suitable Calling for Women?," *The Dental Digest*, Vol. 10, 1904, pgs. 649-656.

85. Charles C. Kelsey, ed., "Ida Gray, Class of 1890: First Black Woman to Graduate from UM School of Dentistry," *Alumni Bulletin School of Dentistry*, (University of Michigan), 1977-78, pgs. 50-52.

86. John T. Toland, "Editorial: Ladies in the Dental Profession," *Cincinnati Dental Reporter*, 1, 1859, pg. 196.

87. *The Dental Register*, Vol. 30. 1876, pgs. 409-410 and Vol. 41, 1887, pgs. 525-528. A good source for articles on women in dentistry is Constance Boquist and Jeannette V. Haase, *An Historical Review of Women in Dentistry*. (Washington, D.C.: U.S. Department of Health, Education and Welfare), 1977.

88. Motley, *History of the American Dental Hygienists' Association*, pg. 7.

89. Chapin Harris, *A Dictionary of Dental Science*. (Philadelphia: Lindsay and Blakiston, 1899), 6th ed.

90. Kidd, *Profile of the Negro in American Dentistry*, pg. 53.

91. Motley, *History of the American Dental Hygienists' Association*, pg. 18. E. Allan Lieban, "Historical Portraits in Dental Culture: M.L. Rhein (1860-1928)," *New York Journal of Dentistry*, Vol. 32, 1962, pgs. 182-184.

92. Ibid., pg. 6.

93. Rodriguez Ottolengui, 'Office and Laboratory," *Items of Interest*, Vol. 19, 1897, pg. 133.

94. Ibid., pg. 133.

95. Ibid. See also on the importance of dental cabinets Bernhard Wolf Weinberger, "The Evolution of the Dental Cabinet," *Dental Survey*, 1936, pgs. 45-47.

96. Charles Edmund Kells, "Office and Laboratory," *Items of Interest*, Vol. 19, 1897, pgs. 52-56.

97. F.P. Cronkhite, "Office and Laboratory," *Items of Interest*, Vol. 21, 1897, pg. 587.

98. C. Edmund Kells, *Three Score Years and Nine*. (New Orleans, C. Edmund Kells, 1926), pgs. 11-12.

99. Charles C. Kelsey, "History Through Our Elder Alumni, Edward Cook Mills—Class of 1889," *Alumni Bulletin*, School of Dentistry, (University of Michigan), 1975-76, pg. 5.

101. C. Edmund Kells, *Three Score Years and Nine*, pg. 12. C. Edmund Kells, "Office and Laboratory," pg. 52.

102. C. Edmund Kells, *Three Score and Nine*, pg. 403.

103. A new design for the Medical Sciences Exhibitions is in progress and it is likely that these offices will be replaced with other exhibits in the next decade.

104. C. Edmund Kells, *The Dentist's Own Book*. (St. Louis: The C.V. Mosby Co., 1925), pgs. 225-242.

105. Olaf E. Langland, A. Peter Fortier, "C. Edmund Kells," *Oral Surgery*, 34, 1972, pgs. 680-689. James F. Gardiner, "C. Edmund Kells: New Orleans Gift to Dentistry," *Bulletin of the History of Dentistry*, Vol. 29, 1982, pgs. 2-7.

106. H. Colin Davis, "The Waiting Room: History, Function and Design," *British Dental Journal*, 120, 1966, pg. 405.

107. Ritter Dental Manufacturing Co., *When is a Dentist a Success?*, (Rochester: Ritter, 1920), pgs. 18-19.

108. Ibid., pg. 27.

109. C. Edmund Kells, *The Dentist's Own Book*, pg. 229.

110. William Wolf, "A History of Personal Oral Hygiene—Customs, Methods and Instruments—Yesterday, Today and Tomorrow," *Bulletin of the History of Dentistry*, Vol. 14, 1966, pg. 60.

111. Motley, *History of the American Hygienists' Association*, pg. 9.

112. Rodriguez Ottolengui, "Office and Laboratory," *Items of Interest*, Vol. 19, 1897, pgs. 513-22

113. Rodriguez Ottolengui, "Office of Dr. William B. Finney, Baltimore, Maryland," *Items of Interest*, Vol. 19, 1897, pgs. 856-863.

114. *A History of the Connecticut State Dental Association*, pg. 72.

115. R. Ottolengui, 1897, pg. 857.

116. Ibid., pg. 863.

117. "Office and Laboratory of Thomas P. Hinman, D.D.S., Atlanta, Georgia," *Items of Interest*, Vol. 20, 1898, pgs. 505-512.

118. Ralph R. Byrnes, J. Ben Robinson, Frederic R. Henshaw, "Thomas Philip Hinman, D.D.S., F.A.C.D., Sc. D., (March 4, 1870-March 19, 1931)," *Proceedings of the Eighth Annual Meeting of the American Association of Dental Schools*, 1931, pgs. 304-306. "Obituary," *The Dental Cosmos*, 73, 1931, pg. 528.

119. Hinman, "Office and Laboratory," pg. 505.

120. Charles F. Allan, "Office and Laboratory," *Items of Interest*, Vol. 19, 1897, pgs. 53-56.

121. E.M.S. Fernandez, "Proceedings," pg. 495.

122. A.B. McVay, "A Well-Arranged Dental Office," *Northwestern Dental Journal*, 6, 1908, pg. 25.

123. Henry Arthur King, "Office and Laboratory," *Items of Interest*, Vol. 20, 1898, pg. 663.

124. Ibid., pg. 666.

125. C.J.B. Stephens, "Office," pg. 600.

126. Ibid., pg. 604.

127. Obituary, "Dr. Thomas Louis Gilmer 1849-1931," *Dental Cosmos*, 1931, pg. 305.

128. E.S. Fuller, "Dental Office of Dr. E.S. Fuller, Piqua, Ohio," *Items of Interest*, Vol. 20, 1898, pgs. 385-88.

129. Ritter, *When Is a Dentist a Success?*, pg. 16.

130. "Dental Office of Dr. E.S. Fuller', pg. 388.

131. A.B. McVay, "A Well-Arranged Dental Office," pg. 25.

132. Thomas L. Gilmer, *The Dental Review*, 7, 1893, pg. 488.

133. H.B. Hinman, "Office and Laboratory," *Items of Interest*, 1898, pgs. 130-134.

134. Glenner, *The Dental Office*, pg. 26.

135. J. Allen Osmun, "A Unique Operating Room," *Items of Interest*, Vol. 20, 1898, pgs. 51-58.

136. Cronkhite, "Office," pgs. 587-588.

137. Eugene Maginnis, "A Dentist's Office," *Northwestern Dental Journal*, 5, 1908, pgs. 141-145.

138. Ibid., pg. 145.

139. T.M. Jamison, "The Equipment of a Country Dental Office," *Items of Interest*, Vol. 20, 1898, pgs. 211-213

140. Ibid., pg. 213.

141. Edward S. Barber, "A City Dental Office," *Northwestern Dental Journal*, 6, 1908, pgs. 93-101.

142. Rodriguez Ottolengui, "The Finest Dental Office in the World," *Items of Interest*, Vol. 35, 1913, pg. 641.

143. Obituary, "Alfred C. Fones," *JADA* and *Dental Cosmos*, 1938, pgs. 798-799.

144. Motley, *History of the American Hygienists' Association*, pgs. 20-21, 23.

145. Ibid., pg. 4.

146. Ibid., pg. 30.

147. Tufts Centennial Issue, *Bulletin of the History of Dentistry*, 1980, pgs. 64-65.

148. Motley, *History of the American Hygienists' Association*, pg. 26.

149. Ibid., pg. 27.

150. Ibid., pg. 14.

151. Ibid., pg. 31.

152. Ottolengui, "The Finest Dental Office," pg. 153. Charles C. Kelsey, "Percy C. Lowery—Distinguished Alumnus," *University of Michigan School of Dentistry Alumni Bulletin*, 1973, pg. 100.

154. F.H. Houghton, "A Dental House Boat," *Items of Interest*, Vol. 21, 1899, pgs. 329-333.

155. Wilnon Menard, "Lady with a Mission," *TIC*, 35, 1976, pgs. 7-11.

156. Charles B. Cartwright, "An Experience with Project Hope," *Alumni Bulletin*, School of Dentistry, (Univ. of Michigan) 1972, pgs. 9-10.

157. Briggs, "Office and Laboratory," pgs. 296-303.

158. George Randorf, "Office of Alexander Vasilovitch," *Items of Interest*, Vol. 19, 1897.

159. Cephas Whitney, "Time-Saving Horse-Shoe Bench," *Items of Interest*, Vol. 21, 1899, pgs. 411-12.

160. Robert Marcus, "Office and Laboratory, Dental Office of Dr. Robert Marcus, Frankfurt-on-Main, Germany," *Items of Interest*, Vol. 20, 1898, pg. 453. (pgs. 450-56)

161. Frank R. Faber, "Office of Dr. Frank R. Faber, Constantinople, Turkey," *Items of Interest*, Vol. 21, 1899, pgs. 244-245.

180. J. Gray Macaulay, "Dentistry in the Confederate Armies," *South Carolina Dental Journal*, 3, 1950, pg. 5.

181. Ibid., pgs. 5, 7, 9.

182. William Hodgkin, "Dentistry in the Confederacy," *Journal of the American Dental Association*, 50, 1951, pg. 350.

183. John M. Hyson, "William Saunders: The United States Army's First Dentist—West Point's Forgotten Man," *Military Medicine*, 149, 1984, pgs. 436-37.

184. Anonymous, *The Dental Corps of the United States Navy: A Chronology, 1912-1962*. (Washington, D.C.: Department of the Navy Bureau of Medicine and Surgery), 1962, pg. 4

185. Taylor, pgs. 209-10.

186. Ibid., pg. 210.

187. Ibid., pg. 211.

188. Robert T. Oliver, Three Years Service in the Philippines," *Dental Cosmos*, 48, 1906, pgs. 208-209.

189. Ibid., pg. 209.

190. Ibid.

191. *Dental Chronology*, pgs. 7, 11, 15.

192. Jeffcott, pg. 225.

193. M. Asbell, pgs. 117-118.

194. Jeffcott, pg. 35.

195. *Dental Chronology*, pg. 19.
196. Jeffcott, pg. 231-232, 313-314.
197. K.F. Smith, "The Practice of Dentistry in the Army and in Civil Life: A Comparison," *The Dental Cosmos*, 60, 1919, pgs. 504-05.
198. Edwin N. Kent, "Dentistry After the War: A Promising Professional Field for Young Men," *Dental Cosmos*, 60, 1919, pg. 806.
199. S.W. Foster, "The Influence of the War on Dentistry and Dental Colleges," *Dental Cosmos*, 60, 1919, pg. 1003.
200. C.N. Johnson, *Success in Dental Practice*. (Philadelphia: J.B. Lippincott, 1913), pg. 11.
201. Ritter, *Practice Building Suggestions*, pg. 22.
202. Richard Glenner, conversation with Dr. Chubin, 1987.
203. Ritter, *When is a Dentist a Success?*, pg. 6.
204. Ibid., pg. 8.
205. Ibid., pg. 9.
206. Ibid., pg. 15.
207. Ibid., pgs. 23-24.
208. Ibid.
209. Bremner, *The Story of Dentistry*, pg. 159.
210. Richard Glenner information gathered by interview with dentists, associates and families.
211. *A History of the Connecticut State Dental Association*, pg. 126.
212. Ibid., and information from former assistant to Dr. Chapman, Berith Gotstedt.
213. Ritter, *When is a Dentist a Success?*, pg.
214. *A History of the Connecticut State Dental Association*, pg. 78.
215. "Tufts Centennial Issue," 1970, pg. 23.
216. *A History of the Connecticut State Dental Assoc.* pg. 135.
217. Jeffcott, pg. 204.
218. Ibid., pg. 225.
219. Ibid., pg. 213.
220. Ibid., pg. 99.
221. Ibid., pg. 63.
222. Ibid., pgs. 98, 213.
223. Ibid., pg. 223.
224. Ibid., pgs. 153, 315.
225. Ibid., pg. 219.
226. Ibid., pg. 232.
227. Ibid., pgs. 220-221.
228. Ibid., pgs. 153, 157.
229. Obituary, "Alfred W. Chandler, Former Navy Dental Chief, Dies at 88," *Journal of the American Dental Association*, 97, 1978, pg. 887.
230. Jeffcott, pgs. 167, 176.
231. Ibid., pg. 176.
232. Ibid., pg. 197.
233. Ibid., pgs. 182-83.
234. Ibid., pg. 160.
235. Ibid., pg. 321.
236. Ibid., pg. 236.
237. Ibid., pg. 236.
238. Bremner, *The Story of Dentistry*, pg. 326.
239. Harold C. Kirkpatrick, *High Speed and Ultra Speed in Dentistry: Equipment and Procedures*. (Philadelphia and London: W.B. Saunders Co., 1960), pg. 4.
240. Ibid.
241. Ibid., and Jerry J. Herschfeld, "Robert J. Nelsen and the Development of the High Speed Handpiece," *Bulletin of the History of Dentistry*, 35, 1987, pgs. 37-42.
242. Ibid., pg. 166.
243. Malvin Ring, "The True Discoverer of the Dental Air Turbine Handpiece, Sir John Walsh of New Zealand," *Bulletin of the History of Dentistry*, 35, 1987, pg. 108. "Notes and Queries: Further Discussion Regarding Discovery of the Turbine Handpiece," *Bulletin of the History of Dentistry*, 36, 1988, pgs. 59-61.
244. M. Ring, pg. 108.
245. Kirkpatrick, *High Speed and Ultra Speed*, pgs. 50-55.
246. Ibid., pgs. 73-74.
247. Ibid., pg. 246.
248. Marvin Mundel, "Motion and Time Study in Dentistry," *JADA*, 57, 1958, pgs. 520-24.
249. E.J. Green and M.E. Brown, "Body Mechanics Applied to the Practice of Dentistry," *JADA*, 67, 1963, pgs. 679-97.
250. *Sigma Instrument System*, Ritter Dental Manufacturing Co., 1972, pgs. 1-4.
251. Micheal Uzelac, "Modern Dental Offices: Compact, Efficient Design—Yet Open and Warm," *Dental Survey*, January 1969, pgs. 42-48.
252. Daniel F. Spect, "Modern Dental Offices: Mood and Effect Created for a Practical Purpose," *Dental Survey*, February, 1970, pgs. 60-66.
253. "The Dentist and Professional Buildings," *Dental Economics*, March 1970: pgs. 34-35.
254. Richard V. Palmer, "Modern Dental Offices: Father, Grandfathers were Dentists—But His Ideas Aren't Traditional," *Dental Survey*, July 1972, pgs. 59-61.
255. N.J. Browne, "Modern Dental Offices: 'Open Look' Adapted to General Practice," *Dental Survey*, August 1972, pgs. 48-49.
256. Thomas O. Ballard, "Offices of San Francisco Dentist are Designed on a Nautical Theme," *JADA*, 81, 1970, pgs. 1292-96.
257. Mundel, "Motion and Time Study in Dentistry," pg. 524.
258. Charles H. Boney, "All Aboard for the Dentist's Office," *Dental Economics*, February 1971, pgs. 24-26.
259. Owen (Rick) Herold, "Modern Dental Offices: Smooth Traffic Pattern Serves Staff of Seven," *Dental Survey*, May 1969, pgs. 58-63.
260. Ollie J. Weigel, "Modern Offices: 'Dream' Design: for Father, Son," *Dental Survey*, August 1970, pgs. 37-39.
261. James H. Drummond, "Building for Tomorrow," *Professional Budget Plan*, 1970, pgs. 12-15.
262. Edwin M. Thomas, "Single-Ownership Group Practice: 'The Best of Two Worlds,' " *Dental Survey*, March 1972, pgs. 39-44.
263. Laren W. Teutsch, "Modern Offices: Teutsch's Law: 'Practice Expands to Fill the Space Available,' " *Dental Survey*, July 1970, pgs. 46-51.
264. Gerald P. Hirsch, et al, "Group Practice/An Inside

View," *Dental Survey*, June 1971, pgs. 24-28.

265. I. Norton Brotman, Howard L. Rothschild, "Modern Offices: 'Co-ordination and Control' Put Fun Back in Practice," *Dental Survey*, January 1971, pgs. 37-40.

266. R.P. McGraw, "The Corporate Group...A Better Way to Practice?," *Dental Survey*, January 1972, pgs. 19-26.

267. H. Ronald Combs, "The Business Side of Design," *Dental Economics*, 77, 1987, pgs. 43-46.

268. B. Holly Smith, "Recreation and the Dentist," *Dental Cosmos*, 49, 1907, pg. 717.

269. R.O. Williams, "Little Things," *Dental Cosmos*, 44, 1902: pgs. 587, 589.

270. Kenneth Macgowan, *Behind the Screen: The History and Techniques of the Motion Picture*. (New York: Dell Publishing Co.), 1965, pg. 87.

271. David Shipman, *The Story of Cinema*. (New York: St. Martin's Press), 1982, pgs. 23, 55. Kenneth Macgowan, *Behind the Screen: The History and Techniques of the Motion Picture*, pg. 105.

272. Gerald D. MacDonald, *The Films of Charlie Chaplin*. (New York: Bonanza Books, Crown), 1965, pg. 57. David Robinson, *Chaplin His Life and Art*. (New York: McGraw-Hill Book Co.), 1985, pgs. 125, 208.

273. Evelyn Mack Truitt, *Who Was Who on the Screen*. (New York and London: R.R. Boker Co.), 1983, pg. 585.

274. Herman G. Weinberg, compiler, *The Complete Greed of Erich von Stroheim*. (New York: E.P. Dutton and Co.), 1973, unpaginated foreword.

275. Frank Norris, *McTeague A Story of San Francisco*. (New York: Grosset and Dunlap), 1899.

276. Eric Rhode, *A History of the Cinema from its Origins to 1970*. (New York: Da Capo Paperback), 1976, pg. 230.

277. Kenneth W. Leisch, *Cinema*. (New York: Newsweek Books), 1974, pg. 268. Kenneth Macgowan, *Behind the Screen*, pg. 268. Herman G. Weinberg and Joel W. Finler, ed., *Greed a film by Erich von Stroheim*. (New York: Simon and Schuster), 1972, pg. 14.

278. E. Rhode, pg. 231.

279. Herman G. Weinberg, compiler, *The Complete Greed*, unpaginated.

280. Joel W. Finler, *Greed a film by Erich von Stroheim*. (New York: Simon and Schuster), 1972, pgs. 10, 13, 16.

281. Leonard Maltin, *Movie Comedy Teams*. (New York: A Plume Book, New American Library), 1985, pg. 1. John Mc-Cabe, *Laurel and Hardy*. (New York: Bonanza Books), 1965.

282. L. Maltin, pg. 4

283. Ibid., pgs. 8-9.

284. Ibid., pg. 11.

285. Ibid., pg. 186.

286. Ephraim Katz, *The Film Encyclopedia*. (New York: Perigee Books), 1979.

287. L. Maltin, pg. 197.

288. E. Katz, *The Film Encyclopedia*, pg. 1099.

289. William K. Everson, *The Art of W.C. Fields*. (New York: Bonanza Books [Crown]), 1967, pgs. 79-85.

290. Leslie Halliwell, *Halliwell's Film Guide*, (New York: Charles Scribner's Sons), 1985, 4th ed., pg. 1333.

291. Ibid., pgs. 1375-76.

292. E. Katz, *The Film Encyclopedia*, pg. 178.

293. L. Halliwell, pg.

294. L. Halliwell, pg. 1246. Leonard Maltin, *The Great Movie Comedians*. (New York: Crown), 1978, pg. 191.

295. Ibid., pgs. 906-7. Lawrence Olivier, "The Entertainer," *American Film*, 1986: pg. 68.

296. Richard Glenner compiled the list of films in which the role of the dentist has been portrayed.

297. Al Di Lauro and Gerald Calkin, *Dirty Movies: An Illustrated History of the Stag Film 1915-1970*. (New York: Chelsea House), 1976, pg. 93.

298. *The Complete Greed*, scenes of film, unpaginated.

299. Editorial, "Pleasant Street vs Dingy Lane," *Items of Interest*, Vol. 17, 1895, pg. 369.

300. J.M. Weems, "Cleanliness in the Dental Office," *Dental Cosmos*, Vol. 52, 1910, pg. 1268.

301. D.W. Barker, "Neatness in the Dental Office," *Items of Interest*, Vol. 15, 1893, pg. 717.

302. O.W. Randall, "A Plea for Porcelain Floors in the Operatory Room," *Items of Interest*, Vol. 24, 1902, pgs. 487-88.

303. Marvin Stone, "Was it Something I Said?," *American Bar Association Journal*, August 1987, pg. 34.

304. Motley, *History of the American Hygienists' Association*, pg. 57.

305. Johnson, *Success in Dental Practice*, pgs. 111-12.

306. F.O. Hetrick, "Our Offices and Appearance," *Items of Interest*, Vol. 17, 1895, pg. 675.

307. "Dentists at the Top of the List," *The Chicago Dental Society Review*, 80, June 1987.

308. J. Stanley Clark, *Open Wider, Please, The Story of Dentistry in Oklahoma*. (Norman: University of Oklahoma), 1955, pgs. 221-2.

309. Ruth Harris, *Dental Science in a New Age: A History of the National Institute of Dental Research.* (GPO, 1989).

Index

THE DR. JOHN HARRIS DENTAL MUSEUM

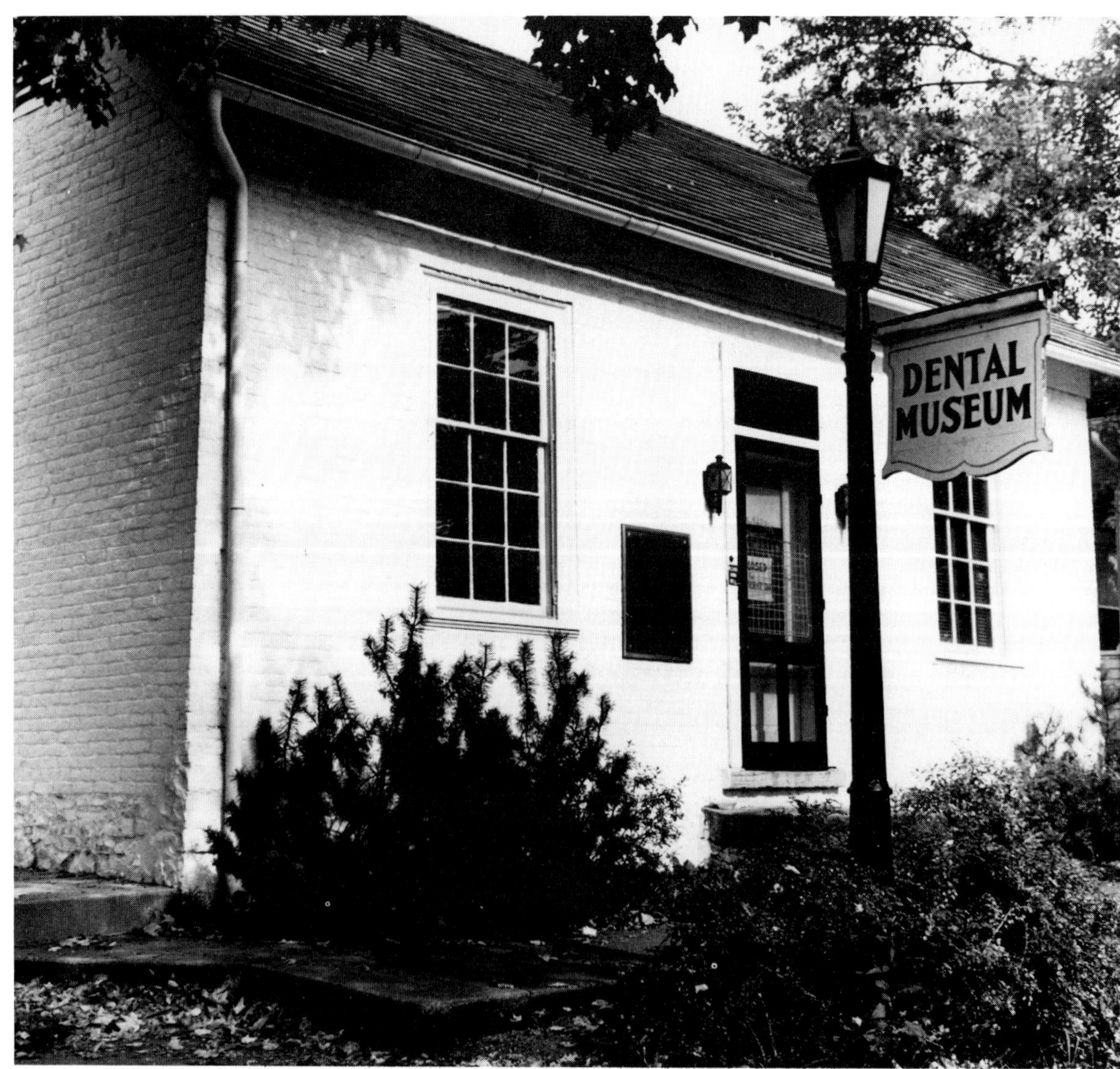

Exterior of the Dr. John Harris Dental Museum, site of the first proprietary dental school in the U.S. Located in Bainbridge, Ohio, the Museum displays, through equipment and furniture of the period, what the school may have looked like when the physician, John Harris, taught a small group of students medicine and dentistry from 1827 to 1830.